"It is a pleasure to write about *Ayurveda for Depression* and Dr. Eduardo Cardona-Sanclemente. His scientific and medical training combined with his Ayurveda knowledge enable him to apply his research to one of the paramount conditions of our time, with a keen eye guided by deep human understanding. This book is a significant contribution to the bridging of Western and Eastern medicine."

—PROF SIR SALVADOR MONCADA, FRS, FMedSci, HonFBPhS, Manchester Cancer Research Centre, University of Manchester

"Dr. Eduardo Cardona-Sanclemente has produced an excellent, detailed, and many-sided account of the Ayurvedic treatment of depression with reference to modern medicine as well. An important contribution in the field of deeper Ayurvedic studies that is worthy of deep examination."

—DR. DAVID FRAWLEY, author of *Yoga and Ayurveda*

"What a beautiful book that elegantly integrates the modern biomedical understanding of depression with the wellness and healing of Ayurveda. Dr. Cardona-Sanclemente invites the reader into his personal story and offers wellness and healing strategies that restore balance and health using an individualized Ayurvedic approach to diet, lifestyle, herbs, and the emotions. *Ayurveda for Depression* provides an insightful and novel approach for those suffering from depression that is compassionate and achievable."

—DIANA I. LURIE, PhD, professor of Neuropharmacology at the University of Montana and certified Ayurvedic practitioner

"Dr. Cardona-Sanclemente deserves our thanks, both for the thoroughness of this exposition of how depression can be seen through the lens of Ayurveda and for the courage he shows in speaking of his own encounters with the condition. The darkness of depression is a reality for many, and this book is a welcome guide to how Ayurveda can shine a light on this condition and how to dispel the disabling shadow that it casts."

—DR. ROBERT SVOBODA, BAMS (Ayurvedacharya), author of *Prakriti: Your Ayurvedic Constitution*

"The incidence of depression is surging worldwide. One reason has been the attempt to drown depression in pharmaceuticals that have little effect and that often increase vulnerability to depression. *Ayurveda for Depression* offers a proven-effective prescription for emotional wellness that rebalances body and mind with an individualized program targeting lifestyle, diet, body systems, and emotions. This is the book that anyone struggling with depression must read."

—MATTHEW MCKAY, PhD, professor at
The Wright Institute and coauthor of *Thoughts & Feelings*

"It is rare to find someone adept in both Western science and Eastern medicine. It is rarer for one well versed in both to apply them to their own crises and healing and demonstrate how we might do the same. Dr. Cardona-Sanclemente speaks to us heart to heart, helping us synthesize much information into personal understanding and providing tools for devising a personal plan toward wellness. I believe this authoritative exploration can touch and benefit many."

—CLAUDIA WELCH, DOM, author of
Balance Your Hormones, Balance Your Life

"Way beyond depression, the essential principles of Ayurveda expressed in this book will be helpful to anyone interested in this remarkable traditional way toward human healthy balance. Dr. Cardona-Sanclemente sees with his heart and radiates that through his unique perspective on science, health, and humanity."

—ALEXANDER DE SALZMANN, MD, Internal Medicine,
Paris France

"Sometimes one encounters a colleague with unique insights and sensitivity who takes a refreshingly forensic view of what we have come to accept as norms. Dr. Cardona-Sanclemente is such a colleague. I know from decades of professional collaboration that this book will be of great support to those experiencing depression and other mental health conditions."

—DR. SABINE GRIGLIO, DSc, research director of the
National Institute for Medical Research (INSERM), France

Ayurveda *for* Depression

Ayurveda *for* Depression

AN INTEGRATIVE APPROACH TO RESTORING
BALANCE AND RECLAIMING YOUR HEALTH

L. Eduardo Cardona-Sanclemente, DSc, PhD, MSc

North Atlantic Books
Berkeley, California

Published by   Cover art © gettyimages.com/AllNikArt
North Atlantic Books   Cover design by Jasmine Hromjak
Berkeley, California   Book design by Happenstance Type-O-Rama

Printed in Canada

Ayurveda for Depression: An Integrative Approach to Restoring Balance and Reclaiming Your Health is sponsored and published by the Society for the Study of Native Arts and Sciences (dba North Atlantic Books), an educational nonprofit based in Berkeley, California, that collaborates with partners to develop cross-cultural perspectives, nurture holistic views of art, science, the humanities, and healing, and seed personal and global transformation by publishing work on the relationship of body, spirit, and nature.

North Atlantic Books' publications are available through most bookstores. For further information, visit our website at www.northatlanticbooks.com or call 800-733-3000.

The following information is intended for general information purposes only.

This book does not intend to be diagnostic in any way and is not a substitute for a thorough clinical assessment or professional treatment. If you are reading this book and feel that any of the problems herein apply to you personally, you are encouraged to seek out an assessment from a qualified professional as soon as possible. If you are at medical risk of withdrawal or in a serious psychiatric emergency (e.g., suicidal or homicidal ideations), you are encouraged to present for medical attention immediately.

Library of Congress Cataloging-in-Publication Data
Names: Cardona-Sanclemente L., Eduardo, 1955- author.
Title: Ayurveda for Depression : An Integrative Approach to Restoring
   Balance and Reclaiming Your Health / Dr. L. Eduardo Cardona-Sanclemente.
Description: Berkeley, California : North Atlantic Books, [2020]
Identifiers: LCCN 2020009291 (print) | LCCN 2020009292 (ebook) | ISBN
   9781623175368 (trade paperback) | ISBN 9781623175375 (ebook)
Subjects: LCSH: Depression, Mental—Alternative treatment. | Medicine,
   Ayurvedic.
Classification: LCC RC537 .C2738 2020 (print) | LCC RC537 (ebook) | DDC
   616.85/27—dc23
LC record available at https://lccn.loc.gov/2020009291
LC ebook record available at https://lccn.loc.gov/2020009292

1 2 3 4 5 6 7 8 9 MARQUIS 24 23 22 21 20

This book includes recycled material and material from well-managed forests. North Atlantic Books is committed to the protection of our environment. We print on recycled paper whenever possible and partner with printers who strive to use environmentally responsible practices.

Thanks,
dearest Joan M. E. Buffotot.

To these blessed, mysterious,
multidimensional paths of life
allowing us to fly.

CONTENTS

ACKNOWLEDGMENTS

I AM GRATEFUL TO ALL of life's experiences that have expanded my viewpoint in one way or another. They helped me learn about my own nature and glimpse the vast, profound nature around all of us.

It is necessary to acknowledge in particular the presence of my great teachers: death, suffering, depression, fear, anxiety, and adversity. They, with their companions—life, joy, love, hope, and humility—showed me that through effort, light prevails over darkness. Their continuous presence is a daily challenge to see and accept conditions under a new light, inviting us to embark on a journey of discovering new body-mind connections.

In terms of expressing gratitude to specific individuals for making this book possible, there are too many kind, warm souls to recall throughout the years. However, I do wish to thank the following people who have marked my life either as mentors or friends: Michel de Salzmann, Vasant Lad, Carlos Corredor, Gustav Born, Sabine Griglio, Catherine Guettet, and Patrick Byrne.

Of course, I also want to thank all the clients, patients, and students I have met throughout the years. You put your trust in me and gave me the opportunity to help you—and thereby learn from you—by listening to your bodies and minds searching for balance. You were my true sources of practical integration of the profound principles of Ayurveda with modern medicine, and of the possibility that I could develop procedures and discover my mission.

Lastly, my thanks and gratitude to Matt McKay for introducing me to Tim McKee and the entire NAB team. Thanks to you all for your warm and professional support in the preparation and presentation of this book.

PART I

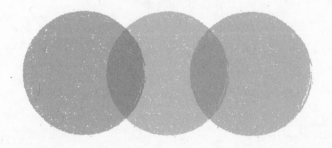

Who Are You, Ayurveda?

INTRODUCTION

The Origins of Ayurveda

AYURVEDA, WHICH MEANS "sacred knowledge of life," is an approximately five-thousand-year-old system of natural health care. Originally transmitted as an oral tradition, its earliest documentation is found in the ancient books of wisdom known as the Vedas, a profound part of Indian history and culture. However, in the Western world Ayurveda is still considered to be a complementary or alternative medicine, despite its long-documented history and daily practice in India for thousands of years. The World Health Organization (WHO) has recognized Ayurveda as a safe traditional medicine based on an extensive body of scientific evidence.[1]

AYURVEDA'S OBJECTIVE

Ayurveda has one objective: to restore balance in you. It is that simple, and the simplicity of this objective will be constantly reinforced throughout this book, because all components of Ayurvedic medicine align to achieve this goal within you. Ayurveda emphasizes the wholeness of each of us. It defines wellness as a state in which all bodily tissues, organs, systems, and functions are acting together interdependently to maintain the delicate balance between body, mind, and consciousness (spirit) in order to promote good health and wellness, in spite of many negative influences around us.

AYURVEDA'S APPROACH TO TREATING DEPRESSION

Depression is a mood disorder manifesting as a loss of interest in life and its enjoyments. Ayurveda calls depression *manovasada,* and this system treats depression by using individually tailored treatment plans. Note carefully that we say "individually tailored" and not "tailored for depression." Unlike Western medicine, Ayurveda does not see you as separate from your condition. The tailoring of treatments to individuals is based on the core Ayurvedic concept of *prakruti*—Ayurveda's name for our unique, individual constitution. If an Ayurvedic doctor has ten patients, there will be ten individual treatment plans.

In addition to addressing physical health, Ayurveda has long-established techniques for meeting the challenges of mental health issues in patients. Ayurveda invites the patient to participate actively in the process of healing rather than passively waiting for potential recovery, such as when taking a new drug regime. Crucial to the Ayurvedic approach is the recognition that if balance is not restored, there will always be ill health. For example, reducing the extreme manifestations of depression in a patient while keeping the patient in a depressive but manageable state is still ill health in Ayurveda. In this respect, Ayurveda rejects the maintenance of ill health and promotes curative pathways.

In contrast, the modern medical system most of us use often attempts to treat the symptoms of disease instead of addressing the roots of the condition. This system usually tackles mental health separately from the physical body. In some way we accept this when we choose to use this system. How often are we willing to accept an over-the-counter solution because it is quick and we want to get on with our busy day? Modern medical practice defines wellness as "the absence of defined disease" and prescribes treatment to attack or kill the disease, often using drugs and medicines that may have side effects. The same treatments are frequently applied to a given set of symptoms irrespective of the individual's requirements, as is often the case with depression.

We do not need to dwell here on the merits and demerits of such a system. Ayurveda is our focus, and it seeks to chart an altogether different path.

MAINSTREAM CLASSIFICATION OF DEPRESSION AND TREATMENTS

Depression is defined as a group of mental disorders associated with the decrease in the quality of a person's mood, causing impairments in daily life. Within this broad definition fall a number of subdefinitions:

- Major depressive disorder or clinical depression: persistently depressed mood, lack of interest in normal activities, fatigue, difficulty concentrating, feeling of worthlessness and guilt, suicidal thoughts, or changes in body weight and sleep.

- Persistent depressive disorder: mild signs of depression that last for two years or longer.

- Bipolar disorder or manic depression: mood episodes that range from extremes of high energy with an "up" mood to low depressive periods.

- Premenstrual dysphoric disorder: signs appear a week or two before an individual's period starts and usually go away two to three days after the period starts.

- Postpartum depression: occurs in the weeks and months after childbirth.

- Seasonal affective disorder: often occurs during winter months or when there is less sunlight.

- Situational depression or stress response syndrome: occurs when having trouble managing a stressful event in life, such as a death in the family, a divorce, or losing a job.

- Atypical depression: different from the persistent sadness of typical depression. A depressed mood can become bright or cheerful in response to positive events.

Antidepressants have been the mainstay of depression treatment, aiming to reduce the manifestation of the condition, but other therapies are also available and are attracting increasing interest as patients seek out effective alternative treatments. The aim of this book is to present to you one such effective alternative treatment that is becoming more widely accessible in the Western world: Ayurveda.

THIS BOOK'S OBJECTIVES

The key objectives of this book are to do the following:

- Provide an essential exploration of Ayurvedic concepts, diagnostics, and treatments and how these are becoming more accessible to you today.

- Share the knowledge and benefits of Ayurvedic medicine and its application to rebalancing the body-mind-consciousness function in individuals living with depression or who are on their way to developing a depressive condition as a result of imbalances growing within them.

- Pioneer a new approach that integrates Ayurveda with corresponding components in modern medicine. This is based on physiological, biochemical, pharmacological, and clinical research on its therapies using accessible, modern, scientific terminology. Previously, most Ayurvedic instruction was rooted in the canons of the ancient Ayurvedic texts, which relate strictly to how Ayurveda should be delivered. These have remained intact and largely unchanged for thousands of years, but they are very difficult for the ordinary patient to use in asking not just whether it works but also how it works. This book takes a novel approach by matching components of Ayurveda with Western medical science, using the technological tools of biomedical science to translate and affirm the remarkable wisdom and effectiveness of Ayurveda. This approach will also help you understand Ayurvedic concepts in everyday medical terms.

- Provide you with fresh perspectives for understanding your body-mind-consciousness function. This understanding will support you as you seek to rebalance your physical and mental health to either treat an existing depressive condition or prevent an emerging condition from progressing.

The book provides references for the scientific studies cited as well as tables, figures, and images to support your understanding of Ayurvedic principles. Specialized Ayurvedic terminology is defined in a glossary in the back of the book.

The book also provides many quotations and citations from classical Ayurvedic Sanskrit verses (*slokas*) or references. When these classical works are cited, we use the following conventional abbreviations to refer to them:

- *As. Hr. Su.*—*Ashtanga Hrudhaya Sutrasthana*
- *As. Hr. Ni.*—*Ashtanga Hrudhaya Nidanasthana*
- *Ca. Su.*—*Charaka Samhita Suthrasthana*
- *Su. Chi.*—*Sushruta Chikitsasthana*
- *Su. Sa.*—*Sushruta Shareerasthana*
- *Su. Sū.*—*Sushruta Suthrasthana*

My Journey
through Depression

MY FIRST, SECOND, AND THIRD CALLING

First Wake-Up Call

When I was in my early twenties, I had the opportunity to explore the west coast of South America with my partner. I was already a young scientist, working on a master's degree at medical school and devoted to studying nutrition, metabolism, and vegetarian diets. It was a magical trip, traveling thousands of miles in a jeep with the feeling of discovering a new world. Our plan was to visit every country along that coast, traveling as close as possible to the South Pole. We traveled for five months, visiting the most picturesque areas of Colombia, Ecuador, Peru, Chile, and Argentina. We crossed very dry deserts, such as the Atacama, to reach the green mountains where the Incan civilization developed incredible towns in the area around Machu Picchu. We encountered amazing flora and fauna along the way—llamas, penguins, and more.

Eventually, after this profound experience of the astounding beauty of nature and the warmth of the local people, our obligations required that we begin our long journey home toward the north. It was time to return to our day-to-day reality. We had driven for weeks, sometimes several hundred miles per day, and we were very much under pressure to return home to face professional, family, and personal commitments. Exhaustion was about to take its toll.

Toward the end of the journey, while driving in the early morning along a steep mountainside road close to the border between Ecuador and Colombia, I lost control of the car. We tumbled down the mountainside. I have a vague memory of feeling the car turning and seeing bright colors as I caught fleeting glimpses of the beautiful green mountains and blue sky while we twisted in the air. Finally, our tumbling stopped. I don't know how long we were there, but I do remember that an elder woman dressed in black spotted us and shouted for help to "bring up the bodies." I knew what it felt like not to be here anymore, between my unresponsive body and a mind trying to understand what we were going through at that shocking moment. I had a vague sense of shapes that were constantly morphing.

Taken for dead, we were transported to the nearest hospital and transferred to the morgue, until one member of the staff realized that we were both actually alive. The astonishment of the doctors and nurses was only matched by my amazement that, as I fluctuated between consciousness and unconsciousness, I felt the strong presence of one of the doctors. I recognized her. She was my peer from first-year medical school, and by extraordinary coincidence she was fulfilling part of her internship in that small town. She didn't recognize me due to my many wounds.

Eventually I became able to communicate and identify myself. In consideration of the gravity of our injuries, we were transferred to a major hospital. Upon recovering consciousness at the new hospital, I finally understood the seriousness of our condition. As a result of the long period of time between the accident and being transferred to the larger hospital, I had developed a gangrene infection in my broken right arm, which had suffered an open fracture. I also had several contusions on my skull and my dorsal spine, a broken leg, and broken foot bones. The medical recommendation was to amputate my infected right arm.

I was in my early twenties, and I resisted this. Against considerable pressure from the medical team, I did not consent to proceeding with the amputation. Instead, trusting in my body's ability to heal such a serious condition, I requested that we take a chance and treat my severe arm infection using plant protocols. This leap of faith was the beginning of something. Between this novel herbal treatment approach and my strong conviction that this was the right route to take, my right arm is still with me, fully functional after all these years. It is a great daily reminder and companion, especially when I practice my regular activities of yoga and swimming.

It is very difficult to describe the emotional and psychological impacts this experience caused for two young people with so much of our lives still ahead of us. Facing my death brought me an instant sense of clarity and purpose. Our destinies changed completely as a result of the serious damage we suffered. Fortunately, my partner was taken to another hospital, where she recovered fully after some months. However, the confusion and emotions I experienced, including regret and a sense of guilt for losing control of the car, left me under the shadow of depression for years to come. This massive impact that affected me on many levels has been a great and difficult lesson that continues to nourish me and challenge me positively to this very day.

Learning that I had the strength to stand on my own two feet, trust my decisions, and listen to my heart has been critical in how I've made life decisions under stressful circumstances since that car accident. This learning hasn't reduced the possibility of accidents or mishaps along the way, but it has helped me handle stressful events more effectively. I understood that even as I was aware of immense physical pain, I had the opportunity to participate in managing it with natural protocols—and this proved to be crucial in the years to come.

Learning how to deal with mental, emotional, and spiritual states became the main focus of how I addressed my depression. Of course, painkillers, anti-inflammatories, antibiotics, and other medications were enthusiastically offered to me. But on some level I knew it was possible to handle such a difficult condition without depending on these medications, by accepting my condition and connecting with it. For now, that is all I need to share with you here. In the following chapters, I will describe in detail what I did to help my condition improve.

I knew that accepting medications was the easy option. I also understood that we all can produce our own natural chemicals, internally. I will be sharing medical and scientific information about that process with you, especially as we consider the metabolic modifications associated with the condition of depression.

Second Wake-Up Call

Years later, after finishing my master's degree, I worked as a professor of medical biochemistry at my medical school for a couple of years, and then I moved to France to complete my biomedical PhD and postdoctoral degrees. After completing those obligations, I relocated to London. While teaching medical students and continuing my career as an academic and medical research scientist at Bart's Hospital Medical School, I received another "gift" by way of life lesson number two.

Again, this lesson came from a major accident. On a warm spring day, I was happily leaving my office at midday to go to the hospital doctors' canteen to meet a colleague for lunch. While walking along the crosswalk between the two buildings, one of those traditional London black cabs came flying toward me and swerved with its side door swinging open, catapulting me against stainless-steel scaffolding. I was knocked unconscious for a long period, and I cannot recall the series of events immediately after the accident.

After recovering consciousness, I found myself in another hospital receiving emergency treatment. There were lesions in my neck and back, just as in my first very serious accident. Gradually I became aware of the seriousness of my injuries. They caused subsequent bifrontal headaches, which a consulting neurologist diagnosed as posttraumatic muscle tension headaches. I started suffering panic attacks, possibly due to cognitive issues, including severe memory loss. I also became unable to communicate properly. I suffered strong neck discomfort and abnormal sensations (dysesthesia) in the right thumb and the index and middle fingers, and I experienced pain from a tear in the supraspinatus muscle, which runs from the shoulder blade to the greater tubercle of the humerus bone.

I was eventually able to walk again, and I visited my doctor to discuss my condition. Based on all my X-rays and CT scans, he was quite concerned about the impact of my injuries, not only physically but mentally. In this respect, I was fortunate to have a doctor who could piece the puzzle together. The MRIs showed serious disc root compression at C3/C4 and C6/C7 of my spine. I was advised to wear a soft neck collar and to take nonsteroidal anti-inflammatory drugs for pain. In my next visit, about a month later, I reported many symptoms: persistent headaches, sensitivity to light and sound, mood swings, depression, poor concentration, tearfulness, loss of motivation, and becoming withdrawn and subdued. My doctor recommended a session with a consulting psychiatrist. After that session, the psychiatrist recommended that I take Prozac and painkillers (amitriptyline, typically used with depression patients). The psychiatrist said my possibilities for carrying on a normal life had been drastically reduced and I would never be the same again. Further examination revealed significant and surprising cognitive deficits.

My ego was very much affected by this accident and its aftermath. From the outside, my professional life looked fulfilled and successful. At the same time, I carried within myself a persistent feeling that something important was missing from the mainstream medical approach I and millions of others were using. I saw things from my two perspectives—as a medical scientist and as a patient. Despite all the technological and pharmacological advances available in modern society, something was absent, and I was now experiencing that absence as a patient because of this second accident. My doctors told me my career was coming to an end because I would be unable to perform as before. They also said I might be taking powerful medications for the rest of my days. The idea of depending on such strong drugs for many years to come made me feel even worse.

Third Wake-Up Call

In search of alternative approaches to secure my full recovery, I found myself experimenting with various techniques to treat my condition. Among them, I was very impressed with the positive effects of craniosacral therapy, so I decided to integrate it into my daily program of recovery by studying craniosacral therapy in parallel with academic studies of Ayurveda to improve my health.

Well into my process of recovery, I was invited to practice at the Upledger Institute Clinic in Florida. I traveled to the United States with serious motivations to further understand craniosacral therapy and incorporate the technique into what would become my clinical practice later on. As a result, I took a sabbatical to offer my services full time while in the midst of my own recovery.

One night, while someone was driving me from the clinic to a colleague's party, we were on the highway when we collided with another car at high speed. I was sitting in the front passenger seat, and I was hit from the side. The impact damaged my door so badly that I had to be very carefully extracted from the car. The airbag—which saved my life—exploded in my face, causing serious facial trauma.

After the accident I experienced continuous right-arm numbness, wrist pain due to ulnar nerve damage, delay in feeling sensation and movement in my arm and knee due to a kind of fusion with the metallic structure of the door, headaches, soft-tissue pain, dysfunction in the neck, issues with my temporomandibular junction, broken teeth, cracked ribs, knee impairments, a tongue injury, and so on. Once again I was confined to bed for several weeks until I was able to walk with the help of a cane. I had to wear a splint and a Minerva collar 24/7 to control pain and prevent the exacerbation of my injuries.

Once again, doctors were recommending that I take various drug cocktails to ease my symptoms, but once more I felt the limitations of a medical system that had the goal of obliterating my physical pain rather than focusing on healing my damaged tissues. Not surprisingly, I had a startling recollection of the previous accident some months back, along with visions of the previous eagerly proffered cycle of drug dependency. At this moment I firmly and resolutely chose—again—to take another path.

You might ask yourself: with such trauma and physical and mental damage, what other pathway could be possible? The answer is contained in this book. I recovered by fully engaging in the academic and practical study of Ayurvedic medicine and integrating into my healing program it in parallel with the valuable knowledge and experiences I learned from my career in biomedicine.

From the beginning of my professional life, my main motivation had always been to comprehend metabolic processes at both the digestive and the mental levels. My primary interest had been the importance of lipids (one of the main constituents of all cells) such as cholesterol—both the "good" and "bad" types—for diet and metabolism, as well as their potential causative role in the development of cardiovascular diseases and related conditions such as obesity, stress, and other metabolic disorders. I was also interested in the role played by neurotransmitters, such as adrenaline and acetylcholine. Now imagine my deep dissatisfaction with the mainstream medical system and the way I was participating in it when life kept placing me in situations where I became the patient rather than the medical investigator.

For some people, one major accident is enough to jolt them into a change of path in an effort to become true to oneself. I am not proud of needing three such shocks to understand the importance of seeking alternatives to mainstream medicine, but eventually I decided to devote all my time to integrating mainstream medicine with alternative, complementary medical modalities.

Perhaps I needed to confront death several times to understand my ordinary life. I have often considered the aptness of that old saying: "Without death, there is no resurrection." Someone or something needed to "die" within me so I could explore beyond the conventional scientific box I was in.

Life generously gave me the opportunity to recover at a time when I'd been spending several years studying Ayurveda in India and other countries. You may ask: why Ayurveda and not some other modality?

Well, to answer that I have to go backward. After achieving the highest academic degrees at Sorbonne University in Paris, I took a six-month trip to India. The inspiration for this trip was my father, an admirer of Gandhi and his principles of nonviolence *(ahimsa)*. I was mesmerized by the beauty of the country, the people, the food, and the profound culture. While in India, I witnessed what in the West we would call medical "miracles," which for me were simply the result of a profound understanding of the body-mind-consciousness connection that allows healing to happen. That is what Ayurveda is all about. As a result of the many such experiences I've had, my motto is:

....

Ayurveda a day keeps the doctor away!

....

That first accident, occurring in my earlier twenties, left me with the impression that I was a drop of water in a flowing river. When that drop reached a point where the waters divided, that powerful situation presented the moment when I really attained adulthood. I have faced my own death three times. Life in its mysterious way offered me a challenge in the face of my mortality and kindly took me into another stream, another way forward. At that moment, my "I" entered the stream that fed into the river of life.

All rivers seek the same destination: the ocean. I have faith that we can all eventually reach that ocean of inner knowledge.

MY CONNECTION WITH YOU

I faced firsthand the prospect of unending drug dependency, but I took another path. This may not appear to be a pathway open to you, but I believe that with the right guidance, presence of thought, and connecting to the sensation of your body you can reset your entire organism without the need to acquire new dependencies. What I am presenting here is a completely different perspective from what is offered today by so much of mainstream medicine. It is my aim to show you how you can benefit from my many years' experience of approaching the body-mind-consciousness paradigm as a scientist, patient, and healer. In all humility, I can say I've approached this paradigm as a healer because I was the first patient I healed on my journey of discovery.

The very real body-mind suffering I underwent to avoid drug dependency and to develop inner support helped me build a connection to something deeper within myself, in parallel with the integration of beneficial Eastern practices into my life. Alongside my own evolution, I see how widely yoga, the sister science of Ayurveda, and related health modalities have been fully embraced in our Western lives. I will share with you my forty years of experience combining mainstream medicine and alternative medicine, particularly Ayurvedic medicine and related modalities, with the purpose of showing you how these methods can be integrated into treatment plans for individuals experiencing depression. This book will show you how these techniques work and how to put them into practice. I will use the skills, insights, and scientific rigor gained from many years of conventional medical research to convey an understanding of the validity and cohesion of Ayurveda.

The framework of Ayurveda allows us to identify our individual constitutions, which permits us to tailor treatments to the individual's condition and particular state of ill health with the objective of restoring balance. Ayurveda is as useful and valid in addressing ill health today as it was thousands of years ago. Here I will show you how the current biomedical understanding of our remarkably beautiful and complex physiology corresponds with Ayurvedic understanding. Your cells perform millions of metabolic activities per second, although you are not aware of them. My aim throughout this book is to bring you, dear reader, closer to understanding—even if only in an abstract way—how extraordinary the human body is and to help you successfully integrate new components into your daily life and feel the physiological changes within.

For readers directly confronting depression, anxiety, or dependency, this book presents practical applications and specific protocols of Ayurveda to support and encourage you as you face your challenge. I hope to inspire you to overcome obstacles and deal with issues in a completely new way. For those who may be reading this book on behalf of a family member, partner, or friend who is suffering from some form of depression, I trust you will relay this information and approach to your loved one in their search for help. For any readers who are professionals who work with patients encountering depression, you should find—irrespective of the particular discipline or modality in which you work—that you and your patients can benefit from the ideas and techniques described here.

. . . .

Pain is inevitable; suffering is optional.
It is up to each of us to make a choice.

. . . .

I still have a scientific and inquisitive mind, actively cultivating its search for knowledge. I also continue as best I can to be connected in a balanced way to my thoughts and feelings. A serious scientist is and always will be a student—always learning. That is what I am and would like to remain. I invite you to keep your eyes, mind, and feelings fully open. From that place we can start our journey together.

2

Introduction to Ayurveda for the First-Time Reader

AYURVEDA'S GLOBAL REVIVAL

Ayurveda originally spread through India as an oral tradition, later being written down in the Sanskrit language in the ancient Hindu scriptures known as the Vedas, which are among the oldest texts in the world. Ayurveda did not begin with the Vedas; it has always existed, just as gravity did not start with Isaac Newton or genetics with the discovery of DNA. For thousands of years the Vedas have given us the philosophy, mechanics, treatment strategies, and detailed descriptions of Ayurvedic medicine. According to Vedic science, the deep inner Self (pure consciousness) triggers the inner faculty (working consciousness), which in turn triggers the physical body. This schema provides the context for Ayurveda's conceptualization of ill health and imbalance, both physical and mental.

As you start to incorporate Ayurveda into your depression management program, you are immediately presented with a challenge: coming to grips with its terminology. Let me assure you, once you get the hang of the basic terms and their meanings, they will become second nature. There is even a joy in using this newly acquired vocabulary to describe who we are, how we feel, and how we perceive ourselves. We will limit ourselves to only the essential terms required to show how Ayurveda assesses and supports the specific treatment of depression, and to those terms that describe more generally how Ayurveda helps us manage our daily well-being. We are going to need these terms to evaluate your body-mind constitutions and body-mind imbalances, in order to recommend specific practices that match your constitution and type of depression.

Ayurvedic terms can communicate several meanings from their basic root meanings. The meanings that apply in a given instance will depend on context, and you will see that we have several uses for certain key words relative to the context being described. The terms we will use are derived from Vedic Sanskrit, the oldest form of Sanskrit, and the language of the Vedic sciences. We transliterate these terms into English and then translate them into modern medical and social meanings.

As with any translation, it is not always possible to capture an exact match in our language for each Ayurvedic term; however, our working definitions are more than sufficient for our understanding and practical use. As a simple example, the Sanskrit word *sattva* is said to have one hundred meanings. This is not true; it almost certainly has more, depending on the context it is used in! It is essential to work with the ancient Sanskrit texts because of their richness and precision in describing mental conditions, and how we can relate these descriptions to the treatment of depression and related conditions. Where possible, we will match the translated terms to words you may be familiar with from modern medicine.

Let's dive straight in and start with fourteen essential terms and their meanings, as presented in the table 2.1.

Table 2.1. Essential Ayurvedic terms

AYURVEDIC TERM	WORKING TRANSLATION
Prakruti	*Pra* = primary/first; *kruti* = creation/formation; DNA; your primary constitution
Vikruti	State of imbalance in your primary constitution
Doshas	Three physio-psychological body-energy principles: *vata, pitta, kapha*
Vata	Movement, bodily activities
Pitta	Energy for metabolism
Kapha	Body structure, cohesion
Dhatus	Seven bodily tissues
Agni	Digestive fire; food transformer
Ama	Undigested food; incomplete mental thoughts or emotions
Malas	Bodily waste products that need to be removed
Atma	The Self, Soul, Consciousness
Manas	Mind; can be individual or universal
Gunas	Three qualities of the mind: *sattva, rajas, tamas*
Sattva	Truth, equanimity, contentment, consciousness
Rajas	Action, energy, movement, dynamism, alertness
Tamas	Inertia, heaviness, unconsciousness, imbalance

We will integrate these terms gradually, in particular the terms *prakruti* and *gunas*. These terms are fundamental to Ayurveda, and learning them now will make it easier to expand your knowledge of Ayurveda in the future if you would like to explore deeper.

The term *Ayurveda* combines two Sanskrit words: *ayur* (life) and *veda* (knowledge or science). Thus, Ayurveda means "the knowledge or science of life" (*As. Hr. Su. 1/3; Su. Sū. 1/12*). Ayurveda distinguishes itself from modern medicine by treating each individual holistically, addressing body, mind, and consciousness together. Ayurveda's systematized knowledge of health care acknowledges your state of health and longevity from your unique viewpoint, serving you via a threefold purpose—preventive, psychological, and curative.

The Ayurvedic treatment of depression involves a number of factors: lifestyle, diet, attitude, beliefs, natural Ayurvedic medicines, and tailored Ayurvedic physical therapies. In assessing your body's degree of imbalance, Ayurveda draws on a combination of factors, including the origin of disease, your strengths and weaknesses, and the seriousness of symptoms you are experiencing.

This system then formulates a comprehensive plan, individually tailored to target the root causes of the problem and bring you back to balance. This balance is achieved by understanding the relationship between the origins of depression and the causes within the entire person. Ayurveda's psychological approach is based on a philosophy of life that focuses on essential aspects of our existence. It harmonizes your body-mind-consciousness systems and brings you back to your natural state of biological stability and strength, providing relief from symptoms—in essence *rebalancing you.*

We will be using here the term "consciousness" instead of spirit or soul. It is important to define the concept of consciousness by clarifying that Ayurveda looks at all sources and manifestations of imbalances as something more than body-mind biological exchanges and transformational energies that result from biochemical reactions. Mainstream medicine has difficulty with the definitions of consciousness and mind. "Mind" conjures up a variety of concepts: minding in the sense of emotional caring, objecting to something, the rational mind of thought and language-based reasoning, mindfulness or focused concentration, absentmindedness, clear-mindedness, small-mindedness, and the mindless blunders many of us make despite ourselves.

Consciousness can mean the perceptive awareness and responsiveness to one's surroundings, or the uncertain boundary between subconscious or unconscious processing and conscious cognition, or the restrictive idea of self-consciousness, i.e., knowing that you know. "A conscious state is one which has a higher-order accompanying thought which is about the state in question," a philosopher once said.[1]

However, with today's astrophysical knowledge, we cannot deny the existence of higher-order or cosmic energies and their role in our galaxy, solar system, planet, and organism. Just as the tides ebb and flow, so do we under the same natural laws. Ayurveda understood those concepts thousands of years ago and saw our whole body as an instrument that works only with the application of force or energy, and it considered consciousness to be a higher cosmic energy. Higher consciousness is required for the body to work. Our bodily nature has a plan, and bodily balance is maintained by a superior energy or consciousness keeping our organism healthy. Higher consciousness is the part of the human being that is capable of transcending animal instincts. Thus, we can say that all of us have a common consciousness, but a higher consciousness also exists.

AYURVEDA, WHERE HAVE YOU BEEN?

How old is Ayurveda? It has existed since the beginning of time, in the sense that Ayurveda is a reflection of nature's way of managing the micro and macro cosmos into balance. However hard we try—and sometimes we try very hard—it is an inescapable fact that we are only visitors. As a drop in the ocean, humankind has been and always will be governed by nature's laws. Thus, we are nature, and we all respond to nature's way.

Historical records show us that in our seven regions commonly regarded as continents, every civilization has had its own medicinal tradition based on its integration with nature. Regrettably, all of them suffered invasions and colonization in one way or another, resulting in the destruction of most or all of the accumulated knowledge of the colonized people, such as when the Spanish burned Mexico's libraries. The Indus Valley, which today includes India, was no exception to plunder. Despite this, Ayurvedic traditional medical knowledge remains alive today, more or less unchanged over the centuries due to its well-documented treatises. Ayurveda's authentic framework of knowledge describes the way we know things and the way things are. The Rig Veda and Atharvaveda, originating from oral traditions at least five thousand years old, were eventually written down, providing about four thousand years' worth of documented data collected by sages and scientists of each era, and describing a tradition of healthy living rooted in a profound observation of natural sciences.[2,3]

RELEVANT TEXTS

As we embark on our journey into Ayurveda, I will draw your attention to a number of key texts. These texts are called *samhitas* in Sanskrit, which translates approximately to "treatise" or "compendium." I quote from the *samhitas* partly because they capture in the written word the breadth and depth of Ayurvedic scientific practices that have remained largely intact for thousands of years and that are highly relevant to how we address depression from the Ayurvedic perspective. I also quote from the *samhitas* because they contain the most profound, timeless wisdom. One sentence from a *samhita* can capture the entire essence of a topic. The *samhitas* are of course originally written in Vedic Sanskrit, and here I will use widely adopted English translations that hopefully are faithful enough to the original meaning.

I will be quoting from two authors who have written canonical Ayurvedic *samhitas,* and from a third who has written pivotal yoga texts: Charaka, Sushruta, and Patanjali.

Charaka

Charaka, who lived and worked circa third century BCE, was a master physician and is considered by many scholars to be the father of medicine. Charaka compiled much of the Indian medical tradition in the form of *samhitas.* These eight books, containing twelve thousand metered verses and alongside paragraphs written in prose, are the bedrock of Ayurvedic practice. Systematically they cover physiology, anatomy, several branches of internal medicine, the causes and symptoms of disease, diagnosis, treatment, prescriptions, preventions, and longevity. The *Charaka Samhita* contains 341 recipes of plant origin, 177 using animal products, and 64 using minerals and metals.[4]

> *Every individual is different from another and hence should be considered as a different identity. As many variations are in the Universe, all are seen in human beings.*
>
> —*Ca. Su.*[5]

Sushruta

Sushruta's name is synonymous with India's surgical inheritance. He is believed to have lived and taught in Benares, India, several centuries before the Buddha. Sushruta composed the *Sushruta Samhita,* a six-book, 186-chapter analysis of the human condition in health and disease, with an emphasis on surgical procedures. Sushruta is acknowledged in the West as the father of plastic surgery, and he was the first to develop novel techniques in reconstructive surgery, such as skin grafts and total nasal reconstruction. *Sushruta Samhita* discusses 1,120 illnesses, including those related to mental health. These discussions cover seven hundred healing plants, 57 preparations obtained from animal sources, and 64 preparations obtained from minerals.[6,7]

Patanjali

The Ayurvedic perspective on treating depression also encompasses yoga. While being a fashionable fitness routine for many, yoga is also an ancient practice developed in India more than five thousand years ago. The word "yoga" derives from the Sanskrit word *yuj,* which means "join" or "unite," signifying this practice's ability to expand physical, mental, emotional, and spiritual well-being.

The earliest written record of yoga appeared as aphorisms *(sutras)* written by the Indian author Patanjali around 400 BCE. Patanjali is to yoga what Buddha is to Buddhism. The many interpretations of his *sutras*—defined literally as "the path to transcendence"—provide the means for self-realization through body poses, breathing exercises, and spiritual and meditative practices.[8]

Yoga is a science closely related to Ayurveda. Before the recent revival of these modalities, those viewing yoga and Ayurveda from the Western medical-scientific mindset often disparaged them for their ambiguity and seemingly inexplicable philosophical principles. This resulted in a dearth of interest in investigating what Ayurveda had to offer Western medicine, depriving many patients of the practical, cost-effective benefits of this traditional health care system. However, Ayurveda and yoga continuously revive themselves and adapt without ever abandoning their original structure.

For example, we can see the emergence and vitality of yoga over the past ten years. Now practiced by millions in gyms and homes all over the world, few doubt the efficacy of yoga in helping to maintain good physical and mental health. What is striking about the explosion of yoga in the West is the precision and purity of practice that yoga students and teachers embrace. Many yoga practitioners are remaining true to yoga's ancient scientific essence. There is little appetite to water yoga down. It remains intact. Similarly, meditative techniques now fashionably called "mindfulness" are also growing in popularity and acceptance. These are all part of Ayurveda's tool kit for rebalancing health without using toxic and unnatural substances. Both yoga and mindfulness share a common practical point with Ayurveda: they are very cost-effective, requiring minimal expense to fully engage with.

With the increased interest in these related holistic systems comes an openness on the part of many people who are interested in incorporating Ayurveda into their health program. Ayurveda has lagged behind in Western popularity, partly because there is a lack of qualified Western Ayurveda practitioners to advise the growing number of patients. The good news is that this interest is almost always self-generated by individual patients with positive perspectives on tried and tested systems such as Ayurveda, in an effort to regain control of their health and restore balance. However, in our eagerness to plow ahead we must first pause to do some preparatory study of the Ayurvedic framework as a whole, so we can understand how Ayurveda sees us and learn how we can use it to help ourselves rebalance.

Ayurveda aims to maintain good health in a healthy person and to help us attain the four principal aims of life: *dharma,* right livelihood and moral values; *artha,* the means to achieve your life's purpose; *kama,* nonattachment to desires; and *moksha,* self-realization of who you are.

My aim at this stage is to walk you through a gentle introduction to Ayurveda, together with a comparative look at conventional medicine. I will briefly describe how both systems approach health, disease, and well-being, paying particular attention to the physiological, biochemical, and psychological factors involved in depression. In this way, you will understand the uniqueness of Ayurveda's approach to balancing the body-mind-consciousness trilogy.

Additionally, I aim to kindle deepening interest in you to see the beauty and simplicity of the Ayurvedic approach and how it offers easy and achievable alternatives to improve the management of your complete health—including treatment of depression. Ayurveda offers every patient a warm welcome.

AYURVEDIC HEALTH

The essence of Ayurveda is the maintenance of a state of dynamic balance among the three body energies called *doshas (vata, pitta,* and *kapha)* within the tissues *(dhatus)* constituted by the *gunas* (universal qualities/attributes).

Ayurveda considers the human body to be in good health based on the equilibrium of body, mind, and consciousness. For each of us, this results from a dynamic balancing of our:

- three *doshas: vata, pitta,* and *kapha* (which are body energies or constitutions, also known as biomaterials or humors);
- metabolic and/or digestive fire *(agni);*

- seven bodily tissues *(dhatus)*; and
- waste products such as feces, urine, and sweat *(malas)*.

The body is composed of no more than doshas, dhatus, *and* malas.

—*Su. Sū.* 15/3

This is the way that Ayurveda has presented good health for millennia:

He is healthy whose doshas, agni, *and the functions of* dhatus *and* malas *are in equilibrium; whose mind, intellect, and sense organs are bright and cheerful.*

—*Su. Sū.* 15/40

I am pleased to report that the WHO agrees with Ayurveda's emphasis on harmony. The WHO defines human good health as "a state of complete physical, mental, and social well-being and not merely the absence of disease or infirmity."[9]

AYURVEDIC BALANCE

The Ayurvedic approach to achieving a dynamic balance for you, the patient, that I will set out here draws on a number of strands:

- A medical system balancing body, mind, and consciousness
- A detailed scientific disposition at the cellular and molecular level
- Foundation in the psychosomatics of ill health and diseases
- Emphasis on systems, not symptoms
- Medicines that function as energizers or rejuvenators
- Natural, simple, affordable remedies
- Emphasis on diet and food compatibility
- Focus on improving the immune system
- Orientation toward rehabilitation and palliative care

CONCEPT OF LIFE: THE THREE UNIVERSAL QUALITIES

Ayurveda regards all creatures as an aspect of nature, and all are governed by the laws of nature. Ayurveda describes three universal qualities of nature that permeate everything. These three qualities, together known as the *triguna*, may be thought of as highly refined potentials that convey direction, organization, and a unique character to that which they permeate. According to the Indian *Samkhya* philosophy,[10] your *prakruti* (body constitution) is composed of these three basic *gunas*.

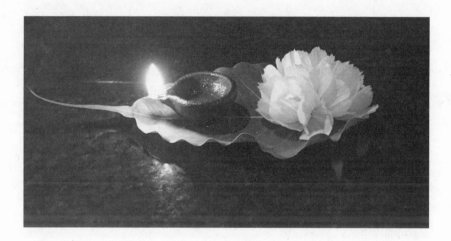

Table 2.2. Typical properties of *triguna* and their examples

TRIGUNA	QUALITY	EXAMPLES
Sattva	Truth, equanimity, contentment, consciousness	Sunlight
Rajas	Action, energy, dynamism, alertness	Atomic movements
Tamas	Inertia, heaviness, unconsciousness, imbalance	Stone

These three qualities function together much as the different parts of a candle do:

- *Sattva* (pure energy required for creation): light
- *Rajas* (activity of movements): flame
- *Tamas* (inert material for conversion into energy): wax

THE FIVE ELEMENTS: SPACE, AIR, FIRE, WATER, AND EARTH

Genetic Constitution: *Purusha* and *Prakriti*

Ayurveda describes every human being as a creation of the universe, through the pure cosmic consciousness that is represented by two kinds of energies: *purusha* (passive awareness or passive potential energy, historically referred to as "male" energy), and *prakriti* (creative potential or divine creative will, historically referred to as "female" energy). It is interesting that modern biomedicine has found that in sexual reproduction, the mitochondria (the source of our cellular energy) are normally inherited mostly or totally from the mother; the mitochondria in mammalian sperm are usually destroyed by the egg cell after fertilization.[11,12]

Purusha doesn't take part in creation. *Prakriti*, on the other hand, does the dance of conception and formation. In creation, *prakriti* is first evolved or manifested as supreme intelligence. The supreme intelligence is the individual intellect, which further manifests as ego or self-identity *(ahamkara)* and is influenced by the *triguna: sattva, rajas,* and *tamas.*

- *Sattva* represents truth and clarity of perception.
- *Rajas* represents action and movement.
- *Tamas* represents inertia and heaviness.

Ayurveda contends that life begins with components that are imperceptible to the naked eye and that pass through various intermediate stages to reach a physically visible appearance. It calls these components *panchamahabhuta* (*pancha* = five, *maha* = big, *bhuta* = first form of existence), which are the five basic elements. In Indian philosophy, every object in the universe is composed of *panchamahabhuta*. In addition, each of the five elements has its own quality *(guna)* and a corresponding sensory organ in your body.

The study of the nature and physical basis of consciousness remains the central enigma of the scientific description of reality for many scientists. It is extraordinary how Ayurveda described the principles of consciousness thousands of years ago. Here I cite a reference to an article that examines the phenomenal nature of subjective consciousness and elucidates a possible biophysical basis for its existence, in terms of a form of quantum (unity of energy) anticipation.[13]

Table 2.3. The five *mahabhutas* (elements) and their attributes, modalities, and associated organs of perception

ELEMENT	PHYSICAL ATTRIBUTE	MODALITY	ORGAN
Ether/Field	Space	Hearing	Ear
Air	Movement	Touch	Skin
Fire	Transformation	Vision	Eye
Water	Fluidity	Taste	Tongue
Earth	Crystallization	Smell	Nose

I will now describe these five elements as manifestations of consciousness *(panchamahabhutas)* with some examples, but first let me quote Sushruta:

The moon wets the earth, the sun dries it; joined to both, air sustains life.

—*Su. Sū. 4/7*

Space/Ether: The Quantum Field

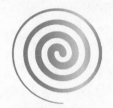 Space/ether is all-inclusive and is an expansion of consciousness. Everything needs space to exist—every molecule of oxygen or drop of water. Space is the vessel for the other four elements to exist and stay in relation with each other. Your body's visceral cavities provide space for your organs and tissues to perform their normal physiological functions, in the same way that the space between two cells allows communication. In other words, everything is interconnected between our many trillions of cells. For example, consider the microscopically small intercellular space between two neurons or a neuron and a muscular cell. This space facilitates molecular and submolecular communication, functionality, and movement.

In the nineteenth century, the scientist Michael Faraday called that connection the "ether field," a term that lacked scientific credibility, and his studies were considered invalid by the mainstream scientific community. However, after nearly two hundred years, new experiments found that the field exists, and most physicists now believe it to be a physical reality. Instead of the "ether field" it is now called the field, the quantum field, the source, the matrix, or the divine matrix, and some people call this field God.[14] The fields—now referred to in the plural because seventeen fields have been described in the scientific literature—are understood as the container for all things present in the universe, the bridge between our inner world (feelings, emotions, beliefs) and the outer world, and the mirror in the world all around us for what we consider to be true in our deepest subconscious beliefs.

It is a theoretical debate in physics today whether there really are no particles at all, only fields. On this theory, particles are merely waves in the field, and the vacuum of space is alive with these fields. Finally, science now acknowledges the interconnection understood and described by the Ayurvedic scholars. The question is: how deeply connected are we to the fields? How much influence does the way I behave, think, and feel about myself and the world around me have on my personal health and my environment? To complete this section, let me quote a *sutra* from the Mahayana Buddhist tradition:

Reality exists only where the mind creates a proper focus of attention.

—Source Unknown

Air

Ayurveda discerns that air, the second manifestation of consciousness, is a universal magnetic field responsible for the movement of the earth, wind, and water. Today, in conventional scientific terms, we understand air as a mixture of invisible, odorless, tasteless gases composed of 78 percent nitrogen, 21 percent oxygen, and small amounts of other elements. These gases direct all things that move and circulate: pumping blood and oxygen to every cell, the rhythmic exchange of air inside our lungs, and impulses from the central nervous system responsible for movement, such as neurons sending and receiving information between themselves or to organs due to the generation of minute molecular "gases." Similarly, the principle of breathing moves the diaphragm, allowing us to take air in and breathe air out, feeding our body with seventeen thousand to thirty thousand cycles per day.[15]

Your intestinal movements and other subtle cellular movements such as thought, desire, and will are also governed by the biological principle of air, which, due to technological advances, is much better understood today at a molecular level.

Fire

With movement comes friction. Friction generates combustion and heat. Consequently, the third manifestation of consciousness is fire or energy, the source of heat. The fire element is the energy of accelerated change or dissolution. The influx of heat transforms matter from solid to liquid to gas, and by eradicating heat the process can be reversed. Your body's fire is represented in various ways. The umbilical area (solar plexus) is considered the seat of fire, regulating body temperature. Fire is similarly responsible for your metabolic processes, such as digestion, absorption, and assimilation, energy that you can feel with your hands by touching your abdomen during the process of digestion. The processes of mental comprehension and appreciation also require the energy or fire of the central nervous system for healthy cerebral function to attain understanding or when transferring information to others.

Water

Water is liquefaction of consciousness, with the characteristic of adaptation to all vessels it occupies. From the heat of fire, consciousness melts into H_2O, the chemical representation of water (hydrogen and oxygen). The water element is the protector of the body and governs biological fluids, representing approximately 60 percent of your body. This "fluid ocean" keeps your body tissues healthy and functioning in many different forms, such as interstitial fluids, cytoplasmic volume, blood, saliva, nasal secretions, orbital secretions, digestive secretions, and cerebrospinal fluid. We eliminate excess water in the form of urine and sweat in order to remove the toxins and products of metabolic waste. Water is essential for nutrition and to maintain the electrolytic balance in the body. In conditions where there is insufficient water circulation, complications arise, resulting in body-mind disorders.

Earth

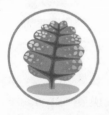

The fifth manifestation of consciousness is the earth element. Earth molecules are the crystallizations of consciousness, according to Ayurveda. Earth enters our body through the foods we consume, and it develops as part of our body. All dense, hard, firm, and compact tissues result from the earth element.

Earth becomes intimately present in all structures of our body: bones, muscles, cartilage, nails, hair, and teeth. Crystallization occurs due to the heat of fire and water. Matter created from earth is more stable, and its particles move slower, providing the required structure and stability for all forms of the world.

These five elements or *mahabhutas* form the energy and matter of our existence, and their interplay results in life.

OUR GENETIC CONSTITUTION REVEALED IN MICROCOSM AND MACROCOSM

According to Ayurvedic scholars, humanity is a creation of universal consciousness, and every human cell manifests all five elements. What is present in the macrocosm is equally present in the body, the microcosm. As a consequence, we can see ourselves as nothing more than a small-scale manifestation of nature, where fundamental physiological processes and properties keep us alive.

Modern biomedicine has helped us to understand at a deeper molecular level the underlying mechanism of our bodies. Each of the major systems—circulatory, digestive, endocrine, etc.—has been studied in great detail, thanks to today's biomedical technology, and much is known about the biochemical pathways of the body's innumerable processes. If we study our cells in light of Ayurveda's five elements, we can see that the cell membrane is earth, cellular vacuoles (storage compartments in cells) are space, cytoplasm is water, nucleic acid (DNA) and other chemical components such as the enzymes of the cell are fire, and cellular movement is air.

Cellular life involves cellular communication, transportation, circulation, energy transformation, replication, repair, maintenance, waste elimination, and defense, among other processes. These functions are influenced by the environment we occupy, as well as our genes or DNA. They follow laws of nature or mathematical formulas, such as the Fibonacci sequence or "golden spiral," which frequently appears in nature, from the macroscopic realm (e.g., snails, flowers) down to the microscopic realm, including our own DNA.[16]

It is important to remember that although many of the scourges of civilization, such as poor hygiene and infectious disease, have been greatly reduced by advances in public health, our modern societies are exposing us to other kinds of environmental issues. These include the quality of air, water, and food available to us; the types of food we cook and eat; the physical activities and psychosocial factors in our personal lives; the traumas we may have experienced; and the toxins we have to eliminate, all of which affect our DNA and *prakruti*. When these factors are out of balance, they can endanger the constant balancing act taking place within your body. By damaging or destroying our habitat (the microcosmos where we are living), we generate the same effects in our bodies, becoming less resourceful and more susceptible to certain conditions.

It was formerly believed that genetic predisposition led to inevitable, unavoidable outcomes for our lives. Today, geneticists are exploring and explaining how our genes are *not* the only factor in shaping our individual constitution. Epigenetics is an emerging science that studies the biological mechanisms by which genes switch on and off. Your DNA gives the instructions for various functional proteins to be produced inside the cell. The functions of epigenetics affect how genes are read by cells and whether the cells should produce relevant proteins. Due to the study of epigenetics, we know now that our environment can influence and modify the way the twenty-five thousand genes in our DNA are regulated and expressed, and our practices, attitudes, and beliefs play a very important role in that process as well.[17] When these environmental factors are imbalanced by our lack of cooperation with nature, that imbalance could lead to disease. It should come as no surprise that Ayurveda understood and incorporated this knowledge thousands of years ago through the understanding that by developing awareness, we can actively help shift an imbalanced state of health to a balanced one.

You will see how Ayurveda can explain epigenetics through its clear conceptualizations and understandings of the causes of imbalance and inherited or noninherited disease factors.[18] Ayurvedic medicine's understanding of our uniqueness plays a very important role by offering tailored recommendations concerning your routine, what you eat, where you live, who you interact with, when you sleep, how you exercise, and even how you age.[19]

3

Fundamentals of Ayurveda

WE ARE ALL THE SAME, YET DIFFERENT

We arrive in this world with much the same physical form as each other, but in a matter of just a few years the differences in our shapes and sizes are striking. Our cellular DNA creates muscles at different rates, burns fat from some parts and not others, and builds varying bone structures. Some of us are taller than others, some have long legs and a short torso, some have short legs and a long torso, some have a barrel-shaped chest, others a sunken chest. Various body types not only look different but also function differently. You may have encountered descriptions of body or mind typologies such as that developed by the Greek physician Hippocrates (ca. 460 BCE–ca. 370 BCE), who is often credited with developing the theory of the four humors—blood, yellow bile, black bile, and phlegm—and their influence on the body and its emotions. Another body typology is the scheme of ectomorphic, mesomorphic, and endomorphic somatotypes presented by Sheldon in 1940.[1]

There exist other classifications beyond the physical form, including variations in mental function (multiple kinds of intelligence), emotional response (levels of emotional reactivity or sensation-seeking), social relationships (level of need for attachment or solitude), and behavioral tendencies (level of stress reactivity).[2] The concept of predetermined destiny can be frustrating for those of us who seek to maintain and improve our lives through diet, nutrition, and exercise. If your body is naturally inclined to be lean, for example, you will find it harder to build muscle and bulk up. Conversely, if you are inclined to store a quantity of fat, you will find it more challenging to lose excess weight.[3]

In Ayurveda, those same conditions equally apply to your mind, a concept we will explore to understand how metabolic, hormonal, and mental processes work with your particular *prakruti* and your condition of depression and how you can become an active participant in its improvement. To do this, we map out the fundamental framework of Ayurveda, which is centered on the concept of the *tridosha*, or qualitative energetic field types, that express your distinctive *prakruti*, or constitutional nature.

Ayurveda also describes three vital, subtle essences called *prana, tejas,* and *ojas,* which correspond to the *vata, pitta,* and *kapha doshas,* respectively.

- *Prana:* vital force without which life cannot exist, primarily taken in through the breath

- *Tejas:* essence of fire *(agni)* and *pitta dosha,* conducting all bodily fires, such as digestion, intelligence, and muscular contraction

- *Ojas:* promotes and sustains physical vitality, mental clarity, and overall health

The concepts of *doshas* and *prakruti* are fundamental to Ayurvedic medical science. *Prakruti* assessment is addressed in three classic Ayurvedic texts: *Charaka Samhita* (focusing on internal medicine), *Ashtanga Sangraha* (focusing on physiology and therapeutics), and *Sushruta Samhita* (focusing on surgery). The evaluation of *prakruti* involves a variety of methods employed by the Ayurvedic physician, such as:

- a thorough physical sensory examination involving visual, tactile, olfactory, and auditory evaluations;

- extrapolation based on information collected by indirect means, including questions asked of the patient; and
- conclusions based on available data, knowledge, and experience.

To understand the unique approach Ayurveda takes to the treatment and management of depression-related conditions, we must first understand *prakruti*.

LIFE IN 3D: THE THREE MAJOR BODY TYPES *(TRIDOSHA)*

Prakruti (pra = primary or first, *kruti* = creation or formation) is the starting point in our exploration of Ayurveda. This word describes in Ayurvedic terms the individuality of every human being. To avoid future confusion, here is a brief description of how Ayurveda classifies the constitutions or *prakruti:*

- Genetic constitution *(janma prakruti):* recorded in the genes (DNA) at the moment of conception
- Mental constitution *(manas prakruti):* interpreted in terms of the three *gunas (sattva, rajas,* and *tamas);* manifesting in unequal proportions expressing the person's individual consciousness
- Bodily constitution *(deha prakruti):* the changes that arise between conception and birth
- Biological *prakruti (dosha prakruti):* biological energy at birth expressed in terms of *vata, pitta,* and *kapha*

In Ayurveda, innate disposition, providence, time, chance, cosmic order, and evolution are regarded as prakruti.

—*Su. Sa.* 1/11

The structural aspect of our bodies is made up of the five elements, but our functional aspects are governed by three anatomic-physiological expressions of these elements *(doshas),* sometimes referred to as biological humors (which, as an aside, we can also see as distinctive functional

41

electromagnetic fields; but we will not delve into this perspective here, as our goal is to describe briefly the concept and implications of *prakruti* for treating depression and related conditions). The concept of *prakruti* corresponds to the modern medical concept of genetic material or DNA. In ancient India, the explicit naming of a molecule like DNA or cellular terminology did not exist as we understand it today, but the role that such substances played in the life process was fully captured and described in Ayurvedic texts.[4]

Even though the discoveries of DNA and functional genomics lay more than three thousand years in the future, scientists of those days described extracellular and intracellular energies, functions, and concepts that align with modern scientific understanding. Ayurveda considers our complex, intricate human body to be controlled by varying combinations of three fundamental biological energies, or *doshas*, in an intensive interplay that governs all the molecular and biochemical mechanisms in the body and mind. Although we cannot translate certain Sanskrit words exactly, it is useful to know that *dosha* originates from the word *dushya*, which means "disturbance" or "that which is vitiated."

The three biological energies, or *doshas*, can be described as:

- **Breezy**: subtle energy or active forces related to activation of movement *(vata)*
- **Fiery**: the body's metabolic system for transformation or chemical activity *(pitta)*
- **Earthy**: energy that creates the body's structure or solid material form *(kapha)*

There is a fundamental correlation between the five elements and the *doshas:* space and air together constitute *vata dosha*, fire and water constitute *pitta dosha*, and water and earth constitute *kapha dosha* (*As. Hr. Su.* 1/6). In that way, *vata, pitta,* and *kapha* are the three biological humors present in a variety of combinations that manifest as different organic body-mind constitutions (see table 3.1).

Table 3.1. The *mahabhutas* (elements) and their associated *doshas*

ELEMENTS	ASSOCIATED *DOSHAS*
Space + air	*Vata:* motion
Fire + water	*Pitta:* chemical/metabolic activity
Earth + water	*Kapha:* solid material substrate

In Ayurvedic terms, under normal conditions, the three biological components of your body's constitution coexist in a certain proportion and are constantly collaborating in a harmonious way. In that way, *vata, pitta,* and *kapha* maintain the overall function of the total organism that is you, despite the fact that they combine in a trilogy and have different properties and functions.

. . . .

At the time of fertilization, the combination of your parents'
prakruti *(their DNA) determines your individual constitution,*
and both the ovum and sperm are equally influenced by your
parents' lifestyles, diets, and emotions.

. . . .

The *vata-pitta-kapha* trilogy, which I call our 3D trilogy, is present in every tissue in every human being, from the cellular level up to the body's systems. These three biological energies govern all biological processes, including your physiological and psychological imbalances. Each of us has a unique combination and ratio of these three *doshas,* shaping our characteristic physiological, physical, and mental features, with further classification into subgroups depending on specific *dosha* predominance. The 3D trilogy can change according to lifestyle, diet, and emotions. When those changes are challenging, they can cause body imbalances or diseases.

There are seven types of *prakruti* based on permutations of the three *doshas:*

- The first three types of *prakruti* represent a strong predominance of one of the three *doshas*, with the other two *doshas* present to a lesser extent. We refer to these monotypes as *vata-, pitta-,* or *kapha*-dominant.

- The next three types of *prakruti* represent a strong predominance of two *doshas*, creating dual types: *vata–pitta, pitta–kapha,* or *kapha–vata* dual predominance.

- The last type of *prakruti* is *vata–pitta–kapha,* which occurs when there is an equal proportion of the three *doshas* (*Su. Sa.* 4/61).

Knowledge of your *prakruti* is essential for a better understanding of yourself and to formulate a personalized program to rebalance your health. The three *doshas* are in an intensive interplay of motion *(vata)*, chemical activity *(pitta)*, and solid material structure *(kapha)* among themselves, and that interplay both governs our internal environment and responds to our external environment.[5,6] Their mutual interaction is crucial for maintaining a steady, equilibrated state, even though there may be disturbing influences that operate upon them at all times. The three *doshas* are the tripod upon which life rests. They are your blueprint.

Maintaining a balance in the activity of the *doshas* as determined at conception *(prakruti)* is necessary for good health. Although the three *doshas* coexist in determined proportions and function in a complementary manner to maintain the overall function of the body, they can manifest properties that are opposite one another, and they are always in a perpetual dance. For example, *pitta* has the property of keeping the body warm, based on fire as its major constituent. On the other hand, *vata* cools the body's temperature. The subtle movements of the *doshas'*

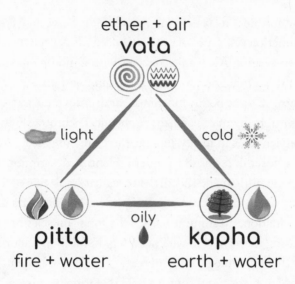

constituents are responsible for the characteristics and functions that shape your unique psychosomatic temperament and body characteristics.

Ayurveda divides each *dosha* into five subdivisions, each one playing a role according to the organs or tissues where it is performing a physiological function. Sushruta described seven basic types of tissues, called *dhatus,* that are crucial in developing, nourishing, and sustaining the body (*Su. Sū.* 15/7). We are not going to delve into this particular topic in any great detail here, because a simplified understanding is sufficient at this introductory stage.[7,8,9]

DESCRIPTIONS OF *VATA, PITTA,* AND *KAPHA* IN THE *PRAKRUTI*

Breezy *(Vata)* Body Constitution

Biological *vata* originates from the five great elements, with the predominance of the elements space and air. *Vata* represents the principle of movement within an organism, or "biological air." Examples of *vata* functions are motor functions manifested by

45

the contraction and relaxation of muscles, digestive movements, and secretory functions.

When comparing Ayurvedic concepts with a modern medical under-standing of those functions, for *vata* the main question is how airy gases could perform all those bodily functions. For decades scholars tried to asso-ciate *vata* with small molecules, like the chemical neurotransmitters adren-aline or acetylcholine. In reality, though, these are not gaseous in nature.

What is closer in terms of a modern scientific description is the very small molecule nitric oxide (NO), the so-called "molecule of life." NO is produced by nearly every type of cell in the human body. Its main func-tion is vasodilation, meaning it relaxes the inner muscles of your blood vessels, causing the vessels to widen. I am grateful to Salvador Moncada, who made the first biological identification of NO, because not only did his discovery transform my conventional scientific research at that time; it also provided me a way to describe the modern medical elucidation of the ancient Ayurvedic concept of *vata*.[10]

. . . .

NO fits like a glove with the Ayurvedic descriptions of vata *in its many important cell functions, including regulation of healthy blood flow and blood pressure levels, communication between cells in the brain, and defending our bodies against pathogens.*

. . . .

Later we will discuss the extraordinary biochemical role of this gas-eous molecule and how it relates to mental health function, starting from the various causes of vitiation of *vata dosha,* the different ways to rebal-ance its function, and its fundamental role in the biology of depression.[11]

Importance of *vata*

- Life exists as long as *vata* continues in the body.
- It controls independent movement and is the source of the body's movements.

- *Vata* mobility keeps *pitta, kapha,* and body tissues in motion.
- It exercises direct control over all bodily functions.[12]

Qualities

- Dryness, lightness, coldness, mobility, roughness, clearness, dispersing (*As. Hr. Su.* 1/11; *Ca. Su.* 1/59)

Function: motion

- *Vata* controls enthusiasm, inspiration, expiration, and all voluntary and involuntary actions of the body, triggering the circulation of all tissues and organs, e.g., blood and plasma circulating throughout the body.
- It is responsible for conception, development of the embryo, and expulsion of the fetus and placenta at birth.
- *Vata* is equally responsible for all sensory and motor functions of the nervous system, as well as the processes of excretion (urine, feces, and sweat).

General comments on *vata prakruti*

- People who have a predominantly *vata* constitution generally tend to have a slender body frame, light muscles, lighter amounts of body fat, cold hands and feet, and poor circulation.
- A *vata* person will have a predisposition to dry hair, dry skin, and a dry colon.
- *Vata* people generally dislike the cold season and prefer warmth, are vivacious, and easily manifest emotions of fear, anxiety, insecurity, and nervousness.
- A balanced *vata* mind is clear, alert, and intelligent, and it pursues many interests and communicates effectively; but it has a tendency to forget things quickly.

Fiery (*Pitta*) Body Constitution

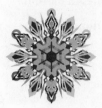 *Pitta* is the result of the combination of the fire and water elements. In order to sustain a balanced life and resist degeneration and decay, we depend on food, which, once digested and assimilated, will nourish and replenish our body tissues. The term *pitta* is derived from a Sanskrit word that means "fire," and in Ayurvedic terms it represents the metabolizing of ingested food for biological transformation and generation of body heat and metabolic energy.

Importance of *pitta*

- The body is the product of food, according to Ayurveda (*Ca. Su.* 28/45).
- Under the principle that everything under the sun manifests by fire, food can be eaten, drunk, licked, and masticated, and it can induce impressions.
- *Pitta* acts in breaking down food and metabolizing it into molecules that integrate into the diverse constituents of our bodies.

Qualities

- Hot, sharp, light, liquid, sour, oily, and spreading (*As. Hr. Su.* 1/11; *Ca. Su.* 1/60).

Function: conversion

- *Pitta* controls all kinds of metabolic processes, including digestion, assimilation, hunger, thirst, and body temperature maintenance. It also controls softness, suppleness, and radiance of the skin.

- *Pitta* also plays a role in attitudes and behavior, e.g., cheerfulness .and courage. It plays a significant role in strong intellect, vision, and lucidity.

General comments on *pitta prakruti*

- The *pitta*-predominant constitution's physical appearance is generally characterized by soft, warm, oily skin and straight, oily hair, with premature hair loss or graying.

- *Pitta* armpit and foot perspiration emits a strong smell, and the feces are oily and liquid.

- *Pitta* individuals enjoy recognition. They are outspoken, have a very sharp mind and memory, and use sharp language. *Pitta* girls start menses earlier than non-*pitta* girls.

- *Pitta* people have strong appetites and digestion. If hungry, they must eat; otherwise they become irritable and hypoglycemic.

- They have penetrating, deep-set eyes and good vision but do not like bright light.

- They love reading and knowledge and have a great capacity for organization and leadership. They are perfectionist, wise, brilliant people.

Earthy (*Kapha*) Body Constitution

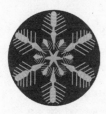

Kapha is constituted by the earth and water elements. It is understood as cohesion or joining.

Importance of *kapha*

- *Kapha dosha* regulates *pitta* and *vata* by providing nourishment (moistness, oiliness, and smoothness) to the whole body.

- *Kapha* heals wounds.

- It improves immunity.

- *Kapha* provides energy for mental and physical labor.

- It regulates patience, wisdom, knowledge, and mental balance.

Qualities

- Heavy, slow, cool, oily, liquid, dense, thick, static, cloudy, sweet, salty (*As. Hr. Su.* 1/12; *Ca. Su.* 1/61)

Function: composition

- *Kapha* is the mechanism for the structural organization of the body.

- *Kapha* represents structure—the cytoskeleton and membranes of the cells, as well as muscular and connective tissues.

- Under imbalanced conditions, *kapha* instigates hypertrophy, replenishment, heaviness of the body, and behavioral modifications.

General comments on *kapha prakruti*

- Predominantly *kapha* constitution people have heavy bones, muscles, and fat, and will tend to put on weight. They have thick, wavy hair, and big, attractive eyes.

- Solidity can manifest as good stamina and strong, well-formed muscles and bones, giving *kapha*-dominant people the ability to endure vigorous exercise when they are motivated.

- All *kapha* movements, digestion, metabolism, speech, and thought tend to be slower than *vata* and *pitta*, but they can work through the day deprived of food.

- *Kapha* is generally cool, but if in the gut then the digestive fire is high, producing a strong appetite.

- The unctuous quality can allow for smooth joint function.

- *Kapha* people have a slow but prolonged, steady memory. They are forgiving, loving, and compassionate, and they have a soft heart that is clearly sensitive.

- *Kapha* people walk slowly, talk slowly, have a sweet tooth, love eating, and tend to be sedentary and do little exercise.

The descriptions of breezy *(vata)*, fiery *(pitta)*, and earthy *(kapha)* give the Ayurvedic classification of the three basic body types. In addition, we observe a correspondence with modern perceptions of the nervous system. The autonomic nervous system works with the endocrine system to control all the automatic or involuntary functions within the body. The autonomic nervous system comprises the sympathetic and parasympathetic nervous systems, and both work involuntarily. The sympathetic nervous system is responsible for what is commonly referred to as "fight or flight," while the parasympathetic system is responsible for what is called "rest and digest." Both systems originate in the spinal cord and branch out from there, working in an opposite yet complementary manner to regulate heart rate and digestive secretions, among other functions.[13]

Based on the above descriptions, we can explain the primordial embryonic layers in the following way:

- Breezy *(vata)* type: ectomorph or sympathetic dominant

- Fiery *(pitta)* type: mesomorph or sympathetic-parasympathetic coregulation

- Earthy *(kapha)* type: endomorph or parasympathetic dominant

. . . .

It is quite extraordinary to appreciate how Ayurveda matches the doshas *with the primordial embryonic layers and the modern scientific description of the autonomic nervous system.*

. . . .

EVALUATING *VATA, PITTA,* AND *KAPHA DOSHAS* TO LEARN ABOUT YOUR *PRAKRUTI*/DNA

Remember that your individual constitution is determined at conception by a particular and unique combination of the three *doshas*—*vata, pitta,* and *kapha*—coming from your parents. Every human is a unique entity, with their individual *prakruti,* just as we each have our own DNA. Your constitution and psychosomatic temperament are primarily genetic in origin. The combination of your parents' constitutions at the moment of conception will be your individual body *prakruti,* and throughout your life this combination will be under the influence of factors such as diet, lifestyle, environment, and emotional experiences.

In addition to the fact that we all have our unique combination of the *doshas vata, pitta,* and *kapha,* each *dosha* also has variations in the twenty qualities *(gunas)* that are predominant in our constitution. Thus, our uniqueness is not only the result of our particular combination of the *doshas* but also the unique combination of the qualities of those *doshas.* To better understand how this works, this chapter provides a *prakruti* evaluation for you to complete. After completing the *prakruti* evaluation, you may find that, for example, you are *pitta* predominant. The interesting question then becomes, which quality of *pitta* is more influential in your constitution—hot, sharp, light, liquid, sour, oily, or spreading? We will address these issues later.

Knowing your personal body constitution is crucial to making Ayurveda work in your daily life and to addressing the condition of depression, because Ayurveda's effectiveness depends on treating people based on their *prakruti*. Knowing your *prakruti* makes it possible to figure out a tailored diet and lifestyle that work for you. Most people have one predominant *dosha*, but sometimes individuals have two predominant *doshas*. Less frequently there are individuals with the same levels of the three *doshas*. If you are a *vata-pitta, vata-kapha,* or *pitta-kapha,* how do you know which *dosha* you have to balance, which nutrients to eat, and which qualities to nurture? To answer those questions, follow the analysis and recommendations in the sections on both of the *doshas* that are co-dominant in you.

The *prakruti* evaluation included here will also help you better understand yourself: why you are the way you are and act the way you act. This evaluation provides an opportunity to answer questions about yourself in a focused way. It may also help you understand why you and others around you react the way they do, and how you can identify and work on different aspects of your relationships by acceptance of other people's *prakruti*.

The *prakruti* evaluation will never be 100 percent accurate. This is partly because, in case of illness, the pathological process affects the body in ways that mask some of the factors evaluated in *prakruti* diagnosis. Also, we all change from good health to reasonable health to bad health and back again at different times in our lives, which will also affect the evaluation. Still, the *prakruti* evaluation teaches you about your inherited *doshic* predominance in a way that allows you to continue learning about yourself, to understand your tendencies better, and to accept them without judging them.

Prakruti Evaluation

This *prakruti* evaluation will reveal your personal distribution of the three *doshas*. If one of the *doshas* is too high, Ayurvedic protocols will guide you to rebalance or fortify the other two constituents by means of diet, lifestyle, and exercises (e.g., yoga, meditation, relaxation, and other activities) in order to harmonize the three constituents and attain a better bodily and mental balance.

Note: in *prakruti* evaluation, you should answer each of the categories based on your typical state of physical and mental health. For example, if your immune system is normally good but you are currently experiencing a weakness in it because of a cold or flu, then your typical immune evaluation would be "good."

For each row of the *prakruti* (*manas prakruti*, *vikruti*) questionnaire, make a tick mark next to the best match to your normal condition. At the end, total up the tick marks for each column and then rank these from highest to lowest scores. The highest total is your predominant *dosha*. The second highest score is your secondary *dosha*, and the lowest score is for your least dominant *dosha*

	VATA (V)	*PITTA (P)*	*KAPHA (K)*
1	**Physique**		
	❏ Thin, bony	❏ Average	❏ Big, sturdy
2	**Height**		
	❏ Very tall or very small	❏ Medium height	❏ Small to medium
3	**Propensity to gain or lose weight**		
	❏ Difficult to gain	❏ Easy to gain or lose	❏ Overweight, difficult to lose
4	**Skin luster**		
	❏ Dull, dusky	❏ Shiny	❏ Lighter than average
5	**Skin texture**		
	❏ Dry/rough/cold, visible veins	❏ Warm/oily	❏ Lubricated, coarse
6	**Body temperature**		
	❏ Cold hands and feet	❏ Warm	❏ Cold or average

		VATA (V)	PITTA (P)	KAPHA (K)
7		Hair quality		
	❏	Dry, thin, brittle	❏ Oily, balding, graying	❏ Strong, glossy
8		Amount of hair		
	❏	Average	❏ Thin to early balding	❏ Full, thick
9		Forehead		
	❏	Small	❏ Moderate, furrows	❏ Large
10		Eyes—appearance		
	❏	Small, darting	❏ Penetrating, light-sensitive	❏ Large, attractive, relaxed
11		Eyes—lubrication		
	❏	Generally dry	❏ Normal lubrication	❏ Well-lubricated, moist
12		Teeth		
	❏	Irregular, small	❏ Regular	❏ Full, well-formed
13		Gums		
	❏	Thin gums	❏ Sensitive/bleed easily	❏ Strong gums
14		Tongue		
	❏	Rough	❏ Soft, pink	❏ Thick
15		Saliva production		
	❏	Dry mouth	❏ Average	❏ Frequent
16		Face		
	❏	Small, dry	❏ Delicate, glowing, acute	❏ Large, pleasant, soft profile
17		Nose moisture		
	❏	Often dry	❏ Unremarkable	❏ Frequently moist

	VATA (V)	*PITTA (P)*	*KAPHA (K)*
18	Thorax		
	❑ Narrow	❑ Moderately developed	❑ Wide, well-developed
19	Bones		
	❑ Thin	❑ Average	❑ Strong
20	Joints		
	❑ Cracking	❑ Loose	❑ Strong
21	Nails		
	❑ Dry, rough, brittle	❑ Soft, pink, flexible	❑ Thick, wide, soft
22	Sleep		
	❑ Light, with interruptions	❑ Not excessive but deep	❑ Deep, excessive
23	Dislikes		
	❑ Cold, dry conditions	❑ Hot places, substances	❑ Cold/oily substances, humidity
24	Appetite		
	❑ Variable/nervous	❑ Strong, must eat on time	❑ Moderate but constant
25	Food temperature preference		
	❑ Warm, oily, moist	❑ Cool or cold	❑ Warm and dry
26	Eating speed		
	❑ Quick, often small meals	❑ Moderately fast	❑ Slowly, big quantities
27	Thirst		
	❑ Changeable	❑ Usually thirsty	❑ Moderate
28	Feces: form and tendency		
	❑ Hard, dry, small, constipation	❑ Soft, loose, diarrhea	❑ Bulky, sluggish

	VATA (V)	*PITTA (P)*	*KAPHA (K)*
29	**Urine frequency**		
	❑ Infrequent	❑ Abundant, yellow	❑ Moderate, clear
30	**Sweating**		
	❑ Reduced, not much smell	❑ Often, strong smell	❑ Moderate
31	**Learning**		
	❑ Fast, tendency to forget	❑ Acute, clear	❑ Slow but constant
32	**Memory/recollection**		
	❑ Best in short term	❑ Well overall	❑ Long term very good
33	**Understanding/grasp**		
	❑ Spontaneous	❑ Average	❑ Takes a while
34	**Reaction to stressful situations**		
	❑ Fear and anxiety	❑ Frustration, irritable, anger	❑ Manage stress well
35	**Resistance to discomfort**		
	❑ Poor	❑ Average	❑ Good
36	**Immune system**		
	❑ Variable	❑ Normal	❑ Good
37	**Ailments**		
	❑ Nervous and mental	❑ Inflammatory, infections	❑ Systemic and respiratory
38	**Frequent illnesses**		
	❑ Neuralgic, joint pain	❑ Skin- and blood-related	❑ Mucus/joint inflammation
39	**Sex drive**		
	❑ Variable, sexual fantasies	❑ High sexual impulse	❑ Regular sexual impulse

	VATA (V)	PITTA (P)	KAPHA (K)
40	**Motivational disposition**		
	❏ Variable (ideas/ mood)	❏ Intense, externalized	❏ Stable, reliable, slow to change
41	**Climate predilection**		
	❏ Hot, sunny, humid	❏ Cold, ventilated	❏ Most climates except humid
42	**Activity**		
	❏ Restless	❏ Moderate, constant	❏ Slow mover
43	**Exercise inclination**		
	❏ Strong: runs, bikes, hiking	❏ Very much (with intensity)	❏ Very little, but appreciative
44	**Walking**		
	❏ Quickly	❏ Moderately fast, determined	❏ Slowly, steady, thoughtful
45	**Work/job activity**		
	❏ Very quick, lots of initiative	❏ Moderate speed, constant	❏ Slowly and methodically
46	**Temperament**		
	❏ Nervous, changeable	❏ Motivated, intense	❏ Relaxed
47	**Sensitive to:**		
	❏ Loud noises, chaotic scenes	❏ Brightness, glaring lights	❏ Strong lights, odors
48	**Positive emotions**		
	❏ Adaptability	❏ Courage, daring	❏ Affectionate, warm
49	**Negative emotions**		
	❏ Fear	❏ Intolerance	❏ Attachment

	VATA (V)	PITTA (P)	KAPHA (K)
50	**Beliefs**		
	❏ Variable, erratic	❏ Strong, determined	❏ Constant, slow to change
51	**Speech/conversation**		
	❏ Fast, not very clear	❏ Strong, clear, penetrating	❏ Slow, prolonged
52	**Tendency to spend money**		
	❏ Unnecessary/ superfluous	❏ On luxuries	❏ Prefer to economize/save
53	**Reaction to difficulties/problems**		
	❏ Anxiety, indecision, worry	❏ Anger, irritation, frustration	❏ Calm, steady/ stable attitude
54	**Others describe me as:**		
	❏ Spacey/indecisive	❏ Intolerant, annoying, intensive	❏ Stubborn, sluggish
55	**Others wish I would be more:**		
	❏ Grounded	❏ Tolerant, less judgmental	❏ Involved, enthusiastic

Total the scores in each column:

Vata:_____ Pitta: _____ Kapha: _____

Highest score _____ Corresponding *dosha*_____

Second-highest score _____ Corresponding *dosha*_____

Lowest score _____ Corresponding *dosha*_____

In descending order: _____

Your *prakruti* profile: _____

DESCRIPTION OF *VATA, PITTA,* AND *KAPHA DOSHAS:* *VIKRUTI* (IMBALANCE)

The vital physiological processes that keep us alive are influenced by the environment and our DNA, and if they become disturbed or imbalanced by our lack of connection with nature due to factors such as diet and stress, that imbalance can manifest as disease if not addressed in time.

Recent studies show that our DNA may be influenced by everything in our environment from the moment of our conception, and it is affected by our experiences, attitudes, and beliefs, causing modifications in the way our genes are expressed. When a person reaches an unnatural or modified state in which they are not aligned with their *prakruti,* Ayurveda calls that state *vikruti.* This is a state in which the body imbalance makes the body-mind state more susceptible to either physical or mental ill health.

We will explore in more detail certain traits or generalities about what *vikruti* imbalance means in terms of abnormal function for *vata, pitta,* and *kapha doshas,* after we consider Charaka's definition of health and disease:

> *Any disturbance in the equilibrium of* dhatus *(tridosha, body tissues, and waste products) is known as disease. The state of their equilibrium is health. Happiness indicates health, and pain indicates disease.*
>
> —*Ca. Su.* 9/4

Vikruti: Abnormal Breezy *(Vata)* Functions

- Increased *vata* activity manifests as excess dryness of the skin and hair, cracking joints, hoarse voice, and dry colon leading to constipation.

- People with too much *vata* may become mentally and physically too mobile, thus creating a state of worry, anxiety, and overwhelming exhaustion, leading ultimately to a type of depression caused by depletion.

- The main symptoms include tics, tremors, insomnia, and/or incessant talking.

- *Vata* aggravation can lead to mood swings, indecisiveness, and impulsive actions. It causes stuttering or harsh speech, emaciation of the skin, body aches, insomnia, debility, and desire for warm objects and substances.

- A decrease in *vata* manifests principally in symptoms of body debility, including loss of physical activity, speech, awareness, and consciousness.

- In terms of ailments, *vata*-predominant people tend to have constipation as well as neurological, muscular, and rheumatic problems.[14]

Vikruti: Abnormal Fiery *(Pitta)* Functions

- The most relevant expressions of decreased *pitta* are poor digestion, cold and clammy feet, and changes in the complexion and radiance of the skin.

- Decreased *pitta* also manifests in bitter and sour tastes, fainting attacks, debility, inflammation/exudation (putrefaction, pus formation), increased yellow coloration (skin, eyes, urine, and feces), excessive hunger, thirst, acid indigestion, loose stools, ulcers, hot rashes, fevers, high blood pressure, and insomnia.

- *Pitta*-dominant people love reading and knowledge and have a great capacity for organization and leadership. They are in general instinctive and gifted people, but they can be also controlling and domineering. *Pitta* people hold strong beliefs and remain open to new information, with a tendency toward comparison, competition, and ambition.

- They are perfectionists, and their aggressiveness disposes them to criticize others or themselves. *Pitta* people tend to get inflammatory diseases.

Vikruti: Abnormal Earthy *(Kapha)* Functions

- *Kapha* is the slowest and steadiest of all three *doshas*.

- Their coolness, moisture, inactivity, and/or consumption of heavy food can push *kapha* constitution out of balance in the direction of lethargy, complacency, obesity, and depression rooted in sentimental attachment to the past.

- The unctuous quality can allow for smooth joint function, but if pronounced can lead to excess fluidity or morbidity.

- Imbalances in the following conditions are likely to be responsible for aggravation: diet, habits, natural tendencies, heredity traits, and seasons.

Your *Vikruti:* Understanding Body Imbalance

To help you better understand *vikruti*, this chapter will now provide a *vikruti* evaluation for you to complete. The *vikruti* evaluation will assess any imbalance of your *doshas* based on your *prakruti* evaluation taken previously. When considering the body imbalance revealed by the results of the *vikruti* evaluation, it is important to rebalance the *dosha* that is most out of balance at the moment. You can determine which *dosha* is most out of balance by determining which *dosha*-relevant qualities are aggravating you the most in different circumstances.

An imbalance in your primary *dosha* is usually the easiest *doshic* imbalance to rectify. You can be imbalanced in any one of the three *doshas*, but you are most likely to be imbalanced in your primary *dosha*.

Here are some short hypothetical examples of how people with a co-dominant *dosha* constitution can address *dosha* imbalances:

- A *vata-kapha* person may emphasize balancing *vata* during periods of travel or when feeling anxious but should shift to balancing *kapha* when feeling unenthusiastic, sleepy, or sluggish, or if putting on some weight.

- A *pitta-vata* person should pay attention to *pitta* when feeling angry, hot, irritated, or harsh toward other people. On days when this person feels jumpy, anxious, nervous, or less grounded, it will be important to focus on balancing *vata dosha*.

- A *kapha-pitta* person could focus on *kapha* foods to reduce body weight and boost vitality, but if the person is manifesting mostly aggressive or irritable feelings, then the focus has to be on balancing *pitta*.

Always remember that all of us have three *doshas* within us, so even our least dominant *dosha* can manifest in an abruptly excessive way, due to various internal or external circumstances.

. . . .

Vikruti, *or your current state of imbalance, can mask your* prakruti.

. . . .

The *vikruti* evaluation will help you better understand your present imbalances and how you have moved away from your *prakruti*. It will also help you understand your own changes as well as changes in people close to you. You could also start to understand why others around you react the way they do as a result of their own imbalances. This is an important tool that could help you identify and work on different aspects of your relationships.

As with the *prakruti* evaluation, the *vikruti* evaluation will not be 100 percent accurate due to physical changes as a result of various health habits, diseases, or mental causes, but it will provide you with a basis for understanding which *doshas* are most misaligned with your nature.

After your *vikruti* evaluation, we will introduce you to the set of tools Ayurveda offers you to regain your mental and physical balance. I hope you will analyze the results of your constitution and imbalance assessments as the starting point in your journey toward good health and balance.

Vikruti Evaluation

Because this *vikruti* test is not intended to provide a static profile, I suggest you do it twice—the first time based on a long period of your recent life, and the second time based on how you've been feeling over the last two or three months—and calculate both scores. This is simply to help you understand whether recent life changes or challenges are affecting your *doshas*. In this way you can be a witness to your own gradual changes and rebalancing. You are encouraged to come back to the *vikruti* test from time to time, as life circumstances change for you.

Note: in *vikruti* evaluation, you should answer each of the categories based on your current medium-term/short-term experience with respect to your physical and mental health. For example, if your weight has recently decreased, not as part of a planned reduction but due to other factors, then your "Weight" response would be "Underweight, undernourished."

		VATA (V)	PITTA (P)	KAPHA (K)
1	**Body appearance**			
		❏ Slim, lean, bony	❏ Average, highly energetic	❏ Big, lethargic
2	**Weight**			
		❏ Underweight, undernourished	❏ Stable	❏ Plump, overweight
3	**Joint manifestation**			
		❏ Cracking, popping, stiffness	❏ Tender, sensitive	❏ Swollen, puffy

	VATA (*V*)	*PITTA* (*P*)	*KAPHA* (*K*)
4	**Joint sensation**		
	❏ Body aches, dryness	❏ Hot/warm, inflammation	❏ Water retention (ankles)
5	**Spine tendency**		
	❏ Sideways curvature	❏ Outward curvature, hunching	❏ Excessive inward curvature
6	**Bone issues**		
	❏ Sore	❏ Sensitive, painful	❏ Heaviness
7	**Muscles**		
	❏ Shivers, twitches, spasms	❏ Tender, inflammation	❏ Swollen
8	**Skin**		
	❏ Rough, dry, scaly	❏ Tender, inflamed, rashes	❏ Oily, smooth, clammy
9	**Lymph nodes**		
	❏ Thin	❏ Sensitive, inflamed	❏ Expanding, congested
10	**Veins**		
	❏ Drained, protruding, weaker	❏ Bruise easily, less visible	❏ Filled, wide, lifeless
11	**Eyes, vision**		
	❏ Dried, agitated, blinking	❏ Redness, light hypersensitivity	❏ Inflamed, viscous, secretions
12	**Ears, sound**		
	❏ Resounding, ringing	❏ Pain, distress, infections	❏ Blocked, secretion
13	**Nose**		
	❏ Dehydrated, crusty	❏ Inflamed, swollen	❏ Blocked

	VATA (V)	*PITTA (P)*	*KAPHA (K)*
14	**Sinuses**		
	❑ Dry	❑ Irritated	❑ Congested
15	**Mouth**		
	❑ Dry, gum disease	❑ Inflamed/sensitive gums, puffy	❑ Extreme salivation
16	**Lips**		
	❑ Dry, cracked	❑ Dehydrated, irritated	❑ Dull, unctuous
17	**Lungs**		
	❑ Dry	❑ Warm, sharp feeling	❑ Excess mucus, breathless
18	**Taste**		
	❑ Lacking taste	❑ Bitter, sour, metal	❑ "Sour" stomach, nausea
19	**Teeth**		
	❑ Cavities, weak enamel/gums	❑ Creamy/yellow, faded enamel	❑ Strong teeth and enamel
20	**Gums**		
	❑ Pale, receding	❑ Irritated	❑ Enlarged
21	**Tongue**		
	❑ Dry, fissured, murky coating	❑ Reddish, irritated, yellowish	❑ Whitish, thick coating
22	**Hair**		
	❑ Dry, weak, brittle	❑ Oily, grayish, baldness	❑ Unctuous
23	**Nails**		
	❑ Dry, brittle, broken, bitten	❑ Soft, sharp, irritated	❑ Whitish, hard, oily

	VATA (V)	PITTA (P)	KAPHA (K)
24	**Food intake**		
	❏ Erratic/compulsive tendency	❏ Excessive tendency	❏ Emotional eating
25	**Digestion**		
	❏ Irregular, ballooning	❏ Fast, heartburn, ulcers, reflux	❏ Gradual, sustained, indigestion
26	**Food absorption**		
	❏ Need warming substances	❏ Reduced	❏ Slow, steady
27	**Food assimilation**		
	❏ Reduced, body debility	❏ Reduced (putrefaction)	❏ Accumulation (obesity)
28	**Elimination**		
	❏ Dry, constipated, irregular	❏ Loose, burning, yellow urine	❏ Large, oily/mucus feces
29	**Liver and spleen**		
	❏ Noticeably enlarged	❏ Noticeably tender	❏ Enlarged and fatty
30	**Thirst**		
	❏ Fluctuating	❏ Heavy, active (feverish)	❏ Low
31	**Breathing**		
	❏ Anxious, worried	❏ Assertive, tightness	❏ Slower, from stomach, apnea
32	**Voice**		
	❏ Dry, hesitating, fiery	❏ Sharp, powerful	❏ Deep, gravelly
33	**Speech**		
	❏ Harsh, rushed, imprecise	❏ Piercing, strong, deliberate	❏ Slow, colorless, dull

	VATA (V)	PITTA (P)	KAPHA (K)
34	**Allergic reactions**		
	❏ Dry, wheeziness, gasping	❏ Rashes, flushes, urticaria	❏ Congestion, nasal secretion
35	**Sleep/napping**		
	❏ Insomnia, disrupted sleep	❏ Slow to sleep, not enough	❏ Excessive, tiredness
36	**Dreams**		
	❏ Frequent, vivid, scary	❏ Intense, deep, brutal	❏ Idealistic, tender, romantic
37	**Sex drive**		
	❏ Low and hurried	❏ High and self-serving	❏ Low but sensual, attachment
38	**Feelings**		
	❏ Worry, distress, frantic	❏ Impatient, rage, hate, envy	❏ Attached, despair, sadness
39	**Motivation level**		
	❏ Restless, quickly exhausted	❏ Intense, drained by thinking	❏ Low, tiredness due to weight
40	**Movement**		
	❏ Faster, agitated, stiff	❏ Fast and insistent	❏ Slow, lethargic, heavy
41	**Memory**		
	❏ Good recent, poor over long term	❏ Adequate, distinguishing	❏ Slow, good over long term
42	**Understanding**		
	❏ Faster but deficient responses	❏ Quicker correct responses	❏ Slower precise responses

VATA (V)	PITTA (P)	KAPHA (K)
Total the scores in each column:		
*Vata:*_____	*Pitta:* _____	*Kapha:* _____
Highest score _____	Corresponding *dosha*_____	
Second-highest score ____	Corresponding *dosha*_____	
Lowest score _____	Corresponding *dosha*_____	
In descending order: _____		
Your *prakruti* profile: _____		

PART II

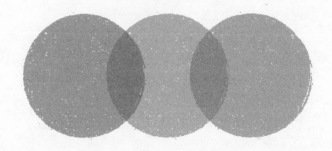

Ayurvedic Tools for Identifying Your Type of Depression

Mental Constitution
(Manas Prakruti)

A SHORT AYURVEDIC DEFINITION of good health is "a balance between body, mind, spirit, and social well-being." When trying to define balanced health in a wider and deeper way for the understanding of mental constitution *(manas prakruti)*, it is more appropriate to define health as the result of:

- Balance between the three *doshas (vata, pitta, kapha)*
- Balanced digestive fire *(agni)*
- Balance among the body tissues (seven *dhatus*)
- Balance of body secretions (feces, urine, sweat)
- Balanced physical and mental activities
- Happy, gratified soul
- Clarity of perception
- Mental purity and integrity, clarity of senses, ability to focus

The best way to understand mental constitution according to the Ayurvedic definition of balanced health requires the analysis of the above factors. All factors are directly related to the interactions between the *tridosha (vata-pitta-kapha)* and the *triguna (sattva-rajas-tamas)*.

As previously discussed, our mental constitution is also part of our DNA. From the moment of fertilization, the three constitutions *(vata, pitta,* and *kapha)* transmitted from the parents at conception bring a unique combination of *sattva, rajas,* and *tamas* characteristics from the universal mind to form the individual mind. The integration of these principles conveys us to a very interesting Ayurvedic concept of the heart as the seat of the mind, an idea discussed by philosophers and scientists for centuries until today.[1]

If that is the case, mental constitution expresses from the third month of pregnancy, when the embryo's heart starts developing. Ayurveda also holds that even before that period, there is an embryonic subconscious mind formed at the moment of conception that carries past-life memory and has the capacity of thought.

STUDYING YOUR BODY *DOSHA* CONSTITUTION AND TYPE OF DEPRESSION

The physical body and the mind are closely connected by the three biological constitutions described as *vata, pitta,* and *kapha,* and by the subtle qualities of the three *doshas* continuously acting upon and react- ing to the mental faculties. Ayurveda stipulates that psychological disor- ders arise as a result of an exacerbation of the three constitutions, either individually or in combination, triggering unbalancing changes in the way we normally act, think, feel, or perceive.

For instance, you know how poorly you can feel when you have con- ditions such as flu, or how irritable you are when you have a high fever or a bad headache. In these circumstances, if the physical manifestations continue for longer periods, they are going to manifest in a more serious physical imbalance affecting your thoughts, emotions, and desires more severely, which may lead to mental ill health.

Based on our previous descriptions of the three *doshas*, depression can be characterized as the breezy *(vata)* type, the fiery *(pitta)* type, the earthy *(kapha)* type, or in certain cases as a type that combines two *doshas*. Let's try to see which of these categories fits you best.

Breezy *(Vata)* Depression

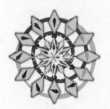 Since *vata* represents the volatile air and space elements, it tends to unground us, separating us from the heavier elements of earth and water. A general description of the *vata* kind of depression is that it is like a wind. It is an expression of the air element, transitory and changeable, in the form of a current of air blowing back and forth. *Vata* normally pushes the other two *doshas*, *pitta* and *kapha*, which cannot move without its power. *Vata dosha* is very much connected to nervous system imbalances and psychological disorders. *Vata dosha* exacerbation will manifest as agitation, imbalance, pain, and physical and mental dysfunctions.

Main Manifestations and Causes

MENTAL/EMOTIONAL MANIFESTATIONS:

- Agitation (severe)
- Anxiety
- Fear
- Feelings of worthlessness
- Fluctuation
- Hallucinations (auditory)
- Hyperactivity
- Impatience
- Indecision
- Insecurity
- Insomnia (three to four hours of sleep, sleepwalking)

- Mood changes (dusk and dawn)
- Reduced eye contact
- Silent lamentation
- Talk (unfocused and excessive)
- Unhappiness

PHYSICAL MANIFESTATIONS:

- Amenorrhea (women)
- Backaches
- Constipation
- Dehydration (dry tongue, thirst)
- Headaches (migraines)
- Lack of appetite
- Loss of body weight
- Malnourishment
- Reduced sexual desire
- Stooped posture

CAUSES:

- Certain medications or drugs
- Departure
- Disappointment
- Loss of a dear person or pet
- Shock
- Trauma

Let me give you an example: Lisa, a forty-nine-year-old woman, slim and tall, actively working, came for a consultation concerning anxious depression. After evaluation of her *prakruti*, which showed the characteristics of a *vata dosha* person, we discussed her symptoms. She was manifesting signs of insecurity, inability to concentrate properly, anxiety, low self-esteem, emptiness, fear, oversensitivity to stimuli, slow thoughts with sometimes sudden rushing reactions, feelings of being overwhelmed or unable to cope, nervousness, restlessness, insomnia, loss of appetite, dryness, and chilliness. Her main concern was to find a way to stop the oppressive chest pain she typically experienced in the late afternoons and evenings, caused by her depression.

As you can see, some of Lisa's symptoms are related to movement. The empty quality of the space and gaseous elements induced an imbalance from her original state of *vata dosha* constitution *(prakruti),* moving her to a state of imbalance *(vikruti).* That shift created a despair she was unable to overcome. Her basic normal physical or emotional needs triggered an agitated mind.

Fiery *(Pitta)* Depression

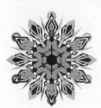 Depression related to the fire element manifests as severe depression or depressive psychosis, mostly due to a rigid and overconfident personality facing disappointment resulting from a failure or traumatic and shocking events.

Main Manifestations and Causes

MENTAL/EMOTIONAL MANIFESTATIONS:

- Aggression
- Anger
- Competitiveness
- Feelings of failure
- Feelings of worthlessness
- Fieriness
- Guilt
- Irritability

- Judgmental attitudes
- Misconduct
- Presumptuousness
- Sadness (inside)
- Self-censuring
- Suicidal thoughts

PHYSICAL MANIFESTATIONS:

- Diarrhea
- Heartburn (stomachache)
- High fever
- Hypersensitivity (light)
- Skin outbreaks (rashes)
- Urticaria

CAUSES:

- Business difficulties
- Dependency on aggravating drugs or medications
- Divorce
- End of a close relationship
- Loss of a very important relative
- Midlife crisis

Carlo, a thirty-five-year-old man working as a consultant for a biotech company, came to see me for treatment of his depression. His main concern was the stress caused by his inability to "fix" a particular professional situation in the face of a demanding schedule and a feeling that his depression was affecting his personal life. The main observed traits were damaged pride, loss of self-esteem, and his perceived impression of injustice at his workplace. When asked to describe his feelings in more detail, he manifested irritability, resentment, chronic frustration, and anger. Carlo's physical manifestations were skin rashes, waking up regularly between midnight and three a.m., disturbed digestion, hyperacidity, and loose stools.

Earthy *(Kapha)* Depression

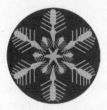 This type of depression is linked to the earth element. It is usually chronic, manifesting as melancholia and sadness.

Main Manifestations and Causes

MENTAL/EMOTIONAL MANIFESTATIONS:

- Excessive sleep
- Feeling of heaviness
- Lack of motivation
- Melancholic
- Morbid temperament
- Obesity
- Overeating
- Sluggish activity
- Social retraction
- Speech is slow, silent, or reduced
- Unvaried comportment

PHYSICAL MANIFESTATIONS:

- Lethargy
- Obesity
- Overeating (without hunger)

CAUSES:

- Contraceptives
- Corticosteroids
- Hypertensive drugs
- Overeating (eating heavy food and undue consumption of sweets)
- Oversleeping

Philippe, a fifty-four-year-old man working for a law firm as a clerk, booked an appointment over the phone to discuss his condition of being "slightly overweight and occasionally lacking energy." During our consultation, he described himself as a bit overweight, despite his medical records and my evaluations showing a condition of obesity. His denial of his condition and a certain need to hide essential information from his medical records quickly became clear. In reality, he was feeling very depressed and traumatized by his body weight.

During our discussion, Philippe finally manifested his state of sadness, lack of will and motivation, pessimism, despair, indifference to life, excessive lethargy, low energy, and slow metabolism. His case clearly fit the description of a *kapha*-depression profile, so I recommended that he investigate possible metabolic causes of provoked *kapha*, such as low thyroid, seasonal affective disorder, or estrogen dominance.

So far we have considered mental constitution for three different types of depression according to predominance of a single *dosha*. However, it is equally possible for patients to present a dual or *tridoshic* constitution. For instance, in the case of *vata-pitta* depression, the manifestation is of manic-depressive or a bipolar condition, where episodes of excitement and hyperactivity alternate with periods of depressive lows. When the depression is more of the *vata-kapha* type, there are periods when the person feels anxious and fragile, but in general the person feels dull and lethargic, seeking refuge in sweets and other kinds of unhealthy foods and substances.

There are also cases of *tridoshic* depression. You can imagine that this condition is the most threatening and the most difficult to treat, since the person manifests agitation, paranoia, anger, irritability, and lethargy more or less at the same time.

AYURVEDIC TYPES OF MENTAL CONSTITUTION (*MANAS PRAKRUTI*)

Let's now address the three universal *gunas* or qualities of consciousness manifesting under the form of three mental or psychic constitutions described in Ayurveda as *sattva, rajas,* and *tamas* and known as *manas prakruti.* Ayurveda uses these three constituents to help us understand the various types of psyches and the potential imbalances that could manifest as mental disorders such as depression.

Vedic philosophy classifies human personalities one step further by analyzing the psychological and moral temperaments in terms of three basic qualities *(triguna):*

- Truth/purity mental constitution *(sattvic)*
- Action/movement mental constitution *(rajasic)*
- Inertia/heaviness mental constitution *(tamasic)*

As we've discussed, *manas prakruti* is part of your DNA. Your father's sperm and mother's ovum both carried the three *doshas* in different proportions, creating the fertilized zygote that, from that moment, carries the combination of both partners' *prakruti.* According to Ayurveda, the zygote also carries *sattva* from the universal or cosmic mind as well as a unique permutation of the other two qualities, *rajas* and *tamas,* from the parents' minds. In this way, these qualities create the individual mind, which becomes *manas prakruti* or mental constitution.[2]

The cosmic mind maintains qualitative and quantitative equilibrium of *sattva, rajas,* and *tamas* as part of the cosmic laws of order. The classic texts describe how cosmic *tamas* creates darkness, cosmic *rajas* creates the movement of the earth, and cosmic *sattva* creates the rising of the sun. According to the laws of destiny (karma), at the time of conception a particular combination of the three *gunas* arises in the consciousness of the fertilized ovum. Different philosophical schools describe those processes in diverse ways, but according to the *Samkhya* philosophy, the mind is derived from the pure essence of *sattva*. *Rajas* and *tamas* are called *gunas* of the mind, but without *rajas* and *tamas,* the mind cannot function.[3]

These individual differences in psychological and moral dispositions, and their reactions to sociocultural and physical environments, are very well described in the classical texts of Ayurveda as principles in nature that govern the mind and emotions. The three *gunas* are essential drivers of the mind that differentiate individuals on the basis of their psychological constitutions.

Ayurveda looks at imbalances related to body-mind biological interactions and transformational energies as the result of innumerable biochemical reactions. The totality of the trilogy *sattva, rajas,* and *tamas* is defined as *consciousness,* rather than spirit or soul, because we are exploring awareness of our surroundings. Modern science has demonstrated the existence of higher cosmic energies. Results of studies conducted by the European Organization for Nuclear Research using the Large Hadron Collider may finally put this matter to rest, even though early scientific experiments concluded that the field previously called "ether" does exist.[4]

Ancient texts say everyone is connected through an enigmatic net, or field, that bridges time and space through consciousness. Ayurveda included these concepts of consciousness thousands of years ago, visualizing our whole body as an instrument that works only with the application of force or energy and conceptualizing consciousness as a higher cosmic energy. Similarly, higher consciousness is required for the body to work. We don't see it, but it is always there.

Our body, composed of trillions of cells, has a plan. Body balance is maintained by a superior energy or cellular consciousness that keeps our organism healthy. Proper functional harmony is extremely important; if that harmony is somehow disturbed by our lack of care or awareness of our basic needs, proper body-mind functioning is not possible. Higher consciousness is that potential part of the human being that is capable of transcending animal instincts. We can say that in a natural way all of us have a common, material, or lower consciousness, but a higher consciousness also exists.

Ayurvedic scholars subclassified *manas prakruti* (psychic body constitution) into sixteen subtypes: seven for *sattva*, six for *rajas*, and three for *tamas*. Our current purposes only require us to discuss the three main classifications. For further study there is additional literature available.[5]

The three types of psyche are described as born from virtue, anger, and delusion, and are said to be superior, medium, and inferior, respectively. The main qualities *(triguna)* of the three mental constitutions are described as follows:

SATTVA

- Components: truth, purity, understanding, balance, harmony, positive attitude
- Constitutions: constructive, righteous, peaceful, compassionate, loving, good

RAJAS

- Components: alert, dynamic, driven, overactive mind, overconfident, irritable
- Constitutions: competitive, passionate, controlling, individualist, self-centered

TAMAS

- Components: inertia, ignorance, imbalance, distorted mind, skepticism
- Constitutions: lazy, inactive, ignorant, disordered, reckless, selfish

A remarkable insight from Ayurveda is its understanding of the constant interplay between these three universal qualities *(triguna)* in the individual consciousness. Ayurveda teaches that the relative predominance of either *sattva*, *rajas*, or *tamas* is responsible for individual psychological constitutions as part of our genetic code. Let me give you a detailed example of each of the differences in psychological and moral dispositions for the three main kinds of manifestations, as follows:

MENTAL CONSTITUTION: KNOWLEDGE/PURITY *(SATTVIC)*

- If you are the kind of person with *sattvic* qualities, you will have the tendency to be caring; have good manners, behavior, and conduct; and be slow to get upset or angry.

- Although people with this constitution work hard mentally, they do not get mental fatigue and don't require too much sleep.

- They look happy, fresh, alert, aware, shining with luster, and joyful.

- They are intelligent, creative, humble, respectful of their teachers, and follow truth and morality.

- They are spiritual, intuitive, humanitarian, and compassionate toward all kinds of life and existence.

- If you are just *sattva* and meditate day and night with no food or sleep, that is imbalanced.

MENTAL CONSTITUTION: MOVEMENT/ACTIVITY *(RAJASIC)*

- If you are more of the movement/activity type *(rajasic),* your principal tendencies are toward having a life of sensual enjoyment, seeking pleasure, avoiding pain and effort, and experiencing restlessness.

- People with the *rajasic* constitution are often perfectionists who enjoy power, prestige, and position.

- They are egoistic, proud, and competitive, and they tend to control others.

- *Rajasic* people work hard, but without proper planning and direction, they may become ungrounded, active, and restless.

- Emotionally, they are angry, jealous, and ambitious, creating stress and fear of failure, and they soon lose their mental energy.

- They are loving, friendly, faithful, calm, and patient to those who are helpful to them.

- They are not always truthful to their inner awareness.

MENTAL CONSTITUTION: INERTIA/HEAVINESS *(TAMASIC)*

- If you have the characteristics of inertia/heaviness *(tamasic)*, your main tendencies will be toward laziness, lethargy, and excess sleep, even during the day.

- Thoughts tend toward focusing on oneself and how to acquire possessions.

- Work activities quickly tire those with the *tamasic* constitution.

- These people prefer jobs with less responsibility, requiring a short attention span, and they love to eat, drink, sleep, and have sex.

- They are greedy, possessive, attached, irritable, uncaring for others, and able to harm others in self-interest.

The soul is essentially devoid of all deformities. The soul is the cause of consciousness through the mind and the specific qualities of the basic elements (touch, shape, smell, taste, and sound). He is eternal. He is an observer. He observes all activities.

—Ca. Su. 1/56

According to Ayurveda, no one person is only *sattvic* or only *rajasic* or only *tamasic.* Our nature and behavior are a complex interplay among all three qualities *(triguna)* in varying degrees. In some, the demeanor is *rajasic* with significant influence of *sattvic guna;* in others it is *rajasic* with significant influence of *tamasic guna.* For example, the *rajasic* manifestation of safety is dependent on an outside influence, specifically the attention of others. The reaction of the *rajasic* mind will be self-protection by assuming *rajasic* activities, like ambition and self-serving endeavors. As young people we realize that through accomplishment and acknowledgment from others it is possible to feel safe again. Thus, the initial *sattvic* experience of a full heart and a free mind is replaced by the drive toward sensory stimulation of different kinds. The fact is that we are stuck in the material world of *rajas* and *tamas*. We need to have release from *tamas* and *rajas* by self-monitoring states such as lethargy, agitation, desire, and temptation.

As a result of becoming satisfied through *rajasic* activities and drive, our mind can burn out, and by collecting temporary satisfactions through the senses, we retreat into a safe, protective cocoon. If individuals with a *rajasic* constitution follow that path again and again, they could become lonely, bitter, and angry, and they eventually may seek drugs, alcohol, or other dependencies to maintain the illusion of the safe cocoon, manifesting a *tamasic* constitution. By living in that state of inertia and dependency, it becomes difficult to leave and requires the cultivation of *sattva* qualities to offer a sight of the lost experience of truth, joy, and happiness, along with the restoration of *rajas* to provide the energy needed for action and change.

IDENTIFYING YOUR *MANAS PRAKRUTI*

Assessment of *Manas* Constitution

In the same way you were able to evaluate and understand your *prakruti* evaluation and potential imbalances by using the *vikruti* constitution test, we can similarly evaluate and understand the state of balance of the mental constitution of an individual by evaluating *manas prakruti*. This chapter will provide a questionnaire that will allow you to perform this evaluation yourself. When you take this test, answer the questions based on your regular state over a number of years and not just a recent state, since we are seeking to measure your normal mental state. Be as accurate as you can with respect to your feelings as you answer the questions. What counts is to capture your real nature, not what you would like it to be.

Ayurveda describes your mental constitution in a similar way to its description of your bodily constitution, by giving a numeric value to each of the three *gunas* in an individual's constitution. For instance, you may be *sattva* 3, *rajas* 2, *tamas* 1 (S3:R2:T1), while another person may be *tamas* 3, *sattva* 2, *rajas* 1 (S2:R1:T3). These measures give us an idea of what mental characteristics a person will tend to have at a particular period of life.

To give an illustration, somebody could complete an evaluation that shows they have a regular mental constitution *(manas prakruti)* ratio of S2:R3:T1. Nevertheless, if they complete another evaluation days or weeks later based on their state at that moment, it may show a different mental constitution *(manas vikruti)* ratio of S2:R3:T2, where *tamas* has a higher proportion (28.6 percent) than it had in the previous evaluation (16.7 percent). *Tamas* may have increased because the person recently has been disrespecting diet, drinking too much alcohol, or working longer hours. Imbalanced mental constitution can change very quickly, even over a short period of time. One day a person might have more *sattva* mind after listening to an uplifting or inspiring talk; some days later, the same person could be more *rajasic* due to a hectic working day.

We can quickly improve our mental state by relaxing or employing meditative activities, bringing more awareness to all we do. Someone who is born with a predominantly *rajasic* or *tamasic* quality can make their mental *prakruti* more *sattvic* through meditation, yoga, noncompetitive activities such as exercise, and proper guidance.

Always remember, the *triguna* is constantly changing; thus, this questionnaire is not intended to provide a static assessment. The purpose of being aware of the three *gunas'* qualities is to attain greater awareness of your tendencies or state of depression. This will help open your eyes to your protective patterns of behavior stemming from influences in your childhood or other stages of your life that created strong and lasting impressions, such as shocks or traumas. According to Ayurveda, these protective patterns affect your body-mind constitution.

For a clearer observation of your state of depression, you need to determine your *manas prakruti*. If, after evaluating your mental constitution, the test describes you as a *tamasic* person, you can acknowledge this in yourself: "Yes, I'm *tamasic*. That's fine." Once you make the effort to observe and become aware of your *tamasic* qualities, then the *tamas* begins to gradually modify due to your practice of self-observation. We are mostly not really aware of who we are; we do not ordinarily take the time to reflect on this. Ayurveda recommends that emotions be observed with detachment and then allowed to dissipate. When emotions are unexpressed or repressed, that repression will cause disturbances in the mind and eventually in the functioning of the body.

A person who has been repressing feelings and who then experiences bouts of anger does not necessarily know they are angry. It is only when they observe their anger "from outside themselves" that they can begin to let this anger dissipate. This example of repressed feelings has physical consequences: it could change the flora of the gallbladder, bile duct, and small intestine, and it could aggravate *pitta*, which causes inflamed patches on the mucous membranes of the stomach and small intestine, as we will observe in later sections. By practicing self-observation and using the *manas prakruti* evaluation from time to time, you will learn to navigate toward creating a more *sattvic* experience of life for yourself.

Manas Prakruti Evaluation

The *manas prakruti* evaluation is an invitation to make helpful changes based on how Ayurveda uses its understanding of the governing principles of *sattva, rajas,* and *tamas.*

Let us briefly consider the three dispositions of the mind in Ayurvedic terms. A truly *sattvic* nature is deep in contentment and truth—in other words, free of desire. A *rajasic* state of mind is active and needs stimulation, usually through the senses, in order to be satisfied. A *tamasic* type is more vulnerable due to their lethargic tendency and the likelihood of being more under the influence of inertia.

Ayurveda encourages us to become aware of our state of mind by observing our imbalances. In this particular case, we are addressing people with depressive tendencies and supporting them in improving from a *tamasic* to a *rajasic* state or from a *rajasic* to a *sattvic* state. For most of us, answers to this evaluation will generally fit in the middle or the *rajasic* area, which is the main state in our active and outgoing culture today.

We all carry psychological issues from the past, and we deal with situations and problems daily. The goal of studying these three mental types is to offer a greater sense of self-awareness of your state of depression or anxiety by opening your eyes to the protective patterns of behavior that perhaps were stages of your coping strategies. According to Ayurveda, it is these protective patterns that negatively affect your body, for example in your gut (digestive fire and its helpful bacteria) and in your mind (stress and anxiety), resulting in an impact that generates imbalances that in the long term could manifest as increased depression or other ill health.

Remember that the *gunas* are always changing; therefore, this questionnaire is not intended to provide a static profile. For that reason, I suggest doing this evaluation at least twice: first based on a long period of your life, certainly the past few years, and then later based on how you have been feeling in the last month or so. Calculate your profile in both cases to help you understand whether recent life changes or challenges are affecting your usual state and how much out of balance you could be. This will help you observe your own gradual changes and rebalancing. You are encouraged to come back to the *manas prakruti* evaluation from time to time, as life circumstances change for you.

Note: in *manas prakruti* evaluation, you should answer based on the time period you are observing—which might be the past five years, or the past three months—with respect to your physical and mental health.

	SATTVA (S)	*RAJAS (R)*	*TAMAS (T)*
1	**Mental lucidity**		
	❏ Good, prolonged	❏ Moderate	❏ Poor
2	**Mental harmony**		
	❏ Peaceful	❏ Reasonable	❏ Rare
3	**Satisfaction**		
	❏ Usually	❏ Partly	❏ Occasionally
4	**Conduct**		
	❏ Compassionate, loving	❏ Assertive, controlling	❏ Destructive

	SATTVA (S)	RAJAS (R)	TAMAS (T)
5	**Work**		
	❑ Selfless	❑ Self-centered tendency	❑ Lazy
6	**Communication**		
	❑ Good	❑ Variable	❑ Difficult
7	**Speech**		
	❑ Clear, peaceful, soft	❑ Fast, agitated	❑ Slow, dull
8	**Concentration**		
	❑ Good	❑ Wavering	❑ Poor
9	**Willpower**		
	❑ Good	❑ Fluctuating	❑ Weak
10	**Creativity**		
	❑ High	❑ Moderate	❑ Low
11	**Knowledge**		
	❑ Deep	❑ Reasonable	❑ Poor
12	**Memory**		
	❑ Good	❑ Variable	❑ Poor
13	**Self-awareness**		
	❑ Complete	❑ Uncertain	❑ Weak
14	**Sense of service**		
	❑ Whole	❑ Variable	❑ Rarely
15	**Emotions**		
	❑ Authentic	❑ Contradictory	❑ Suppressed
16	**Anger**		
	❑ Rarely	❑ Occasional	❑ Frequent

	SATTVA (S)	RAJAS (R)	TAMAS (T)
17	**Hate**		
	❑ Rarely	❑ Occasional	❑ Frequent
18	**Violence**		
	❑ Never	❑ Occasional	❑ Frequent
19	**Grief**		
	❑ Uncommon	❑ Occasional	❑ Frequent
20	**Fear**		
	❑ Hardly	❑ Sometimes	❑ Frequently
21	**Pride**		
	❑ Little	❑ Some	❑ Much
22	**Desires**		
	❑ Rarely, brief	❑ Moderate, frequent	❑ Long-standing
23	**Attachment**		
	❑ Rarely, brief	❑ Moderate, frequent	❑ Long-standing
24	**Greed**		
	❑ Rarely, brief	❑ Moderate, frequent	❑ Long-standing
25	**Uncertainty**		
	❑ Rarely, brief	❑ Moderate, frequent	❑ Long-standing
26	**Feeling down**		
	❑ Rarely, brief	❑ Moderate, frequent	❑ Long-standing
27	**Contentment**		
	❑ Regularly	❑ Occasionally	❑ Rarely

	SATTVA (S)	RAJAS (R)	TAMAS (T)
28	**Forgiveness**		
	❏ Easily	❏ With effort	❏ Begrudgingly
29	**Consideration**		
	❏ Mainly to others	❏ Self and friends	❏ Slight, self-considering
30	**Honesty**		
	❏ Constantly	❏ Quite often	❏ Infrequently
31	**Commitment**		
	❏ Total	❏ Limited	❏ Poor
32	**Truthfulness**		
	❏ Always	❏ Most of the time	❏ Rarely
33	**Enjoyment**		
	❏ Regular	❏ Moderate	❏ Occasional
34	**Love**		
	❏ Unconditional, giver	❏ Selfish, taker	❏ Needy, obsessed
35	**Peace of mind**		
	❏ Generally	❏ Relatively	❏ Rarely
36	**Spiritual power**		
	❏ Humankind	❏ Self-interest	❏ Unengaging
37	**Mindfulness**		
	❏ Daily	❏ Occasionally	❏ Rarely/never
38	**Movement**		
	❏ With awareness	❏ Fast, active	❏ Sluggish, heavy, dull
39	**Orderliness**		
	❏ Always	❏ Makes efforts	❏ Generally lazy

	SATTVA (S)	RAJAS (R)	TAMAS (T)
40	**Exercise**		
	❏ Gentle, daily	❏ Competitive	❏ Rarely
41	**Sexual activity**		
	❏ Infrequent, soulful	❏ Variable, pleasurable	❏ Excessive, lusty
42	**Sleep**		
	❏ Sound, satisfying	❏ Interrupted, unsatisfying	❏ Excessive, heavy
43	**Diet**		
	❏ Light, wholesome	❏ Mainly wholesome	❏ Unwholesome
44	**Digestion**		
	❏ Good	❏ Variable	❏ Slow
45	**Elimination**		
	❏ Regular	❏ Mainly regular	❏ Irregular, heavy
46	**Drugs/alcohol**		
	❏ Rarely	❏ Sometimes, socially	❏ Frequent
47	**Money focus**		
	❏ Rarely	❏ Some	❏ Strong

Total up the scores in each column:

Sattva _____ *Rajas* _____ *Tamas* _____

Highest score _____ Corresponding *guna* _____

Second-highest score ____ Corresponding *guna* _____

Lowest score _____ Corresponding *guna* _____

In descending order: _____

Your *manas prakruti* profile: _____

Ayurveda and the Mind: How Ayurveda Treats Depression

AWAKEN THE DOCTOR WITHIN YOU

How to Address Depression

The physical body and the mind are closely connected by the unique three biological constitutions described as *vata, pitta,* and *kapha.* The subtle qualities of these three *doshas* are continuously acting and reacting with the mental faculties. In Ayurveda terms, psychological disorders could arise as a result of an exacerbation of the three constitutions, either individually or in combination, triggering unbalancing changes in the ways we normally act, think, feel, or perceive.

What Is Dis-ease?

I consider disease to be a warning signal from our bodies telling us a change of attitude or lifestyle is needed. If you were driving your car and suddenly a warning light started to flash on the dashboard, you might take a detour to the closest garage. Once there, I don't think you'd like it if the mechanic said, "I've solved the problem: I removed the fuse for that warning light, so it won't flash anymore." He is certainly not an Ayurvedic mechanic!

The fact is that our bodies give us signals, and we do not fully pay attention to them. Can you think of times when you preferred to do something to mask the problem (disable the warning light) rather than listening to your body (investigate why the light is flashing)? Is it acceptable to ignore body-mind imbalances until they manifest in a condition that is incapacitating or even life-threatening? That choice is yours, and the results of that choice are also yours.

No matter which mental health issues we are discussing, Ayurveda is consistent in how it approaches them: what is the causation, given the patient's imbalance in body-mind constitution? For ease of explanation, when I refer in this book to depression or anxiety disorders, I am seeking to encompass many conditions within the subclassifications in this broad field. Where instructive, I will be more specific, but rest assured that we are addressing an entire family of conditions and using Ayurveda to identify the main culprit: your individual body-mind-consciousness imbalance.

Perhaps you are interested in understanding how Ayurvedic doctors diagnosed body imbalances thousands of years ago. For example, how was diabetes diagnosed during the early days of Ayurveda? Well, as early as 1500 BCE, Ayurvedic doctors used a sophisticated biotechnological analysis method to diagnose diabetes. As well as practitioners evaluating patients' urine samples by sight (turbidity) and smell (sweetness), they employed an additional diagnostic system that was easily available, always accurate, and extremely handy for transportation. It provided great satisfaction to the Ayurvedic doctor and the patient.

Are you thinking about ancient versions of urine test strips or glucose monitors? No, this piece of equipment is wholly natural: ants. The doctor would take small urine samples of potentially diabetic individuals and put them next to a sample of a young healthy person, and the doctor would then allow ants to choose between the different samples. The ants would head quickly to the diabetic sample, bypassing the healthy sample, because of the sweet taste of a diabetic patient's urine.

UNDERSTANDING MENTAL CONSTITUTION AND FUNCTIONING

Doing Less, Being More: My Own Issues

Psychiatrists are trained medical doctors who prescribe a medication management program as a course of treatment. Psychologists focus on psychotherapies and use behavioral interventions to treat patients' emotional and mental issues. In my case, I am not a psychologist or a psychiatrist; rather, I am an Ayurvedic doctor who became a depressive patient as a result of my high-impact accidents affecting me physically, mentally, and emotionally. For this reason, the nature of mental processes has long had a strong resonance for me in my professional work.

After my third accident I became even more drawn to processes related to mind-body-consciousness. The physicians in charge of my medical case described me medically as somebody with potential suicidal depression due to my inability to continue my academic and scientific career as a result of my physical and emotional traumas. They strongly advised that I take allopathic drugs such as Prozac and painkillers to control my conditions of pain, anxiety, and depression, but I refused to do so. Thanks to the agelessness of Ayurveda providing answers to individuals with mental and behavioral disorders, I was able to improve my condition, which led me to this simple but profound observation:

. . . .

The issues are within the tissues!

. . . .

Through my own path of processing traumas and healing, I became aware of how much we have been educated to trust our likes and dislikes. But who is the one who enjoys or hates things within me? In general, we receive little or no education in how to relate to, trust, and

97

respect our sensations and feelings toward ourselves. Perhaps that is the main reason why we have such difficulty in dealing with our own questions and concerns, and with other people's feelings toward us.

Universal Thinking

According to Ayurveda, the process of thinking is not personal; it is a universal phenomenon. Thinking contemplates the existence of the individual mind *(manas)* and a universal or cosmic mind, called *vibhu*. This universal mind is all-pervading, expansive, and permeating. Just like breathing, it undergoes a continual expansion and contraction. But where is the mind physically located?

The common thought in the West is that the mind is located in the brain. Well, Ayurveda sees it differently: mind is present everywhere in the body, all the way down to the single cell and its constituents, including the nucleus and the mitochondria, as well as the intercellular spaces allowing intelligent communication. Each of these components is a center of awareness, with its own mind allowing the cell to continuously exchange with other cells through *prana* (breath), considered to be the continuous stream of intelligence. Yes, each cell is breathing in an intelligent way, and this process extends from cell to cell, then to the tissues, from tissues to organs, from organs to systems, and from systems to our entire body—and even further.

As a scientist conducting research on metabolic processes, I had no difficulty accepting these concepts, even if I did not initially accept the concept of a universal mind because of how materialistic my mindset was in those days.

Personal Thinking

Let's consider: what is thinking? Thinking is an anatomical/physiological function of our bodies. The principal functions of our mind are thinking, focusing, inquiring, locating, and deciding our objectives. The Upanishads, a set of classical Indian treatises of spiritual thinking, describe the mind as an interminable, permanent stream of flowing thoughts.[1]

Generally, we classify the process of thinking that occurs in our personal consciousness as "our thinking," and therefore we become thinkers. As a result of our process of identification, a thinker is shaped within ourselves from our early years of life. As we live our lives, we identify ourselves with our regular, recurrent thoughts; consequently, our thoughts become the object of our thinking. However, we are rarely conscious of the stream of repetitive thoughts and how those thoughts produce consequent actions. That lack of awareness created by repetitive thoughts results in inadequate action, which can cause a progressive imbalance, instigating long-term physical and mental pathological conditions.

I invite you to observe your own mechanism of thinking again and again in a calm way, enjoying what you see without judging. Just be an observer as if you were in front of a screen looking at a movie, with the difference that the movie is a biopic of your actual life—and that your purpose for watching is to introduce some changes to it.

Self-Awareness

Part of the great teaching of Ayurveda is the enormous importance given to observing ourselves in every action—in other words, to self-awareness. From where within myself am I acting? Is it from feelings and emotions resulting from past recollections? Our actions are often dictated and directed by past experiences, and when this happens it is bound to create what Ayurveda calls *ama* (undigested food byproducts or mental impurities).

If we look deeper, we can describe mental *ama* as an act emerging from repressed or inhibited thoughts and emotions, which is just an action resulting from a reaction. According to Ayurveda, all actions are just reactions to situations in the past, created by a performer within us remembering suppressed thoughts again and again, nurturing the ego in one way or another. It is worth repeating: *the issues are within the tissues.* Those unconscious issues are trapped in the cellular memory of our body-mind system. This is why the Ayurvedic practices suggested in later chapters play a very important role in activating your bodily system and cleansing you of the negative consequences of those trapped memories that affect our normal body-mind cellular functions.

The Loop: A Vicious Circle

Soon after my third car accident, a vicious circle of thoughts arose within me. As I shared this loop of trapped thinking with others, I learned that I was not the only one to have this kind of experience. I felt comforted and supported by the attendees at my seminars who shared their own similar experiences of this trapped thinking, based on their pivotal or traumatic experiences.

I saw that strong mental division where part of my mind was preparing for the next car accident to happen (which, by the way, fortunately never came). I was living within a loop of repetitive thinking instead of fully enjoying the moment that was in front of me. What was creating those thoughts? My mind? Yes, "my mind," that stream of continuously flowing thoughts; and in that flow, thoughts were also encouraging fear so that my mind was becoming just fear. Everything was taking on that particular color of fear, and with it, the shadow of depression took form. I observed again and again how the process of fear produced anger as a result of my inability to move away from it. Thought promoted anger, so the mind became anger.

Today, having spent many years doing research on the causes of atherosclerosis (blockage of the arteries), it's easy for me to view this problem in terms of the wrong interaction of different molecules generating compounds or macromolecules that easily precipitate in the arteries, causing obstruction. I visualize mental *ama* as the precipitation of clogging actions originating from repressed thoughts and emotions that trigger stenosis or rigidity of the mind. In the aftermath of my accidents, I realized I needed to learn more about those processes and to act on the real necessity to stop being the slave of my thoughts.

The Process of Developing an Observer

The reality is that all of us are thinkers because we repetitively associate ourselves with specific thoughts, especially when we feel depressed. However, when thinking is generated from a place of awareness, then we are facing a complete action of intelligence, an action that conveys lucidity and compassion. Ayurveda calls this *bhakti* or love. Actions from a place of love, awareness, and intelligence do not create debris. This type of action will touch our hearts in a transcendent way. Walking a path of uncluttered simplicity opens the gates of perception, allowing awareness and the possibility to live life truly as a whole.

I started studying the mind on a daily basis and taking proper care in the recovery of my body, including eating a healthy diet and integrating practices such as meditation and yoga into my daily life in a more serious and systematic way. Among the many benefits I received was the opportunity to just observe the process and progression of my thinking and its divisions, and to try not to get identified with it too much. By objectively observing our thinking, we can go beyond thinking. Yet again, the issues are within the tissues, but the tissues—especially the mental ones—have very subtle manifestations that require a certain level of attention in order to not get trapped in them.

. . . .

Love your mental and physical tissues, and
they will release you from your issues!

. . . .

Doing Less, Being More

Your brain, "the busy organ in the body," is constantly at work in the process we practice the most: thinking. Even during calm situations, normal sleep, or deep sleep, when the brain is supposed to be actively renovating and revitalizing its tissues and functions, it is still working and processing information.[2] If your brain feels overworked, overwhelmed, or overstimulated in your daily life as a result of your active, busy mental-physical state, that may be because you do not know how to let go or calm your mind.

Who Are You?

It is important to discover how our personalities and unconscious pre-conceptions influence the way we engage with ourselves and other people emotionally. In this way we can move beyond our established patterns of "labeling" and "othering" both ourselves and others.

Such patterns may be causing you to feel like it is difficult to connect with yourself and others around you. This situation typically generates moods that require a thoughtful change. Are you living only with the memories of the past, and are you constructing your future from that place? What about trying to live in the present? What is "now"? It is just the present moment! Does that proposition make any sense? Perhaps constructing the future from the present is more productive and less depressive, because that would allow us to stop unconsciously finding refuge in our unpleasant or negative experiences that will not let us act in our own best interests today.

Were You a Blank Sheet of Paper?

When we are born we are like a blank sheet of paper, living totally in the moment, absorbing every impression like a sponge, but with a mission according to the Ayurvedic law of karma: from that ocean of consciousness at the time of conception, an individual soul's past-life karma yields qualities formed by a movement of the three *gunas*. We come here with our *sattva, rajas,* and *tamas* qualities in a particular combination to conquer *tamas* and *rajas* and reach pure *sattva*. However, other people and life's circumstances start coloring this blank sheet with all kinds of writing and imagery. Many factors such as education, morals, information (which we call "knowledge"), feelings of duty, honor, conscience, and so on are written on it, which may cause us to forget our goal—if we ever were aware we had one.

What is inscribed on this sheet is what we later call our unchallengeable "personality," which may be strongly influenced by *rajasic* or *tamasic* qualities. Gradually, with age, we come to believe these writings more and more, and they become so-called "knowledge" of ourselves. This is an example of what we call a "person," to which we often add words such as "talent" or "genius." Sometimes the dirtier the sheet becomes with so-called knowledge, the cleverer the person is considered to be. What kind of qualities are part of that genius? If by any chance our "genius" does not have a good cup of coffee, or has a difficult commute to work, or gets caught in the rain without an umbrella, then the person's mood is spoiled for the whole day, probably manifesting *rajasic* or *tamasic* qualities that are going to play a very important role in the process of depression formation by attachment to identification.

If we try to correlate the above example with our daily life experiences, in one way or another we can identify ourselves there. It's normal for all of us to feel stressed, sad, disappointed, or discouraged at times, especially when we are experiencing difficulties or low points in our life. However, in some people, according to their constitution or personality, under certain circumstances this temporary low mood becomes a persistent one. Instead of evaporating at the end of the day after we have moved on to other life issues, it persists, staying with us. If the process comes with other symptoms, such as lack of motivation to seek out enjoyable activities, a feeling of hopelessness, or thoughts about self-harm, here we have the emergence of a clear picture of depression formation.

As we move on from early childhood and grow, some people quickly "decide" that the outside world is not necessarily as safe as the one at home. Painful experiences will affect our feelings, resulting in the message that the vulnerable experience of trying to keep being *sattvic* is not necessarily safe.

Potential for Change

Changes at the level of your physical body are not so difficult; you can become obese or anorexic by excessive actions in one direction or another. Your mind, being adjustable, indiscernible, and refined, can generate even faster fluctuations in your mental constitution, depending on your lifestyle, conditions, and the environments completing your own cells, tissues, organs, and general constitution, providing as a consequence your actual mental and physical activities and functions.

Many of us experience depression at one time or another. It happens for a variety of reasons, such as the breakup of a relationship, the death of a family member, or a job loss. Depression is a sign that you have reached a point where you cannot easily handle the issues you're facing. Overcoming depression is a process, not an event, and all processes consist of a series of steps.

People experiencing depression often mistakenly believe they cannot be happy in life due to the lack of certain things such as material assets, higher affluence and income, or romantic companionship. Shifting negative thinking patterns by learning acceptance is a tried-and-true way to improve our quality of life. People with depression can use Ayurveda to start the process of knowing themselves by learning about their physical and mental constitutions and using that information to implement a proper diet, make lifestyle changes, and engage in cleansing programs. In this way, you can develop awareness of your own inner processes, particularly of the stream of repetitive negative thinking, lack of acceptance of yourself, and other debilitating patterns, and you can start to rebalance your body-mind equilibrium by understanding that *your issues are within your tissues.*

For Ayurveda, human life's main goal is to attain and inhabit a state of awareness or complete freedom. The practice of assessing and understanding mental constitution *(manas prakruti)* can help people reach beyond their regular mental processes and find a truer, more harmonious inner nature as a result of self-observation, acceptance, and active participation.

Cellular Change Means Mental Change

One other way to change patterns of imbalance is to interact with, listen to, and communicate with others with an open mind. Try to share your impressions and real feelings without sugarcoating them. This suggestion may strike terror in some readers, as one of their problems is difficulty in communicating freely and honestly with others. This difficulty is often rooted in that repetitive loop of negative thinking.

I do not underestimate the difficulties inherent in reaching out to others. I have encountered many patients with precisely this issue. All I can say is that if you embark upon such a sharing experience with others, you will be surprised to find that there is common ground, especially when exploring unknown, unfamiliar, or uncomfortable subjects. When you reach out to others and try to involve your body and mind, there is the possibility of creating clear biological transformations in your body. Those biological changes can take you to deeper levels of empathy, helping you master practical skills to connect with yourself and others around you.

At the core of all depressive states is a need that is not being fulfilled. But how can you meet this need? How does it work in your particular case? We will answer that question by considering the biology of these processes in more detail.

Mental Normality and Mental Health: The Defense Mechanism of Personality

Mental health is a perpetual dance within your individual constitutional *doshic* balance of both trilogies of *vata-pitta-kapha* and *sattva-rajas-tamas*.

In mainstream medicine, if the patient has a sense of well-being and the clinical examination finds no psychological illness, then the patient is usually considered psychologically normal. However, the lack of any psychological illness is not true mental good health. Defense mechanisms are psychological strategies we unconsciously use to protect ourselves from feeling uncomfortable when unacceptable thoughts or feelings such as anxiety or worries arise. We use defense mechanisms to protect ourselves from feelings that arise when we feel endangered or because of our very tough ego. Ego-defense mechanisms are considered natural and normal and are not usually under our conscious control. However, they can spiral out of balance, causing neuroses such as anxiety, obsessions, phobias, or hysteria.

Ayurveda understands that physical *vata*, *pitta*, or *kapha* constitutions can experience modifications that change their internal settings in the mental faculties, in order to help us deal with reality and generate an impression of security and a false sense of safety via mechanisms such as repression, denial, projection, displacement, or sublimation. These *doshic* psychological defense mechanisms operate in a unique way according to our constitution, especially under situations of stress or crisis. The emotional interaction of our physical constitution or *doshas* with our mental faculties can operate as a defense mechanism that can generate serious long-term body-mind imbalances.

Mainstream medicine has studied the concept of replicable personality types in a way that sheds light on the wisdom and applicability of Ayurvedic theories.[3] A recent study of personality types that examined four large data sets comprising more than 1.5 million participants showed that the personality types identified in the study population corresponded to Ayurvedic descriptions.[4] When considering mental disorders and matching them to the concept of the three *doshas,* we can appreciate that a person's predominant constitution affects how a disorder manifests in that individual. Let me give you some examples of mental aggravation or *manas vikruti that can lead to serious conditions:*

- In general, under a condition of aggravated *kapha* at the mental level, certain people are inactive, hopeless, and lacking in desire, potentially revealing a sort of split personality.

- Under a condition of aggravated *pitta* at the mental level, the person will refuse to accept failure. Consequently, the person is incapacitated by feelings of severe anguish and desolation, which in extreme circumstances creates a condition of depressive psychosis.

- In complaints of *vata* disorder in the mind, the individual erroneously thinks of persecution by an ill-intentioned person, potentially developing a condition of paranoia or obsessive reaction.

These examples, which have the potential for extreme outcomes, illustrate the importance of the evaluation, understanding, and recognition of one's personal constitution or *prakruti* and the use of the *manas prakruti* evaluation.

AYURVEDIC VISION OF THE CONSTITUENTS OF THE MIND

Digestion of Food/Digestion of Impressions

To understand better how Ayurveda supports mental health and helps move the mind away from depressive states, we will now explore some basic concepts of the mind as Ayurveda perceives it. They have been very helpful to me under tough circumstances, and I hope they will be equally helpful to you.

We must first acknowledge how much we are part of our enormous universe and its energies, and how much they are part of us. The effect of the moon on the tides of the ocean and the role played by the sun in the production of vitamins in our skin are just two of many examples of our interdependence with the cosmos. Ayurveda says that cosmic energy, called *prana,* reaches the body via our breath, skin, and the food and water we consume. *Prana* conveys sensation through the five senses. In that way, each time the mind experiences the sensations of sound, touch, vision, taste, or smell, it is in contact with *prana.*

The mind has three faculties working together that can be modeled as a sort of digestive process resulting from an emotional impression:

- Intellect *(dhi or buddhi):* digestive faculty of the mind when stimulated by food or thought
- Recollection *(dhruti):* recalling of data/process or the ability to hold information
- Stockroom *(smruti):* ability of accumulation for the purpose of perpetuation of recollection

The process of storing information, which we call memory, is a type of mental energy that allows us to recognize familiar processes within new situations. The same function is performed when we eat food, which is converted into energy storage in our muscles and other organs, mostly in the form of glucose to fuel our bodily functions controlled by

107

our brain. In this way, we see here how body and mind are always in a perpetual dance, supporting each other.

. . . .

If we listen to our body, our mind will be happy;
if we listen to our mind while being in contact with
our body, our mind will be even happier.

. . . .

Ayurveda understands that the mind transfers all feelings to the intellect, and then the intellect transfers information to memory. Discrimination is the duty of the intellect so we can perceive things precisely as they really are. To do this the intellect must be attentive, inquisitive, and focused, which provides appreciation, recognition, and good judgment. Judgment, in turn, depends on memory, since we require previous experience of a specific object or situation in order to associate, compare, and judge. In this way, understanding occurs.

This is a very subtle process of mental ingestion, digestion, and assimilation by which the mind creates objectives and aspirations. This process depends on the state of your *triguna* and what you are cultivating in your life. Like an onion, by peeling off layer after layer we can discover what is at our core and have an experience more connected to our essence, which is distinct from what we call our personality. We can also describe this as erasing some of the scribblings on our life-sheet of paper and seeing things with more clarity.

. . . .

The ability to govern the mind and its emotions in this way
is part of our nature, and it can be cultivated through
self-observation and active participation.

. . . .

I think it is everybody's aspiration to experience more *sattva* qualities, because *sattva* denotes fullness of the heart and freedom of the mind. Most of us live in the world of *rajas*, continually pursuing satisfaction through our senses. I strongly believe based on my own experiences that we can peel that onion and interact with the different layers, experiencing life by connecting more and more to what in Ayurveda we call our *sattva* mind—which I prefer to call our depression-free mind!

Moving from depression toward *sattva* mind is a journey. I invite you to begin that journey by looking at your life and seeing if you can correlate your experience with the Ayurvedic concept of *sattva, rajas,* and *tamas* mental constitution. If you would like to explore these concepts further, I suggest reading more on the subject of the Vedas and Vedantic philosophy.

We will conclude this section with a short description of the important aspects that an Ayurvedic doctor takes into consideration when assessing your depression, so you are at least familiarized with the process.

Ayurvedic Aspects Practitioners Consider When Evaluating and Treating Depression

- Evaluating your primordial constitution by using the *prakruti* evaluation included in this book will allow you to get a better idea of your predominant *dosha.*

- The practitioner will conduct a physical assessment by taking your vital signs, including checking the radial pulse, and performing an Ayurvedic evaluation of your tongue, eyes, body frame, weight, and gait.

- Evaluating your potential *dosha* imbalances by using the *vikruti* evaluation included in this book lets you understand the causes of your modified state.

- Evaluations of diet and nutrition in both Ayurvedic and conventional terms are equally important and will be discussed in subsequent chapters. It is also important to evaluate the most common mind-independent causes of depression in physiological and biochemical terms.

- Evaluating your mental constitution *(manas prakruti)* by using the questionnaire included in this book helps you observe some temporary mental threads that could be associated with depression, such as feeling a lack of pleasure or hopelessness in your activities. For example, *vata* types will manifest anxiety and a tendency to lose weight, *pitta* types will express anger and preoccupation, and *kapha* types will manifest a tendency to sleep excessively and gain weight.

- The practitioner will conduct a behavioral assessment to evaluate your clarity of perception, general interaction style, and social comportment (hyperactive or hypoactive).

- An assessment of the causes of your depression will try to discover the areas in your lifestyle that could instigate depression associated with feelings such as sadness, guilt, fear, failure, or hurt. This assessment will also attempt to establish how long the state of depression has been manifesting.

- Clinicians assess the severity of depression, its impact on quality of life, and the patient's potential for self-harm.

- Through self-inquiry, developing understanding, and experience, Ayurveda offers you an immense abundance of information on the relationships between causes and their effects, whether those relationships are immediately obvious or more subtle in nature. This approach invites you to be an active participant in your own process.

Ayurveda understands that nothing will change unless you change. I am quite sure you feel the same. If that's the case, now is a good time for you to explore and use these concepts with an open mind. After experiencing Ayurvedic treatments both personally and professionally, I can say to you that they are highly applicable to mood disorders such as depression, but they require active participation with regularity, perseverance, and awareness.

Less severe cases of depression can be addressed by a qualified Ayurvedic practitioner. If the condition is more severe, I recommend that the patient and practitioner work in collaboration with a conventional doctor skilled in the modern treatment of severe depression to evaluate and address the category, cause, and type of depression state, with a view to management and positive progress with a reduction in the severity of the condition. This is due both to the life-threatening nature of severe depression and the immediate action that is sometimes required to remove or substantially reduce the threat of self-harm.

It is only with the heart that one can see rightly; what is essential is invisible to the eye.

—ANTOINE DE SAINT-EXUPÉRY

PART III

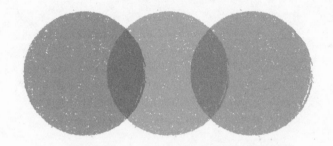

Now You Know Yourself Well: Get Better Using Ayurveda

Improvement through Lifestyle Changes: General Recommendations

TREATMENT IS MORE THAN A PILL

Karen doesn't sleep well or enjoy eating. She is burdened by work problems, health issues, strained family finances, and a host of other seemingly pervasive problems. She has become accustomed to outbreaks of mild depression all her life, but right now she feels abruptly and significantly worse, manifesting as a severe case of what she calls an "anxious depression."

Karen is prescribed an antidepressant; many psychiatrists would recommend that, because it may rapidly address her depression symptoms. Unfortunately for Karen—and virtually everyone in a similar situation—the "treatment" stops there. If she had had a heart attack, her cardiologist would not just prescribe medications for chest pain and leave it at that. There would be continuous follow-up and remedial measures. Any heart-attack patient will get advice on eating better, stopping smoking if relevant, getting more exercise, and learning how to manage their stress. Today's treatment for many patients with depression is very different. Even responsible, caring psychiatrists and general practitioners who know about the links between diet/exercise and depression may not have the tools they need to help patients increase their exercise or to study their patients' lifestyle and diet. These are important factors to consider in constructing a more engaged and uniquely tailored treatment program for patients suffering from depression.

We are all familiar, directly or indirectly, with situations like the one described above. We see very clearly that something is missing in how conventional health systems deal with depression. More than 264 million people around the world have depression, according to the WHO. In the United States, it is estimated that 18.57 percent of adults (45 million people) are experiencing mental illness, with 4.38 percent of adults experiencing severe mental illness.[1] It is also estimated that 13.01 percent of American youth ages twelve to seventeen experienced at least one major depressive disorder during the previous year—and these figures keep growing.[2] Finding appropriate mechanisms that treat depression effectively has never been more important than it is today.

THE AYURVEDIC UNDERSTANDING OF DEPRESSION

Imbalance caused by the accumulation of *ama* at either a physical or mental level is the real root of depression. *Ama* can be defined as toxic substances that harm or weaken body-mind functions. *Ama* can be physical, such as undigested foods, or it can be mental, such as incompletely processed thoughts or emotions resulting from our life experiences. These events can generate sustained negative feelings that sometimes last for decades after the incident as accumulated *ama* in the mind.

> *Disease lodges where the disturbed and mobile* doshas *get stuck due to anomaly in the channels.*
>
> —*Su. Sū.* 24/10

If we are more well-adjusted and we face a difficult situation, we usually overcome those feelings and get on with our lives within a reasonable period of time. Nevertheless, some people find it very difficult to cope with adverse circumstances, and they succumb to depression. Sometimes this can feel like falling into a spider's web. It is as if the network of fine threads we have gradually woven in our lives becomes entangled, preventing us from seeing and handling the complex of interconnected elements promoting depression. Under those circumstances, we become entrenched in a more persistent low state that can last a long time, from weeks to years. This state could manifest along with other hallmark symptoms, such as a lack of motivation to participate in activities we ordinarily enjoy, a feeling of hopelessness, thoughts of self-harm, or even suicidal tendencies. *Ama* in those circumstances becomes a loop of repetitive negative impressions accompanied by all kind of emotions.

Diseases have their seat in the mind and the body.

—*Su. Sū.* 1/26

Ayurveda conceptualizes depression not as a disease but as a symptom of a constitutional imbalance of the three *doshas,* due to external or internal factors such as *ama.* Thus, Ayurveda addresses depression according to the individual's constitutional imbalance.

Ayurveda considers the condition of depression as a mood disorder marked by a loss of pleasure and interest in life. Making an in-depth inquiry into the individual's experience and current state of mind and symptoms considerably helps in understanding when the depression began and possible factors that could be responsible for it. Also, some vital functions change in depression, e.g., breathing can become shallow, and blood pressure drops. In certain conditions, depression can also cause sudden mood swings or shortness of breath (dyspnea), as in major depressive disorders or bipolar disorder.

Ayurveda looks for specific reasons for depression, such as:

- Diet
- Isolation

- Loss of concentration
- Grief
- Sadness
- Reduced working ability
- Crying spells
- Suicidal thoughts

In the Ayurvedic understanding, depression develops from how one feels about and views the world in general and one's own life in particular. It also varies depending on the person's predominant *dosha*. Treating depression is not just about regaining basic functional control with antidepressants. It is more of a matter of rebalancing, which involves resetting the way you look at your whole life. Ayurveda proposes that, as we deal with any struggle in our lives, we can look at depressive situations or states as a real opportunity for profound and positive change in our whole life.[3,4]

ANTIDEPRESSION PROTOCOLS: AN INVITATION TO RETUNE YOUR BODY-MIND SYSTEM

We now address how to manage depression from the Ayurvedic perspective. You will have gathered from the earlier chapters that it is a science of total health care, built on strong pillars, including four aspects that Ayurveda considers essential for sound living:

- Attitude
- Character
- Good interpersonal relations
- Healthy, nourishing diet

Ayurvedic medicine focuses on:

- Understanding our fundamental biological and physiological processes

- Genetic predispositions that influence each individual's experience of health and disease
- Environmental inputs

The way to control diseases is purification, pacification, diet, and conduct, all properly given and observed.

—*Su. Sū.* 1/27

When addressing depression—or any physical or mental health issue—Ayurveda asks which components of your *prakruti* are in excess and how they can be brought into balance. These are the two fundamental questions posed by the Ayurvedic physician during a consultation with a patient.

The Ayurvedic physician manages a process that is based on either depletion or repletion of the tissues, depending on your *prakruti* requirements. Ayurvedic management primarily involves five cleansing procedures, together called *panchakarma*, that address all bodily imbalances. These procedures induce the elimination of endogenous and exogenous toxic products as part of the overall disease management and healing process. We will cover this treatment in more detail later on.

. . . .

The science of Ayurveda focuses on protecting life,
from the cellular level of every living organism up to the
whole human being. Ayurveda looks at life as a
whole and not as a series of fragmented events.

. . . .

The modern method of disease nomenclature and assigning a drug to "fix" depression is being increasingly challenged. People experiencing depression who are conscious of their choices and able to educate themselves in this digital information age are seeking alternatives to conventional treatment pathways. Some of these alternatives, such as Ayurveda, derive from much older health systems that have been in use for thousands of years.

Ayurveda emphasizes the biochemically unique aspects of each patient and the importance of treating illness and promoting wellness by focusing on this uniqueness. Thus, to treat depression, Ayurveda will assess you completely as a whole before individually tailoring modalities to restore your physiological, psychological, and structural balance.

To address depression, Ayurveda follows the same basic principle it uses when addressing any other disease: find the root cause. For depression there are many possible factors involved, and we have to investigate and analyze them all. For example, is the patient's depression caused by a lack of sleep or chronic fatigue syndrome? Or is depression manifesting as a constant tiredness, as it does for many people? If a person doesn't sleep well, their tiredness and fatigue can feel like or be (mis)interpreted as depression. In this particular example, it is very important to analyze sleep patterns in terms of depth, duration, and regularity.

ANTIDEPRESSION LIFESTYLE MODALITIES: NURTURING RECOMMENDATIONS

Daily and Seasonal Routines to Start Reenergizing

The time of day (daily cycle), the yearly seasons (seasonal cycle), and your age (life cycle) influence the balance of your *doshas* and can affect your body-mind *prakruti*. Modern biomedical studies reconfirm these Ayurvedic discoveries.[5,6]

Ayurvedic Life Cycle

Time is self-existing, without beginning, middle, or end. Time is the ultimate destroyer of all living things. From the time of birth to the teenage years, the predominant *dosha* is *kapha* (earth/water predominant elements). Observable manifestations of this are the process of fast growth and the tendency for frequent colds and runny noses we see in young children (and why we take care to dress small children warmly, because they are not always mindful of the need to stay warm).

From the teens to the sixties, *pitta* (fire/water predominant elements) tends to predominate in a period of life containing higher activity and challenge. Later in life, there is a tendency toward *vata* (air/space predominant elements), manifested by disorders such as arthritis, dryness of skin, tremors, emaciation, and memory loss. Independently of your age, no matter what your *prakruti* constitution is, you need to shift your diet and lifestyle to adjust for the *dosha* predominant during the phase of life you are going through, to keep the body-mind complex balanced.

Ayurvedic Seasonal Cycle

Classical Ayurvedic texts describe six yearly seasons instead of the four we are accustomed to. In the same way we know how to keep in good health by adapting our clothing to the seasonal shifts, Ayurvedic scholars understood that our *doshas* get disturbed by strong seasonal changes and require adequate measures to counter the perturbations. When the characteristics of the seasons such as rain, heat, or cold are excessive, deficient, or extreme, they are likely to disturb the three *doshas* in an individual.

Here are some examples of how Ayurvedic scholars describe the seasons, adapted to our conception of four seasons:

- Early spring is the season when *kapha* (phlegm and mucus) becomes liquefied. It is a season of increased colds, flus, and bronchitis as a result of *kapha* aggravation.

- When the sun starts to heat and dry our bodies and environment in late spring and summer, that is the seasonal time for *pitta dosha* aggravation. The most typical examples of exacerbation are mental irritability, heat rashes, sunburn, and burning, swollen feet. In order to reduce *pitta* aggravation, it is recommended to avoid strong, direct contact with the sun (especially at midday) as well as excessive physical exertion.

- Fall is a phase of winds, dropping temperatures, and preparation for winter. During the fall *vata dosha* has a tendency to exacerbate, so naturally it is important to reduce your contact with windy and cold environments.

- Winter is cold and damp. Under those circumstances *kapha* is the *dosha* most susceptible to aggravation. Colds, congestion, and bronchitis are common as a result of phlegm and mucus disorders.

Ayurvedic Daily Cycle and Practices

Ayurveda recommends several daily cleansing practices (*Ca. Su.* 5/72–75). We all have our daily habits, which in some cases are not necessarily good for us. Thousands of years ago, Ayurveda recognized a correlation between an unhealthy lifestyle and depression.

For the improvement of all types of depressive conditions, Ayurveda strongly recommends activities that increase self-confidence and self-esteem instead of competitive activities. In addition, your biological clock or circadian rhythm can be affected by irregularities in your food intake. Your organs need periods of rest without food to allow tissues to repair and for proper function. In general, regular, healthy daily practices are required to bring about changes in your body, mind, and consciousness that will help to keep you in a state of balance or to initiate the process of rebalancing if required.

. . . .

Healthy daily practices normalize your biological clock.
Support digestion, absorption, assimilation, and secretion,
and generate discipline and harmony within yourself.

. . . .

Here we present a general list of suggested activities; we will present more detail describing these therapies and their significances later. When you begin implementing these practices, I suggest starting gradually until you get into the habit of the full routine.

- Morning wake-up: before or around sunrise
- Feeling a sense of gratitude: to life for giving you another day

- Clean the face, mouth, and eyes: use cold water and rinse out your mouth
- Drink water in the morning: drink a glass of room-temperature water to wash your internal organs and stimulate peristalsis
- Tongue scraping: to remove dead bacteria and remnants of food particles
- Clean your teeth: use a soft toothbrush to avoid abrasion of your gums
- Oil pulling or gargling: to strengthen teeth, gums, and jaw
- Nasal drops *(nasya):* applying warm ghee (clarified butter) or oil in the nostrils in the morning
- Ear oil: drops of warm oil in the ear to help disorders such as ringing of the ears, excess earwax, reduced hearing, lockjaw, and temporomandibular joint syndrome
- Oil massage *(abhyanga):* application and rubbing of warm oil over the head and body
- Evacuation: bowel movement once or twice daily, ideally
- Bath/shower: removes sweat, dirt, and fatigue; brings energy to the body, clarity to the mind
- Clothes: wear clean clothes according to the season
- Exercise: to improve strength, movement, and stamina; also to improve your digestion and elimination and support a sound and relaxing sleep
- *Pranayama:* breathing exercises
- Meditation: to bring balance and peace into your day
- Food intake: do not let breakfast escape you

Performing these practices will clear your body of toxic byproducts at various physical levels, providing you with more mental clarity as a result. They can be regularly practiced by all three body constitution types because their intent is general body cleansing.

Diet and Nutrition

If you are feeling depressed, ask yourself: what have you been eating? And then ask yourself: how often do mental health practitioners ask this question? An increasing body of research over the past decade shows that a healthy diet high in fruits, vegetables, whole grains, fish, and unprocessed lean red meat can help people experiencing depression.[7]

There seems to be an infinite number of diets and dietary guidelines out there. We recognize that one size does not fit all when it comes to how, when, why, and what we eat. Modern approaches to fitness regimes/ diets and/or medications are often simply marketing or a superficial life-style fad that may involve adverse actions; and, according to Ayurveda, these adverse actions cause imbalances.

Ayurvedic principles place a high value on the quality of the life we lead by looking for ways to maintain the body in a state of active, functional balance—a combination of processes that enhance longevity. Ayurveda reminds us that we should eat to live instead of living to eat. By knowing and accepting your *prakruti*, you are taking the right path to discover what's best for you at this point in your life. The paramount factor in Ayurvedic medicine is a tailored diet to rebalance your predominant *dosha*, which will restore your *prakruti*. This body-mind rebalancing will assist you in overcoming depression based on integration of the six tastes of food into your daily diet, seasonal adjustments, and food compatibility.

An unhealthy diet that is high in processed foods increases the risk for disease in anyone who eats it. Such a diet may make depression worse while failing to provide the brain with the variety of nutrients it needs. For example, processed or deep-fried foods often contain trans-fatty acids that promote inflammation, which has been shown to be one of the causes of depression. In later chapters you will find detailed nutritional and dietary recommendations and examples of different types of food recommended for your main body constitution.

Fasting

Fasting has been used since ancient times to give the body a break from the demanding task of digestion.[8] In Ayurvedic terms this does not necessarily mean completely depriving yourself of food and tormenting yourself through hunger pains and discomfort. Fortunately, since Ayurveda acknowledges the uniqueness of each individual, there are tools we can use to help each of us use fasting in the way that is best for us.

. . . .

Ayurveda understands that undigested food matter or ama, *occurring as a result of poor digestion, is the root cause of all diseases. To counteract this problem, Ayurveda recommends ensuring a strong digestive fire* (**agni**).

. . . .

Fasting is usually understood to be vastly reduced food intake over an extended period, but it can also involve eating a cleaner, lighter diet appropriate for your constitution or current state of health in order to properly eliminate *ama* from your body. We can practice mini-fasts in our daily routine as a response to a situation where we have been constantly overeating. The body needs time to digest what has been eaten, so a good place to start with our daily food regime is to respect that time.

Only in rare circumstances does Ayurveda recommend a complete fast, or so-called "zero fasting," because it reduces digestive fire *(agni)* and increases your *vata*. Ayurveda has many suggestions and protocols concerning fasting, each related to the patient's particular circumstances. Among them, for example, is the advice that spring is the best season for fasting because it is a heavy and watery, or *kapha,* season.

Remember that our ancestors obtained the benefits of intermittent fasting in a natural way. Since food was scarce and what was harvested in the early spring was very low in fat, the naturally occurring low-fat diet of the spring season forces the body to obtain energy from burning its own body fat. More recently, research has suggested there are major health benefits to caloric restriction, such as reduced risks of cancer, cardiovascular diseases, diabetes, and immune disorders.[9] Still, there is so much conflicting information about fasting that it can be difficult to decide which method to try, if any. What may be suitable for you can actually be detrimental for someone else—and this is the essence of

Ayurveda, which says we need individual attention because we are each different, with our own specific factors.

Your Gut Role

Ayurveda, through its concept of *agni,* sees the gut as a central axis in health and considers that without good gut or bowel strength we will never be able to enjoy proper health. Unfortunately, your gut is under daily pressure to manage chemicals such as antibiotics, hormones, and pesticides in our foods, some of which have a negative impact on your general bodily and gut health. One type of damage caused by these artificial molecules is a reduction in helpful strains of bacteria in our microbiome, harming the gut environment and affecting your mood.

Later we will devote a full chapter to the relationships among the gut, the microbiome, the brain, and depression, but for now I am presenting you a general introduction to the subject. The term *microbiome* refers to all the microorganisms living within us and on us, as well as the genetic material they contain. It is estimated that nearly 30 trillion microorganisms live in or on each of us. The lower part of our bowels contains 99 percent of all the microorganisms in the body. These are mostly bacteria living in a densely populated ecosystem, involving between five hundred and a thousand different species. Within the gut ecosystem there is a balance between what we can call "good" and "bad" bacteria, which is essential for physical and mental health. Several studies show that a balanced, healthy microbiome will reduce depression and anxiety and improve mood. Ninety percent of the neurotransmitter serotonin, known as a contributor to feelings of well-being and happiness, is produced in the digestive system. The probiotic *Lactobacillus rhamnosus* (one of the "good" intestinal bacteria) has been shown to lower the stress hormone cortisol, resulting in reduced anxiety and depression.

Some nutritional psychiatrists affirm that the gut-brain connection is the core of managing anxiety and depression for many people. The balance among various bacteria in the gut is increasingly considered essential for good mental health. Recent studies show that when the microbiome is compromised, gut contents pass through the cellular lining of the gut wall and move into the circulatory system, allowing them to generate a series of reactions that can cause inflammation, potentially manifesting symptoms of mental imbalances. Why does this happen? A new and growing body of research has demonstrated that your gut has its own "nervous system" that operates independently of the cerebral cortex of the brain, which is concerned with your vision and hearing.

. . . .

Your gut mirrors your emotions. Most of your immunity originates in the gut, and the community of microorganisms (microbiome) living in your gut continually reports to the brain on the state of your body.

. . . .

It is the inner community of living microorganisms that keeps up healthy digestion and immune system response, among other valuable functions.

Bacteria cells in your body outnumber your human cells 10 to 1, but because they are much smaller, they account for only about 1 to 2 percent of your body mass—although they do make up about half of your body's waste. For those reasons a proper diet and lifestyle are required to promote a healthy gut if you want to start seeing mental and physical improvements. Let me give you an example:

Peter, a forty-five-year-old with a dynamic personality who suffered episodes of depression, was referred to me. He wanted to stop using antidepressants or reduce his reliance on them and substitute a natural method, if possible. He described no side effects from his medication other than constipation, which concerned him. Peter felt a sense of stability as a result of having found a psychiatrist knowledgeable about depression who prescribed effective medication, so I addressed his only remaining complaint in the Ayurvedic way, with a mild natural laxative and small food intake modifications. Regular evening use gave him the required gastrointestinal motility, and since his medication was doing well, he continued his treatment with the treating physician. This is an example of how mainstream medicine and Ayurveda can work together for the well-being of people suffering from depression.

Awakening the Body by Physical Activities: Exercise/Yoga

Daily exercise is recommended for treating depression. Modalities such as yoga, walking, hiking, swimming, running, and aerobic exercise are generally very supportive in rebalancing the neurochemical activities of the mind-body for all body constitutions.

For example, in a 2016 meta-analysis that examined twenty-three randomized, controlled trials in which exercise was used as treatment for unipolar depression, the researchers found that, compared to no intervention, exercise "yielded a large and significant effect size." This finding led them to conclude that the antidepressant effects of exercise involved these molecular mechanisms:[10,11]

- Kynurenine, a neurotoxic stress chemical produced from the amino acid tryptophan

- Myokines, which are cytokines produced and released by muscle cells in response to muscular contractions

- Brain-derived neurotrophic factor, a growth factor that regulates neuroplasticity and new growth of neurons

- The endocannabinoid system, a system the body uses to help maintain homeostasis

- Beta endorphin, an endogenous opioid neuropeptide and peptide hormone

Physical exercise should be undertaken after due consideration for age, physical capacity, place, time, and food habits; otherwise, it may invite disorders.

—*Su. Chi.* 24/48–48½

We can refer here to a quote attributed to Patanjali, the father of yoga:

Yoga takes you into the present moment, the only place where life exists.

Several reports indicate that the practice of yoga is beneficial for improving numerous medical conditions. Deep breathing is another powerful way to calm both the mind and body, which not only benefits your physical health—particularly cardiovascular health—but is also one of the ways to improve mental health. By practicing yoga postures *(asanas)* and integrating them with your breathing, you increase blood flow and oxygen supply to your brain, encouraging a vigorous increase of nutrients and release of accumulated toxins *(ama)*. Exercise is also one of the best ways to boost the body's endorphins, the so-called "feel good" chemicals our bodies release when we perform stimulating physical activities. Exercise increases neuroplasticity (also called "brain plasticity") by promoting the growth of new brain cells and the formation of new neural connections.

Although we have many temptations to descend into a mostly sedentary lifestyle, I strongly suggest you get your body moving if you want to improve your state of depression and enjoy better health. Of course, I am not suggesting training for a marathon just because you feel depressed; rather, I advise you to find a way to enjoy exercise that suits your *prakruti* and lifestyle.

Generally, yoga is a low-impact exercise that is safe for beginners and open to all ages. There are also different styles of yoga, so it is possible to find the one that best suits your individual needs and abilities. When choosing the style of yoga you want to practice, make sure to take into consideration your actual health condition, state of mind, interests, and fitness level by consulting with a qualified yoga instructor to learn more about the physical demands of any type of yoga.

It may surprise you to learn that the main physical and mental health benefit of yoga practice is to control the thoughts arising from the mind. Some of yoga's other practical benefits include the following:

- Calming your body's stress response and nervous system

- Improving your mood and behavior so you can function better

- Strengthening your self-awareness

- Improving body balance, flexibility, and strength

- Reducing tension and promoting relaxation

*There is always a light within us that is free from all sorrow and grief,
no matter how much we may be experiencing suffering.*

—Patanjali

Yoga has eight phases known as *ashtangas* that are recommended for the purpose of developing peacefulness of the mind *(manas)*. They are:

- *Yama* and *niyama:* rules to be respected for the cleansing of the mind and social behavior

- *Asanas:* physical postures to keep the body healthy and to be used as therapy for certain diseases

- *Pranayama:* breathing exercises

- *Pratyahara:* discrimination between thought and the self

- *Dharana:* fixation of the mind in the ganglionic centers and hypothalamus

- *Dhyana:* the ability of uninterrupted mind to focus on a chosen object or subject

- *Samadhi:* state of complete tranquility of the mind

Here are some yoga-related suggestions based on *prakruti:*

- *Vata* person: the principal region of *vata* in the body is the pelvic cavity. To address that area, postures helping to stretch the pelvic muscles, such as forward bend, backward bend, spinal twist, cobra pose, camel pose, shoulder stand, and plow pose are recommended. They pacify and subside *vata dosha.*

- *Pitta* person: the principal body region of *pitta* is the solar plexus. Postures that stretch the muscles of the abdominal area are recommended to calm down a *pitta* person. The postures are fish, boat, camel, and bow pose.

- *Kapha* person: the principal seat of *kapha* is the chest. The recommended poses to stretch the chest and improve local pulmonary cavity and *kapha* pulmonary circulation are cat pose, cow pose, bow pose, plow pose, and shoulder stand.

- Some general exercise recommendations: you should learn how to practice the different postures with a certified yoga instructor. Jogging is not recommended for *vata*. Swimming is good for *pitta* and *vata* people. Hiking and jogging are good for *kapha* people.

There are four general types of exercise: aerobic exercise (endurance), strength, flexibility, and balance exercises. The practice of yoga offers all four. The positive benefits of yoga have been studied by scientists and now form part of the recommendations of most health organizations. Proposals for treatments and therapies include being active and exercising, in addition to drugs and psychotherapy.[12]

Activity that exerts the whole body is physical exercise.

—*Su. Chi.* 24/38

When comparing exercise with yoga, there is evidence that suggests yoga interventions appear to be equal or superior to other forms of exercise with respect to a number of outcome measures.[13] Emphasis on breath regulation, mindfulness during practice, and maintenance of postures are some of the elements that differentiate yoga practices from other physical exercises.[14]

When studying the effect of yoga on depression, the results show yoga's potential to reduce anxiety and depression and to improve self-esteem.[15] A number of other studies show the role that yoga plays in helping depression.[16] It is interesting that in recent decades society has come to view yoga and Ayurveda less as obscure practices and more as legitimately important parts of Western life and health maintenance.[17,18]

Let me share with you an example from my practice: Joanna, a twenty-six-year-old woman, came to me with severe depression. She was unable to shower or leave her bed for days; at her worst, she couldn't keep her room clean. This condition is called executive dysfunction. She described it as if her brain was not connected to her limbs, resulting in lack of energy and motivation. I suggested creating a routine of gentle physical activity and some important nutritional changes. After presenting her with different options to achieve changes, she agreed to start doing yoga. She started building up the sessions gradually, going from twice a week to daily practice at home. Eventually she told me that her daily yoga practice had created a new dynamic in her life, cutting the time it took her to get up in the morning from half an hour or longer to just a few minutes. Today, in addition to her daily yoga practice, she maintains a very enjoyable connection with food tailored to her constitution.

Connecting to Your Breath: Breathing Exercises *(Pranayama)*

Thoughts come and go like clouds in a windy sky, but a conscious breathing practice like *pranayama* could serve as your anchor. *Pranayama,* a form of breathing exercises within yoga, means "control of the life energy" or "extension of the *prana* or breath." According to Ayurveda, *prana* is the vital force without which life cannot occur. It is also the current of tissular intelligence that controls cellular communication, sensory perception, motor responses, and all subtle electrical impulses of the body—the refined essence of movement. *Pranayama* uses various techniques that regulate and restrain breath, helping to control the mind and improve the quality of perception and awareness.

The practice of yoga requires training and can take time to reach a reasonably proficient level. Breathing, on the other hand, is vital to life, and it happens automatically. For that reason, unfortunately, we take breathing for granted. However, when breathing becomes disturbed or altered, it is very noticeable, and we can participate in that alteration by making intentional changes to our regular breathing patterns. The average human respiratory rate is thirty to sixty breaths per minute at birth, dropping to twelve to twenty breaths per minute in adults. This means we breathe approximately thirty thousand times per day. *Pranayama* can be practiced wherever you are and does not require any particular equipment, and you can witness effective results right away.[19]

Here is a simple technique that a beginner can experiment with. It is an easy practice to do for five to ten minutes before going to bed, known as *sama vritti* or equal durations:

- Begin to breathe deeply. Inhale through your nose and exhale through your mouth, and feel the breath going down into the depths of your belly.

- Keep your breaths gentle, regular, and steady. Count them if that helps you.

- Extend inhalation for a count of one to five. Build up to five over time if it's a bit too much at first.

- Do not hold your breath or force a stop in the breathing process. Easily transition from the inhale to the exhale, letting air flow out of your mouth gently. Count to five if that eases things.

- Practice this method for three to five minutes every day. It is good for releasing tension.

. . . .

Ayurveda indicates which **pranayama** *exercises are suitable to address your condition of depression according to your constitutional type.*

. . . .

Here is a pranayama exercise called alternate nostril breathing *(anuloma viloma* or *nadi shodana),* which has very important physiological effects. To perform this exercise, follow these steps:

1. Inhale through your right nostril, with the left nostril closed by the ring and little fingers.

2. Exhale through your left nostril, with the right nostril closed by your thumb.

3. Inhale through your left nostril, with the right nostril closed by your thumb.

4. Exhale through your right nostril, with the left nostril closed by your ring and little fingers.

Take a short break before your next set of repetitions. Continue for a total of ten cycles of this pattern, inhaling and exhaling with long, deep, slow breaths.

It is recommended that you practice *pranayama* regularly. Once it becomes part of your daily life and you start to feel its benefits, *pranayama* will become like your food. It is a very subtle, balancing nourishment for your entire body-mind-consciousness. You can find information and videos about *pranayama* online, but I advise you to be very careful. Go slowly, be patient, and get expert advice and training. *Pranayama* must never be practiced in a hurry. Avoid strain, and don't try to progress too quickly, because altering your breathing patterns without proper instruction can cause you harm.

Reflection: Meditation

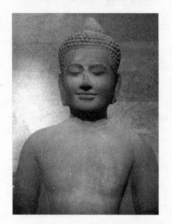

Meditation can be a highly effective method for dealing with mental stress and depression. It has been practiced for thousands of years, and originally it was meant to help deepen understanding of the sacred, mystical forces of life. Today meditation is commonly used for relaxation and stress reduction, and it is considered a type of mind-body complementary medicine.

Meditation helps you bypass restless chattering and permeates deeper levels of consciousness. It creates a significant gradual shift, rewiring the brain to reason and function differently and producing a deep state of relaxation and a tranquil mind. Inhabiting a higher state of perception can keep you from sinking back into negative places. If you are nursing feelings of being uncertain, lost, dissatisfied, or weak, an appropriate meditation technique will offer you the possibility to learn how to come back to yourself, to who you really are, and you will gradually discover your real self.

There are many types of meditation. I encourage you to explore them to find the one that is most appropriate to your needs. Some examples of types of meditations you can explore are guided meditation (guided imagery or visualization), mantra meditation, mindfulness meditation, qigong, tai chi, and yoga. Some of the most common features of meditation include focused attention, relaxed breathing, quiet sitting, comfortable position, and an open attitude. Meditation is one of the tools the ancient Ayurvedic physicians practiced and advised for balancing mind and body and for expanding self-awareness and cultivation of your intrinsic state of balance.

. . . .

In the state of restful awareness created through meditation, your heart rate and breath slow down, your body decreases the production of stress hormones such as cortisol and adrenaline, and you increase the production of neurotransmitters that improve your health, such as endorphins, dopamine, serotonin, and oxytocin.

. . . .

The meditative technique identified today as "mindfulness" has even been shown to have a beneficial effect on genetic expression, promoting a healthy microbiome, which in turn boosts the overall immune system. Meditation has also been found to affect the enzyme telomerase (telomeres and the enzyme telomerase interact with a variety of molecular components to regulate cell-cycle signaling cascades), which some researchers believe is actively involved with the process of aging. Yes, you can use meditation to modulate your genetic expression![20,21]

Some general meditation recommendations depending on your main *prakruti* are:

- *Vata:* meditation on light or fire, focusing on a candle or another light source that is not bright. This type of meditation calms emotions.

- *Pitta:* meditation on spatial expansion/outer awareness with compassion.

- *Kapha:* meditation on the limitless and the shapeless.

Peace can be reached through meditation on the knowledge that dreams give. Peace can also be reached through concentration upon that which is dearest to the heart.

—Patanjali

Potential Precautions or Restrictions for Meditation

Some people with mood disorders find they cannot meditate when they feel depressed. If thoughts are overwhelming, such people can become too anxious or nervous to sit and relax. It can also happen that when some people begin to practice meditation, they realize things about themselves that they are uncomfortable with, which can make their depression feel worse.

Meditation teaches us the benefits of shutting down our inner dialogue, especially when those thoughts tend to be negative. It's not healthy to indulge self-doubt or self-hatred. So if you observe what you're thinking during meditation and it isn't serving you, change the subject. Meditation is a practice, and you won't be perfect at it right away, but it's worth trying and constantly adjusting and noticing what works for you. Meditation provides real insight into why we behave as we do. There can be a shocking realization when you start observing your thoughts. You see what's in there, and it can be very upsetting. With depression, every individual situation is different, so it is very important to seek expert guidance from meditation teachers who have expertise in using meditation with depression.

Without meditation in my daily life, I would have had a much more challenging struggle with depression and stress, and I wholeheartedly recommend it to all patients. I find that it sharpens everything, in particular my appreciation of my surroundings, keeping life fresh.

Meditation does place high demands on us. It requires that we be completely one with the moment. When we experience this oneness, there is deep-seated change in one's psyche. In this moment-to-moment awareness, there is a cleansing of the body, mind, and consciousness. This cleansing brings us to the state of peace, which is happiness and harmony. In that state, life becomes a movement of spontaneous meditation. Think of your practice of meditation as part of your journey to better physical and mental health.

Good Sleep

According to Ayurveda, embracing the natural cycles of the earth and our bodies is of fundamental importance, and Ayurveda offers practical strategies for balancing sleep cycles.[22] We spend roughly a third of our lives asleep, so getting enough sleep at the right time has a huge impact on your brain chemistry.

. . . .

Try to reconnect to a natural sleep cycle,
even if your condition of depression is
incredibly challenging.

. . . .

Most of us experience sleep problems at some point. There is a large part of us that longs for a natural sleep cycle, even if we are not very aware of it, and returning to that type of sleep brings a sense of relief. There is a difference in energy and mood when getting enough sleep compared to being sleep-deprived.

We know from biological research that almost every cell in our body has its own clock. In each of your cells, that clock regulates a different set of genes, instructing them when to turn on and when to turn off. Any disruption of our natural daily cycles (also known as circadian rhythms) can result in loss of sleep, which can be a contributing factor in depression. The association between quality of sleep and depressive illness is complex. The role of sleep is to repair and rejuvenate our bodies. To optimize your health, it's important to pay attention to and honor ancient patterns of waking, sleeping, and eating. In your particular case, depression could cause sleep problems, which in turn may contribute to your depressive disorder. For some people, symptoms of depression happen before the onset of sleep problems; for others sleep problems happen first.

In Ayurveda, sleep disorders are classified according to your main *dosha*. The types of sleep disturbances for *vata*, *pitta*, and *kapha* constitutions manifest differently. Treating them involves strategies tailored for each *dosha* because the *doshas* have a distinct influence on our sleep habits. Your *prakruti* and present state of balance will influence the types of sleep imbalances that are most likely to appear.

People with a predominant *vata prakruti* are more likely to experience *vata* sleep disorders, *pitta*-predominant types are more likely to experience *pitta* sleep complaints, and *kapha*-predominant people manifest mild sleep concerns, if any. Body-mind imbalances (or your potential *vikruti*) can mask your *prakruti* and will influence your condition. If you have not already done so, I advise you to complete your *prakruti* and *vikruti* evaluations in order to understand which *dosha* is more preponderant for you. For example, you can have a *pitta*-predominant *prakruti*, but perhaps as a result of lack of exercise, too much eating to compensate family or work situations, or other issues, you become overweight or obese. Those circumstances can change the spectrum of your sleeping disorder, moving you into a more *kapha* sleep pattern as a result of your body-mind changes.

Alternately, suppose you have a *pitta*-predominant *prakruti*, but as a result of too much work pressure combined with a strong desire to participate in a competitive marathon, you keep losing weight. Your pattern due to those activities is going to create an imbalance in your *pitta*-predominant constitution, moving it into a more *vata* pattern, so the kind of sleep disorders you will manifest will be more related to the *vata prakruti* type.

These next short sections are intended to help you understand how each of the three *doshas* informs your experience of sleep. See which of them you recognize yourself in, either in terms of your sleep predilections and habits or the sorts of imbalances that influence your sleep patterns.

Vata Dosha Sleep and Sleep Imbalances

Vata-predominant *prakruti* individuals' sleep is irregular and light. They can have difficulty falling asleep, but sleep can be very deep when the person is tired. They tend to sleep fewer hours than other constitutions, but they feel better with extra sleep rather than less. When anxious or depressed, the classic *vata*-type sleep imbalance is to awaken during the night between two and six a.m. and find themselves unable to fall asleep again.

Pitta Dosha Sleep and Sleep Imbalances

Pitta-predominant *prakruti* individuals sleep well, though rather lightly, and they require a moderate amount of sleep. The classic *pitta*-type sleep disorder is difficulty in falling asleep if the mind is busy. *Pitta* types can easily skip sleep when they are preoccupied with a project or under deadline pressure, and they can be incredibly productive from around ten p.m. to two a.m. This can activate the mind, stimulate ambition, and completely overwhelm any desire to sleep.

Kapha Dosha Sleep and Sleep Imbalances

Kapha-predominant *prakruti* individuals are heavy sleepers. In general they can sleep soundly everywhere, and they certainly are not easily disturbed or awakened. When out of balance, *kapha* tends to trigger disproportionate sleep, heaviness, sluggishness, and difficulty in waking up.

To calm depression and agitation and to support a proper sleep pattern, Ayurveda proposes the following general recommendations for all three *dosha* types:

- Keep a regular daily routine as recommended in the section of this book concerning daily and seasonal routines.

- Try to get up naturally before or around sunrise and begin the new day with an oil massage, shower, breathing exercises, yoga, and meditation.

- Always try to eat a *vata*-pacifying diet if your mind is very active.

- At least one hour before bedtime eliminate the use of devices with screens (TVs, computers, and smartphones).

- Reduce, moderate, or even eliminate stimulants and depressants (caffeine or nicotine, and alcohol) because they tend to disrupt physiological cycles essential to sound sleep depending on their doses.

- Practice short, gentle *pranayama* to support the mind, the nervous system, and good sleep.

- Meditation before bedtime helps you handle stress, bringing you to a place of peaceful awareness.

- Just before going to bed, give a gentle massage to your feet with *bhringaraj* oil or sesame oil.

- There are a variety of herbs you can take in supplement form to support good sleep, such as ashwagandha, jatamansi, saffron, chamomile, brahmi, tagar, and nutmeg.

- Don't suppress your natural urges.

More specific recommendations for your predominant *dosha* are the following:

- Avoid daytime naps. That will help you to have a better sleep the following night, especially for *kapha* types.

- Eat a light dinner at least three hours before bedtime, followed by a walk, if possible, to reduce the meal's heavy *kapha* qualities, especially for *kapha* and *pitta* types.

- *Pitta* people should eliminate bedtime reading to avoid eye and mind stimulation.

- Make sure a *vata* exercise routine is not overly stimulating, but gentle and grounding instead.

- *Vata* types are advised to engage in slow, relaxing activities two to three hours before going to bed.

- The herb ashwagandha supports the body in resisting stress while calming the *vata* mind.

Numerous studies are suggesting that the microbiome plays a role in insomnia, circadian disturbance, and depression. Studies show the microbiota in your gut are under circadian control, meaning disruptions in sleep can affect the composition and health of your microbiome, which could have substantial impact on your overall health by affecting the actual quality of your sleep. Total microbiome diversity is positively correlated with increased sleep efficiency and total sleep time.[23] We will explore the role of the gut in this process in the chapter on the microbiome.

Positive Mind

Just as everyone has a unique fingerprint, you also have a particular pattern of constitutional energy that has implications for your potential tendency toward depression. Ayurveda and mainstream medicine agree that internal and external dynamics can disturb your balance, causing changes in your mental and physical constitution.

. . . .

Think health, not disease.

. . . .

Negativity is everywhere. Without us even realizing it's happening, negativity can bring you down, drain your energy, impair your productivity, and hinder your creative process. It can even lead to disorders such as depression.

Negativity can also become a pattern. To better understand your negative patterns, it is instructive to examine your habits and routines. If you feel trapped in a negative world and you're ready for a change, you can raise the level of positivity in your life with a few simple steps. Because of our daily routines, most of us don't stop to think about where our habits came from, independently of whether those habits are healthy or unhealthy. In that way, we become more susceptible to negativity, perhaps due to the conditions of life such as our workplace, our friends, or thoughts we have.

Researchers have discovered convincing associations between cardiac health and mental health. For example, accumulated stress, untreated depression, and anxiety disorders increase your odds of having a heart attack or developing heart disease. Stress hormones are again seen as the primary culprit here, but we have to find the physical or mental causes for release of those hormones.[24,25]

When you are inspired by some great purpose, some extraordinary project, all your thoughts break their bonds.

—Patanjali

Positive thinking alone is not the solution to all life's challenges or problems. However, from my professional practice as well as my own challenging experiences, I know that our thoughts inform our aptitude. If you would like to enjoy better health, then make the effort to think about strategies to improve your mental and physical health. Do not concentrate or focus on your depression, however hard that advice may be to follow. Perhaps you are thinking right now: *Yes, that is easy to suggest but difficult to achieve.* Trust me, I have been there. The fact is that your mind is immensely powerful, and it has major contributions to make to your well-being. Use it cleverly and wisely. Your mind is like an adjustable mirror, so adjust it in order to see a better world. I consider reassurance and confidence the first line of management for depression. We then build on that foundation through processes such as self-observation and counseling to gain improvements in our condition.

Mary, a forty-five-year-old woman, came to me with a clear negative approach and a clearly stated desire: she wanted to get rid of her depression. How could she get out of her head and silence all the inner voices? Mary had tried everything, but only at the end of her long working days. She was in a vicious circle and was not integrating health-supporting activities alongside her demanding work routine, which gave her a negative mental approach to changing patterns. After consultation and analysis of her *prakruti* and *vikruti*, I advised her to keep seeing her supervising specialist and in parallel to integrate into her daily life at least two or three of the following modifications:

- Thirty minutes of daily exercise: yoga and/or meditation

- Improving the quality and quantity of sleep

- Reduce consumption of sugar, caffeine contained in diet drinks, and other colas

- Diet modification based on low manufactured fructose, replaced by natural sugars

- Having lunch away from her work environment, preferably with a friend

After a few consultations concerning lifestyle, diet, and physical activity, her negative mental approach changed. She embraced physical activities and diet modifications. She described herself as happier at work and in general, and she even reduced her antidepressant dosage after discussing it with her psychiatrist.

Social Interactions

Your life is a set of interactions and relationships, a perpetual connection between you and the people around you.[26,27]

Aversion is a form of bondage. We are tied to what we hate or fear. That is why, in our lives, the same problem, the same danger or difficulty, will present itself over and over again in various prospects, as long as we continue to resist or run away from it instead of examining it and solving it.

—Patanjali

Ayurveda invites you to connect in a new way with yourself and others searching for harmony, happiness, joy, and bliss. Remember, we all need laughter; it is healing. Laughter releases pressure by opening your mind and heart. A sense of humor and enjoyment helps us avoid taking our personality too seriously, which can reinforce our fear of exposure. If you cannot laugh about yourself from time to time, you will never be able to find freedom. Having a sense of humor about yourself will bring you a quality of consciousness that gives you insight to deal with your inner life, despite experiencing emotions such as hurt, grief, and sadness.

Ayurveda can start you on the pathway to freedom from depression by acceptance that the past is just that: the past, and the only future is the now. Your now is the only one that counts, so enjoy it!

Human Contact

Ayurveda places huge importance on the role of physical contact as part of treatment protocols. Ayurveda offers many techniques of body massage for different ailments, as well as head massages for calming the mind and other techniques (these are described later in this book). I am sure that from your own experience you know the importance of a warm hug, a good handshake, or a congratulatory pat on the shoulder or back. These are all manifestations developed by different cultures representing emotional expressions through supportive physical contact.

> *It is not enough to have intuitions; we must act on them; we must live them.*
>
> —Patanjali

Do not overlook such a valuable therapeutic tool. For centuries, many empirical and scientific studies have shown that humans become almost unrecognizable in the absence of touch, and people who are deprived of physical contact have lower social and developmental capacities.[28]

Pastimes/Hobbies

Hobbies are diversions that can be very supportive for the management of depression, moving you away from a vicious circle of thoughts and boosting self-confidence. They are often an enjoyable and positive investment of your time, especially where they include interactions with others and team work. For that reason, if you don't have a hobby, try to develop one. Invest your time in a positive activity such as dance, gym, swimming, the arts, cooking, reading, or volunteering in your neighborhood or community. This will keep your mind productive and occupied, and it will have positive health benefits for you and others around you. It is never too late to start a new activity.

Supplements: Short-Chain Fatty Acids

Supplements are a vast subject, and here I would like to address only one example that is relevant to the treatment of depression. Your brain is composed of more than 60 percent fat, so a proper intake of adequate amounts of essential fatty acids is important to promote brain cellular regeneration and to cushion and protect neural pathways for your optimal mental health. Over the last decade, a growing number of studies has shown that supplemental short-chain fatty acids (SCFAs) can help with depression if taken in reasonable doses. Some studies have shown a relationship between depression and vitamins B and D, some SCFAs (omega-3 and omega-6), microbiota, and melatonin.[29,30]

Recent studies have found direct links between the health of your gut and the composition of your microbiome on the one hand and the health of your brain on the other. Microbiome composition and SCFAs have been found to directly affect various diseases of the central nervous system, including neurodegenerative, neuroinflammatory, and psychiatric diseases.[31] SCFAs play an important role in overall brain health because they help maintain the blood-brain barrier.

The evidence is becoming clear, but there is still more research to do, so we will keep focusing on the natural assistance that Ayurveda has to offer based on a proper nutritional intake of natural products and diet. However, because there are so many supplements in the marketplace, my main recommendation is to make sure that any supplement you take is organic. Otherwise, you are just ingesting high concentrations of biomaterial that may be contaminated with pesticides, insecticides, and herbicides as a result of their mass production in industrialized facilities. People often ignore this aspect of our nutritional intake, even though it is very important for your health. The majority of supplements available on the market today are made artificially, so if you would like to take supplements, consume those made from whole foods.

Since the main objective of this book is to address natural methods that can be helpful for the conditions of depression and anxiety, later we will present a chapter describing useful herbs and preparations.

A Personal Suggestion: Hydrotherapy (Cold Showers)

The use of hot or cold water for various treatments (hydrotherapy) is as old as humankind.[32] Cold showers have been used for centuries to take advantage of our body's tendency to adapt to strong sensations by becoming more resistant to stress. They should be used as a supplement to traditional treatments but not as a substitute for them. Perhaps cold showers are not a main source of treatment for your particular condition, but they do help to improve symptom relief and general well-being, so let me enumerate some of their benefits:

- Increased endorphin production: taking a cold shower for up to five minutes, two to three times per week, has been shown to help relieve symptoms of depression in a clinical trial. The cold water sends electrical impulses to your brain, stimulating your system to increase alertness, clarity, and energy levels. Endorphins are released, leading to feelings of well-being and optimism.[33]

- Improved metabolism: we have two kinds of fat—white and brown. White fat is associated with obesity and heart disease. Brown fat is activated by exposure to cold temperature and plays an important role in adult health. Healthy levels of brown fat also indicate that white fat will be at a healthy level. Cold water can balance certain hormone levels and heal the gastrointestinal system.[34]

- Improved circulation: bringing the temperature of an area of the body down speeds up the delivery of warmer, freshly oxygenated blood to that area. This is why, when we bruise or tear a muscle, ice applied to the area reduces inflammation, speeding up recovery time. Taken habitually, cold showers can make your circulatory system more proficient. Athletes have known about this for years, even if we have only recently seen data that supports the use of cold water for healing after a sports injury.[35]

- Resisting colds and flu: the shock of cold water in the bloodstream stimulates the production of leukocytes, enhancing your resistance to these common illnesses. Remember, our bodies are designed to become resistant to the elements we are exposed to. For instance, leukocytes help fight infection in the body. One study indicated that cold showers could make the body more resistant to certain types of cancer,[36] and a clinical trial showed that people who took cold showers called in sick to work less often.[37]

How to take up such a practice? The ideal way to form the cold shower habit is to ease into it. Cold showers are beneficial for most people, but the habit takes some getting used to. Begin by slowly lowering the temperature at the end of a usual shower until you start to react to the colder water. Then stay underneath the water for two or three minutes. Breathe deeply to decrease any mental discomfort. Next time make the water slightly colder, trying to last for another minute or two. After doing this several times, you'll find that you even look forward to turning the hot water down. People with long-term clinical depression should not use cold showers as a replacement for what their doctor has prescribed under any circumstances. Discuss any changes to your routine with your medical practitioner.

7

Are You Just
Depressed Bacteria?

THE FABULOUS POWERS OF YOUR BELLY
AND THE PARAMOUNT ROLE OF AYURVEDA

This chapter is important because it connects various themes from previous parts of this book. It is intended to give you a holistic vision and understanding of what is really going on in our body-mind-consciousness processes and how to address depression in a natural way through the support of Ayurveda. I will set out for you scientific information in lay terms so you will have the foundation on which to build a better understanding of your depression from a whole-body perspective.

In Ayurveda the central issue is always our imbalances, either mental or physical, and the status of our *agni:* our digestive fire or metabolic energy that allows us to digest and integrate food components and their energetic powers into our bodies, as well as to properly eliminate waste products. Do we understand how these processes occur in our bodies and how they can affect our bodily balance? Do we know what is required in terms of inputs for our bodily processes to function well?

In reality, we are oblivious to what happens beneath the surface unless it manifests in a problem, such as stomach pain, cramps, or organ failure. We assume, as we do in much of modern life, that everything is all ticking along nicely until a bout of illness stops us in our tracks. Even then we are prone to blame external forces: "it's the cold weather," "I'm under stress," and so on.

Ayurveda possesses unique wisdom in its approach to ill health and imbalance, and it offers corrective steps to restore ourselves to a healthy state. So we must ask: was Ayurveda able to understand these processes and recommend tailored lifestyles to keep people balanced in the absence of today's sophisticated technologies? Let us go a bit deeper with this question, because I believe it can provide a light at the end of our tunnel, and not only in a figurative way.

I will start by posing another question to you, which I will ask you to keep in the back of your mind as you read the following sections: Are we just habits?

The bacteria, viruses, parasites, and phages present in our bodies and concentrated in our intestines are invisible to the naked eye, not just because we cannot see them unaided but also because we deny their existence. Still, modern biomedical technology makes it possible to see them and observe their role in our digestive processes. We have also derived some understanding of their proper function. Most leading nutrition specialists recommend eating more fruits and vegetables to increase the levels of vitamins, fiber, and other beneficial substances we consume. The issue I want to dwell on a little here is this: Is there a link between the presence of bacteria (especially in our gut), the types of foods we eat, and how a wrong combination puts our physical and mental health at risk? Can we improve our physical and mental health by simply varying our eating patterns and the types of foods we eat?

We know that the gut houses more than 70 percent of our immune system, which makes sense given that the lining of your gut is the barrier between your inside and outside world. Are there revelatory connections between the gut, the immune system, and the brain?

To begin answering these questions, we need to shift our focus for the moment to the pioneering studies on the potential correlation between your brain, your food intake/breakdown/absorption, and your depression. In that way we can approach this challenge through the appropriate use of Ayurvedic knowledge.

THE GUT MICROBIOME

From our first breath we are exposed to trillions of bacteria. The majority of our microbial colonization depends on the type of birth delivery we undergo. If we are born via the birth canal, we are colonized by fecal and vaginal bacteria; if we are born via cesarean delivery, we are exposed to a bacterial environment closely related to human skin and the hospital environment, which may have a lasting influence on our microbes. In both cases, when we came into the world these microbes instantaneously colonized the external and internal surfaces of our bodies' tissues and organs, such as the skin, the respiratory system, the urinary tract, the reproductive organs, and our digestive system.

The term *microbiome* refers to all microorganisms (and their genetic material) living in the body; the term *microbiota* refers to populations of microorganisms present in the body's various ecosystems (for example, the gut microbiota and skin microbiota). At the level of the digestive tract or gut, the microbes we used to call our intestinal flora are now known as our microbiota. The microbiota establish themselves deep in our bowels as an inner forest of 10^{14} or 100,000,000,000,000 (100 trillion) microorganisms who enter an agreement with our body for lodging and protection in exchange for mutual health.[1] In other words, the microbiome essentially says: since I am smaller but far more numerous, let's live together in harmony.

We are hybrid beings, composed of trillions of microbial cells and trillions of our own cells working intimately with us, their host, to perform an entire group of functions that are beneficial to our health.

ROLE OF THE MICROBIOME

We, the hosts, exist in a subtle process of symbiosis or interdependency with them. It is postulated that the type of food we eat is responsible for defining 60 percent of gut microbiota variability, while genetics is responsible for only 10 percent. Perhaps you are connecting these comments with terms such as "prebiotics" and "probiotics." We are going to consider these in more detail when we take an objective, trend-free look at them later in this chapter.

Furthermore, from comparing bacteria present in the intestinal flora of hundreds of individuals, we also know that microbiota vary from one individual to another. Despite the fact that microbiota are present everywhere in our bodies, the vast majority of them are found throughout the digestive tract, with an exponential population increase in the colon (also called the large intestine, which is much wider than the small intestine but also shorter—a mere six feet in length compared to approximately twenty-two feet).

Microbiota are involved in the metabolism and digestive absorption of nutrients performing many functions, such as assisting in the digestion of tough carbohydrates (oats, barley, rice, potatoes, and legumes), helping to break down proteins, degrading bile acids, and synthesizing important vitamins and other important bioactive metabolites, such as short-chain fatty acids (SCFAs).[2] Those fatty acids are primary energy sources for the colonic cellular layer, which helps maintain intestinal balance and plays a role in cell differentiation, cell proliferation, and metabolic regulatory processes. With regard to depression, several studies suggest that microbiota act on our brain—and consequently on our mood and temperament—via a gut-brain axis.

Although microbiota were long unknown to Western medicine and only reached prominence in recent years, we have gradually discovered their central importance to well-being, and these discoveries have mobilized thousands of researchers around the world to engage in a new scientific revolution. Not only are the microbes that make us up essential to our well-being; they also open up a new therapeutic area for the understanding of many diseases, including anxiety and depression.

Compare these recent revolutionary discoveries with Ayurveda's understanding of the importance of a natural diet based on wholesome foods from the vegetable kingdom, which has been protecting the homeostasis between microbiota and the body-mind balance of people in India and other Eastern civilizations for thousands of years. Perhaps it is time for the Western patient to start applying these Ayurvedic concepts, which are simple, basic, functional, cost-effective, and readily applicable in support of our mental condition. We should also remember that these approaches were partially in use in the West some generations ago, before the hypnosis of industrialization commandeered our responses to our surroundings, work, and social life.

CATEGORIZATION OF THE GUT MICROBIOME

Whether the belly region is called the gut, the intestines, the bowels, the viscera, or even the "second brain," as some have recently put it, there are fascinating discoveries in this area of research. Advances in biomedicine are providing us more information and clarity. Of particular interest to us is the fact that these discoveries correspond with the Ayurvedic concepts of *agni, prakruti, vikruti,* and *manas* (or digestive fire, individual constitution, individual imbalance, and the mind, respectively).

When categorizing the microbiota, we can visualize the diversity of the microbiome as a multiplicity of small laboratories or factories manufacturing natural drugs for us, which provide innumerable functions to protect and enhance our health. There are several *phyla,* or big families, of bacteria. Within these phyla are contained many species of microorganisms, including bacteria, yeast, and viruses. The dominant gut microbial phyla are Firmicutes, Bacteroidetes, Actinobacteria, Proteobacteria, Fusobacteria, Cyanobacteria, and Verrucomicrobia, with the two large families Firmicutes and Bacteroidetes constituting 90 percent of our gut microbiota.[3]

It is estimated that around five hundred to a thousand species of bacteria live in a healthy human body. You may recognize the names of some genera (plural of "genus") of bacteria, such as *Lactobacillus, Bacillus, Clostridium, Enterococcus,* and *Ruminicoccus,* all of which are part of the Firmicutes phylum. The Bacteroidetes phylum consists of predominant genera such as *Bacteroides* and *Prevotella.* The Actinobacteria phylum is proportionally less abundant and is mainly represented by the *Bifidobacterium* genus.

MICROBIOME DISTRIBUTIONS IN DIFFERENT POPULATIONS

Did you know that most of our understanding of bacteria is the result of analyzing our excrement? Let's discuss this subject a little bit in detail without disturbing you too much.[4]

Since we eat every day, normal bowel movements should occur one to three times a day. Each gut is different, but a healthy gut often has a pattern. In terms of full digestion processing time, it generally takes twenty-four to seventy-two hours for your food to move through your digestive tract. Food doesn't reach your colon for six to eight hours, so bowel movement happens only after that period at least. Don't worry yourself into sitting on the toilet on the clock waiting for the drop, but if your schedule is significantly off or erratic, that can lead to hemorrhoids and other complications in the long run.

Constipation has various possible causes, including stress, dehydration, thyroid issues, and low fiber intake in your diet. For that reason, when you stop being regular, start by checking your diet.

Through studies conducted in two areas completely isolated from the modern world, in the Amazon and Tanzania, the anthropologists Blaser and Dominguez showed that the diet and fecal microbiota of those groups presented a richer and more diverse intestinal flora than those of city dwellers in Japan, China, the United States, and France.[5,6] Those results show that people in these traditional societies have much more diverse gut microbiota, raising concerns about the risk of

disappearance of certain intestinal bacteria that could play very important roles in our well-being, should these communities die out. In fact,
other comparative studies of the microbiome in the United States and
other Western countries make us aware of the fragility of our intestinal flora. It is estimated that the microbiome of one in four people is
impoverished by a decrease in total bacterial load of important groups
such as the *Lactobacillus, Bifidobacterium,* and *Eubacterium* genera as
well as a lower amount of SCFAs.

A hypothesis from these research studies is that the explosion of
conditions such as inflammatory bowel disease, obesity, type 2 diabetes,
depression, and autism may be associated with this impoverishment.[7]

Two questions rise as a result of the scientific data: What if the
future of medicine is played out in our belly, as Ayurveda postulated
thousands of years ago? Can Ayurveda and its recommended practices
such as good fiber consumption address the microbiome imbalance?

THE INTERCONNECTION BETWEEN THE GUT MICROBIOME AND DIETARY FIBER

Studies in humans investigating the effects of whole grains show that
when given whole-grain barley, brown rice, or a mixture of both for a
month, people experienced an increase in bacterial group diversity. Consequently, it may take a broad range of substrates to increase bacterial
diversity, which can be achieved by eating whole plant foods. Additionally, the alterations of gut bacteria in the study coincided with a drop in
systemic inflammation in the body.[8,9,10]

The health of our bodily systems and in particular our digestive tract
depends on our interaction with the environment. The origins and quality of the foods we consume from our youngest age until our death play
an essential role in how our *agni* or metabolic fire is going to process
our food. When we consider the period of time when Ayurveda was
introduced to the world, those populations were living in direct contact
with nature, free of all the pollutants we are "naturally" exposed to today.
Even more important, they were eating *real* natural foods with their full

content of fiber. It is easy to extrapolate that they had a very rich microbiota, as is the case with the recent studies of the isolated populations in Tanzania or the Amazon.

The major food component needed to properly feed our intestinal microbes is fiber. Fiber is the most crucial ingredient for gut health. Having low fiber intake is greater cause for concern than low protein intake. If you decrease dietary fiber, you are depriving your bacteria of its substratum, altering bacterial fermentation, colony size, and species composition. Our symbiotic bacteria are equipped to degrade fiber. An insufficient fiber intake will immediately mean losing richness and diversity of the intestinal microbiome and finding ourselves in a more fragile situation overall.

When we eat fiber, especially the kind present in plants, some bacteria reward us by manufacturing those small SCFA molecules that are very protective against inflammation. We are "infested" by bacteria that require fiber. If we take away their preferred meal, in exchange and indirectly we deprive ourselves of valuable healthy substances they produce for us.

PREBIOTICS AND PROBIOTICS

Before discussing this topic, it is relevant to give a short description of the proper meaning of these two relatively new terms.

- Prebiotics are nondigestible food ingredients that beneficially affect the host by selectively stimulating the growth or activity of one or more beneficial bacteria in the colon that improve host health.

- Probiotics are an oral supplement or food product containing a sufficient number of viable microorganisms to alter the intestinal flora of the host (that's you and your gut), with potential health benefits. Probiotics are live bacteria and yeasts that are by and large beneficial for your digestive system if properly applied. Many types of bacteria with different benefits are classified as probiotics. The most common probiotic is the *Lactobacillus* present in yogurt and other fermented foods. Its different strains can help with diarrhea and could help individuals who cannot digest the sugar in milk (lactose). *Bifidobacterium* is another probiotic present in some dairy products and can be supportive in alleviating the symptoms of irritable bowel syndrome and some other conditions. An example of a yeast found in probiotics is *Saccharomyces boulardii,* helping alleviate digestive issues such as diarrhea and other conditions.

As the importance of the gut microbiota in well-being and illness is increasingly acknowledged, interest in all kind of interventions that can modulate the microbiota and its interactions with its host has rocketed. Separately from diet, prebiotics and probiotics represent the most substances most commonly used in an effort to sustain a healthy microbiome or restore balance when it is believed that bacterial homeostasis has been disturbed by disease. Once again we return to the central theme of Ayurveda: the maintenance of balance through bacterial homeostasis. Although a considerable amount of basic science indicates the ability of various prebiotic molecules and probiotic strains to usefully influence host immune responses, metabolic processes, and neuro-endocrine pathways, the evidence from human studies leaves much to be desired at this stage. Be aware that for many products marketed as probiotics, some of the most fundamental issues relating to quality control, i.e., characterization, formulation, viability, and safety, may be inadequately addressed. It will be of great value to all of us if health departments more actively promoted dietary educational programs. These programs and information are badly needed by patients, consumers, and the general public.[11]

In reality prebiotics are nothing different from the dietary fiber that helps the microorganisms in our intestines to grow, since that is their nutriment. If wholesome foods are integrated into your diet, all those natural, nondigestible fibers in vegetables, legumes, cereal grains, nuts, seeds, and fruits are going to do the job just fine by becoming accessible to the microbiota. In other words, you don't need to take a prebiotic if you are following Ayurvedic dietary principles in your daily life. Probiotics can help keep your gut healthy, but if you already have healthy bacteria in your gut and you're following Ayurvedic dietary principles, then your body does not need these additional probiotics.

Fermented foods and some kinds of cheeses and breads support gut health because they provide healthy, living microorganisms that improve absorption of minerals and add more nutrients to food. The most common fermented foods that naturally contain probiotics or have probiotics added to them include yogurt, kefir, kombucha, sauerkraut, pickles, kimchi, tempeh, miso, sourdough bread, and some cheeses, such as traditionally made cheeses like cheddars, gouda, provolone, and Alpine cheeses like Emmentaler and Gruyère.

OTHER MICROBIOME ISSUES

Modern life improvements such as antimicrobial treatments, vaccinations, intensive use of disinfecting and cleaning products, and unwholesome diets exert a deep and lasting impact on the microbiome. Changes in the gut microbiota may cause *Clostridium difficile* infection, irritable bowel syndrome, pathogen colonization (e.g., vancomycin-resistant *Enterococcus*), autoimmune and allergic diseases, obesity and metabolic disorders, and neuropsychiatric disorders.

Food Additives

The problems associated with today's powerful food industry are not only related to the reduction or absence of fiber in our food. The scientific community is increasingly questioning the ongoing addition of "innovative" artificial chemical molecules to our food and thus our health. The United States provides many opportunities to study the kinds of additives present in processed foods and to track their presence (and persistence) in any transformed product, and many studies have been conducted in this area.

As discussed earlier, processed foods can cause inflammation in the lining of our gut in the areas where food is absorbed. Your gut doesn't have any other choice but to accept what you are providing. Its role is not to recognize if what you have eaten is digestible food or not. Instead, your gut might recognize the presence of artificial food ingredients, such as high-fructose corn syrup, as an invader. This sets off an inflammatory response in which our bodies are literally fighting these foods as if they were an infection. For example, most kinds of chocolate bars contain emulsifiers—additives that are used to stabilize processed foods. Just pause for a second here and consider that the emulsifier is only there in the manufactured food to hold it together long enough to last the length of the supply chain, from the factory to your stomach. It's not there because it's nutritious. Some of these additives are used to allow a mix of fat and nonfat compounds to look fresh and stable in the supermarkets, despite the fact these additives can have other effects on our health.

How do these additives work on our bacteria? Could it be possible that a simple chocolate bar enhanced with additives changes our microbiome? The answer is yes; several laboratory studies conducted on animals and humans have shown these effects.[12] In the following section of this book we will discuss this issue in more detail. Eating wholesome foods such as whole fruits, vegetables, and unprocessed meats can lower the metabolic stress placed upon your body.

Remember, we are the first providers in the perpetual food cycle of nourishment. As a consequence, we are the ones who have to be intelligent and conscious enough; we cannot ask our gut to tell us what to eat—although perhaps we could if we had a real connection with our senses, which we will also discuss later in this book. The real point here is for you to understand that you can do yourself a great service by awakening to the idea that it is time to address lifelong, everyday habits that may be harmful.

Antibiotics

When we take an antibiotic, it may eliminate the toxic bacteria within us, but at the same time we might also forever lose essential bacteria in our gut, since antibiotics have the effect of a bomb. They are designed to destroy bacteria, and they do this by killing them indiscriminately, which causes deforestation of our good bacteria.[13]

I am not against the use of antibiotics—they have saved many lives—but it is time to learn how to use them in a safer way to avoid the high cost of damaging our essential microbiota and consequently our balance. The Pasteurian microbiological approach to disease commanded us to search for a pathogen. In pathologies such as inflammatory bowel disease, modern medicine is following the same approach, blaming certain bacteria or viruses before realizing that the real problem is a systemic loss of healthy bacteria and thus a loss of their protective bodily functions. If you have recently taken antibiotics, you'll need to help your gut by building up new friendships again.

Stress

Stress is a major risk factor for many pathologies, including cardiovascular diseases, as a result of an increase in hormones such as cortisol and neurotransmitters such as adrenaline.[14,15] In our body, everything is interconnected, so these conditions can change your gut, altering your microbiome by turning it into a "butterfly cage" of distress and anxiety.[16] Several studies show that taking the time to meditate and relax can help ease symptoms of gut disorders.[17,18]

Ayurveda understands that the more relaxed you are, the better you will be able to nourish your body, mind, and spirit. In our daily life we are not just addressing digestion of material food.[19] Moment by moment, all kinds of impressions are nourishment for the body, the mind, and our consciousness. When eating, even if it is wholesome food, take the time to chew your food. This helps to start the digestive process by breaking down food into smaller pieces and stimulating release of enzymes present in your saliva that combine with the food, giving signals to the rest of the body that it is time to pay attention to the digestive system.

MIND YOUR GUT: MICROBIOME AND THE BRAIN

A very good example to help us understand the mind-gut connection is a condition called leaky gut syndrome, a digestive condition that affects the lining of the intestines. Under normal conditions, the gaps in the intestinal walls allow water and nutrients to pass through into the bloodstream while keeping substances harmful to the bloodstream out. In leaky gut syndrome, these openings become wider, allowing food particles, bacteria, and toxins to enter directly into the bloodstream. A 2018 study stated that imbalances in the gut microbiota can trigger the body's immune response, which results in gut inflammation and increased intestinal permeability.[20] Other scientific studies suggest that leaky gut may contribute to neuroinflammation that causes many neurodegenerative conditions, such as anxiety and depression.[21,22]

ROLE OF THE MICROBIOTA-GUT-BRAIN AXIS IN DEPRESSION

The gut-brain axis is a bidirectional link between the central nervous system and the enteric or abdominal nervous system. It involves direct and indirect pathways between thoughts and emotional centers in the brain with peripheral intestinal functions. Recent neuroscientific research has shown the importance of the microbiota in the development of brain systems. The gut microbiota is vital to human health and the immune system, and it plays a major part in bidirectional communication between the gut and the brain.

The role that the SCFAs produced by the microbiome play in psychiatric disorders is attracting interest because SCFAs have been found to mediate communication along the gut-brain axis through their impact on various communication channels that your gut and brain use to "talk" to each other, such as the vagus nerve, gut hormones, neurotransmitters, and the endocrine system. This finding has the potential to challenge the way we treat psychiatric conditions such as anxiety and depression.

Disturbances of the gut microbiota caused by unwholesome diet, antibiotic use, stress, and other factors could lead to an atypical microbiome becoming a risk factor for psychiatric and neurodegenerative disorders.[23] Scientific evidence shows that the gut microbiota are associated with metabolic disorders and neuropsychiatric disorders.[24] More recently, scientists studying data involving 26,118 men linked probiotic-rich food consumption with lower prevalence and less severity of depression.[25]

MICROBIOME, DEPRESSION, AND ANXIETY

Scientific studies show that patients with depression or anxiety display distributions and proportions of the organisms in their microbiome that are different from those seen in people not experiencing depression. These studies show that people presenting major depression and anxiety have increased numbers of Bacteroidetes, Proteobacteria, and Actinobacteria, and decreased numbers of Firmicutes (which are normally more abundant). On the other hand, patients diagnosed with generalized anxiety disorder show decreased prevalence of five genera *(Faecalibacterium, Eubacterium, Lachnospira, Butyricicoccus,* and *Sutterella)*. These particular microbes are the ones producing the important SCFA molecules. Because stress can activate inflammation and increase gut permeability, researchers are trying to determine whether a leaky gut allows macromolecules and microorganisms to leave the gut and reach the brain, where they induce neuroinflammation.

Another recent study conducted in unmedicated adolescents found that depression severity was associated with increased intestinal permeability. The study also found that intestinal permeability could mediate the association between sympathetic nervous system activation and depression severity. The evidence suggests that increased intestinal permeability could activate the immune system, promoting the development of depression.[26]

We know now that every emotion starting in the brain will be reflected in the gut, and anything that happens in the gut will be reflected in some way at the brain level. The main reason to keep a healthy gut is because it is the real home of 60 to 80 percent of our immune system and 90 percent of our neurotransmitters (chemical messengers that help control mood).

THE FUTURE OF AYURVEDIC PARTICIPATION IN TREATING DEPRESSION

One of the many questions science is trying to answer is how intestinal bacteria are involved in disease. From the scientific point of view, we still don't understand the exact species of microbiota we really need for good health. Since there are so many different species, we need to understand which ones support our digestion and produce the essential components for the assimilation of our food, and how unwholesome food affects them. We also have to be careful that we do not consider species in isolation. It is possible that some species work best when they cooperate with others, and this relationship may not be easily identifiable if we isolate analysis of certain species of bacteria. Again, as in Ayurveda, it is important to see the whole.

We are on the brink of a potential therapeutic revolution as a result of discoveries from recent microbiome research. These studies reveal that the variety of bacterial species within us and the quality of the exchanges among them are important factors for the development of the immunity of tomorrow's children, and for the maintenance of health among adults. I have the impression that a new bridge is being built, paving the way for more productive communication between the science of Ayurveda and modern biomedical sciences. This bridge is based on the emergence of newer disciplines such as epigenetics, chronobiology, pharmacogenetics, and metabolomics (the scientific study of chemical processes involving metabolites), which are already changing the generalized reductionist view of biomedicine held by some. We are also benefiting from new therapeutic approaches that precisely tailor personalized nutrition treatments according to the patient's phenotypic information, such as age, gender, physical activity, and social conditions. Based on those approaches, my ears are hearing: "Ayurveda, Ayurveda!"

It is encouraging to realize that some Western scientists are trying Ayurveda-based whole-system clinical trials by developing integrative protocols. Hopefully by understanding the microbiota and integrating that knowledge into our daily lives, perhaps one day we will be able to address diseases in a far more holistic way, focusing on the well-being of people suffering from body-mind conditions such as depression and many others.

AYURVEDIC RECOMMENDATIONS

We have discussed the reasons why microbiome diversity is very important for our body-mind balance. We can obtain a diverse, high-quality microbiome by following many of the daily lifestyle recommendations and protocols that Ayurveda recommends. Your body is constantly communicating with you—or at least it is trying to; so let's consider a brief description of some personalized protocols that will allow you to learn and speak the language of your gut:

- Your body and mind are very much interconnected via your gut. Therefore, when eating, relax your mind to reset your gut. Stress changes your microbiome, so respect your body. Eating slowly and steadily will help you win the race.

- Don't always eat the same food; embrace a diversified diet. Keep your diet diverse so your microbiome won't become a ghostly forest. To boost the microbiome's ability to rebuild and thrive, researchers propose that you consume many different fruits and vegetables each week. Ayurveda has been telling us this for thousands of years.

- Avoid heavily processed fast food as much as you can. Instead, eat organic and natural foods that are rich in fiber. Their consumption is essential for certain bacteria that are beneficial to you. Studies have shown that adopting a high-fiber diet for only six weeks improves microbiota diversity by almost 30 percent.

- Avoid eating food packed with additives. Studies in mice have shown that a diet rich in additives causes the microbiota to deplete. The intestinal barrier is also damaged, triggering intestinal inflammation, metabolic deregulation, and weight gain. These additives are the same ones consumed by millions of humans around the world.

- Make sure to monitor your bowel movement schedule to recognize when you might be constipated, which is a major body imbalance. If you're not regular, you could be holding onto food you ate for days and days, which can convert into toxins. Ayurveda describes in great detail how *ama* or undigested food—waste hanging around longer than it should—putrefies in your body, causing numerous body-mind disorders. Again, include a variety of fruits and vegetables in your diet, and drink enough water.

- Don't disconnect from yourself. Learn to keep connected, and accept your present condition if depression is there. Ayurveda offers so many options to anchor yourself if you're feeling stress, anxiety, or depression. Breathing exercises, mental vocalizations, yoga, and walking in nature for fifteen to thirty minutes are simple practices you can use. Polydrug therapy, disruption of biological rhythms, dependency on smoking, heavy drugs, alcohol, and other stressors can only lead to more intractable problems.

- Stay active. Engage in physical activity. It might be difficult to start exercising, but it will repay you a fortune in the long run in terms of body-mind balance. There are so many options, from yoga and stretching to Pilates, swimming, and more.

- Avoid antibiotics, and use them only in case of serious health conditions. The consumption of antibiotics has increased steadily over the past sixty years. They are designed to destroy pathogenic bacteria, but they kill both good and bad bacteria indiscriminately. An active topic of research is whether early exposure to antibiotics plays a role in the global obesity epidemic.

Do not disrespect the microbiota that lodge with you as their host. They require care as well as proper physical and mental food from you. They are living with you—and you are living with them. In exchange for good-quality "food," they will provide you plenty of health benefits on your path to restoring balance.

Caring for Your Depression: Ayurvedic Body Treatments

THE ANCIENT AYURVEDIC TEXTS described a number of acute psychiatric disorders, such as bipolar disorder, severe depression, psychosis, and schizophrenia. Scientists and clinicians in those days designed complete Ayurvedic protocols for the treatment of those disorders.

. . . .

To address psychiatric disorders, toxins (undigested food) or ama *are the real target. The vital aim of an Ayurvedic detoxification is to release* ama *from the body.*

. . . .

Substances in the body and mind that are inefficiently processed or are situated in biological spaces where they are not supposed to be should be removed. Digestive dysfunction and consequent potential brain issues could result from being in a toxic inflammatory state. Just as when you see an external injury getting red and swollen, inside your body inflammation occurs when you are exposed to harmful or unnatural substances that either by themselves or in combination with other substances accumulate in your cells and tissues, where they have toxic properties. Ayurveda refers to this process as *ama*. Below we will discuss Ayurvedic treatments for depression that will help you expel *ama*.

BODY MASSAGE *(ABHYANGA)*

Among many ancient Indian traditional practices, a massage of the body and head with Ayurvedic medicated oil before bathing is popular. Body massage is part of the Ayurvedic procedures. Massage can be given by a trained Ayurvedic therapist, or it can be practiced as a self-massage.

According to Ayurveda, the practice of daily oleation rebuilds the balance of the three *doshas* and enhances well-being and endurance. Oil massage supports the release of toxic metabolic byproducts through the skin and the lymphatic system, which supports your immune system. The skin is the largest organ of your body, and the daily application of Ayurvedic medicated oil can help keep the skin microbiome healthy, thus supporting immunity, extending longevity, and improving vitality. The skin has more than twenty million sensory neurons, which—aside from the microbes they are exposed to—can encounter other irritating environmental factors, such as air, weather, stress, clothes, travel, and pollution.

You can benefit from oil massage, and Ayurveda provides tailored recommendations concerning the proper frequency of massage and type of oil to use, based on your main constitution. Regular body massage is beneficial for all three primordial *doshas,* but it is especially grounding and relaxing for *vata dosha* disturbances of the nervous system.

Here is a short description of the steps for self-massage:

- Warm the oil. It should be comfortably warm, and you should apply it in a warm room.

- Skull: initially apply oil to the crown of your head, working slowly out from there with circular strokes, covering the whole scalp for three to four minutes.

- Face: apply oil in a circular motion on your forehead, temples, cheeks, jaws, and ears. Upward movements are always recommended.

- Limbs: massage your limbs toward the direction of your heart. It is recommended to give long strokes on the arms and legs, and circular strokes on the elbows and knees.

- Torso/abdomen: massage in general circular clockwise motions.

- Finish the process by massaging your feet.

- Allow penetration and absorption of the oil into your skin and further body layers for five to ten minutes. Next, take a warm bath or shower, and dry your body gently.

DETOXIFICATION/CLEANSING PROGRAMS (*PANCHAKARMA*)

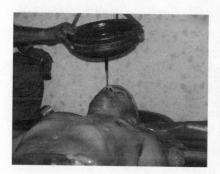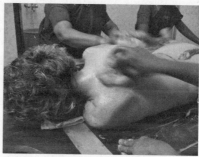

The full Ayurvedic detoxification program is called *panchakarma,* which in Sanskrit means "five actions." *Panchakarma* is a specific set of procedures useful not only for eliminating bodily toxins but also for treating all body-mind conditions. A detox or cleanse provokes the elimination of accumulated irregular metabolic waste toxins both internally and externally, to reestablish balance. It is logical to think that if your mind or body is not eliminating toxins such as undigested mental phenomena (repetitive impressions or thoughts) or physical components such as undigested materials (food, microorganisms, synthetic chemicals, xenobiotics, drugs, etc.), those products will accumulate and over a period of time may contribute to various conditions, including anxiety or depression.

Under ordinary circumstances, your body has a natural ability to efficiently process and remove these waste materials by means of the usual metabolic processes. This is true even when your constitution is in a state of mild imbalance. However, when the constitutional imbalances become more severe, due to issues such as anxiety, depression, poor nutrition, lack of exercise, unhealthy lifestyle, genetic tendencies, disturbed digestive enzymes, lack of metabolic cofactors, or hormonal problems, then the factors that regulate the body's internal homeostasis become affected. This can lead to the accumulation and eventual spread of toxins throughout the body, resulting in *prakruti* imbalances, manifesting as *vikruti* and potentially generating an illness.

This waste material accumulated at the levels of cells, organs, and body systems, known as *ama*, needs to be completely released from the body. Certain health specialists will tell you that it is totally pointless to cleanse or detox because the digestive tract completely rebuilds its cellular lining continuously and because the body has a natural detoxification system. Other health specialists recommend periodic detoxes via various protocols, sometimes going to extremes that cause depletion of minerals, vitamins, and calories. Instead of being beneficial, these kinds of depletions could induce severe cravings, loss of lean muscle mass, hormonal imbalances, mental disorders, and other issues.

. . . .

*The notion that we do not need to detoxify
our bodies is basically incorrect.*

. . . .

It is true that our bodies have a natural detoxification system in place, but today's lifestyle places continuous pressure upon our bodies through the accumulation of toxins coming from the air we breathe, the food and medications we ingest, and the impressions we receive. Our body keeps trying to eliminate those physical, mental, and emotional toxins resulting from conscious or unconscious traumas. We consider it important to regularly change the oil in our cars, but we don't see it the same way when it concerns our own bodies.

The efficacy of the Ayurvedic process of body detoxification or cleansing resides in various means of secretion and excretion of toxic substances from the body and mind. This process consists of tailored protocols that address each of the affected constitutions *(doshas)*. These detoxification protocols are enema, nasal cleansing, bloodletting, therapeutic vomiting (emesis), and laxative therapy. The Ayurvedic scholar Sushruta described these medical procedures in detail in the *Sushruta Samhita*.[1,2]

Each protocol serves a different purpose:

- Laxative therapy/purgation is the best therapy for elimination of excess *pitta*.
- Emesis is the best therapy for elimination of excess *kapha* (mucus).
- An enema is the best therapy for elimination of excess *vata*.
- Bloodletting (by applying leeches or blood donation) removes excess *pitta*.
- Nasal cleansing/inhalation therapy using medicated oils removes *kapha* from the head.

In addition to the cleansing protocols described above, appropriate Ayurvedic medication can be given in order to improve disposition and temperament and to treat anxiety and depression, as well as their associated conditions, such as sleep disturbance and lack of self-confidence. Remember that in Ayurveda all treatments are given according to your own constitution and how the three *doshas* combine within you. In preparation for a *panchakarma* treatment, you may undergo a series of preparatory steps, including *abhyanga* (a broad range of massage treatments, encompassing oil massage).

Medicaments possessing digestive properties have been found to be essential in stimulating and improving body-mind metabolism. For example, cleansing detoxification treatments such as purgation and nasal drops are adopted based on a patient's constitution, especially for the *pitta* type, and according to the patient's particular needs at the time of treatment. Purgation treatments in particular balance *pitta* and *vata* constitutions, which are related to mood and intelligence. Nasal drop treatments strengthen the mind and sense organs.[3,4,5]

Mainstream medicine finds it easy to accept the concept that metabolic byproducts are physical substances that can be toxic to the body, but it is far more difficult to acknowledge that some kind of emotions or thoughts can equally be toxic byproducts. Fortunately, an increasing number of medical specialists and psychologists are coming to understand this concept. Ayurveda doesn't differentiate between toxic body byproducts and toxic mind byproducts, because both affect the whole interconnected body-mind-consciousness complexion.

I have personally experienced the extraordinary effects of a mental cleansing procedure called *shirodhara*, which is an herbal forehead massage. This came about as a treatment for conditions resulting from one of my three accidents, in which I suffered a serious injury at the back of my head from a very strong impact against a stainless-steel post. As I described in chapter 1, after the accident I experienced a combination of tension, worry, fear, continuous headaches, and depression. To achieve some relief for these conditions, I enrolled in a detox program in which I was advised to undergo *shirodhara*. This involves gently and continuously pouring oil over the forehead for around half an hour in parallel with a very gentle head massage. Sesame oil or coconut oil are the traditional oils used, but other oils or liquids such as milk or even buttermilk are sometimes used as well, depending on the patient's condition and constitution.

In my case, the tailored medicated herbal forehead massage helped me relieve all the accumulated symptoms of anxiety, stress, and fatigue as a result of traumatic cell memory accumulated at the skull and cranial level. This gentle, continuous pouring of medicated oil gave me deep feelings of relaxation and pleasure, and it gradually helped me regain mental clarity and relaxation, helping me accept my condition in a positive way.

NASAL CLEANSING

Nasya is a procedure for cleaning the nasal passages that makes use of oils, medicinal herbs, and decoctions. In *nasya,* different types of substances are used to treat various disorders. *Nasya* oils lubricate the nasal cavities and sinuses. Generally, nasal cleaning uses a nurturing, nourishing, and cleansing herb-infused oil that alleviates discomforts that occur above the neck and in the head area.

This protocol is recommended to be administered in the early morning on an empty stomach, and it doesn't take too much time. Here is a short description of the process:

- You can do it yourself by lying down with the head tilted back.

- Gently place three to four drops of oil into each nostril.

- Absorb or inhale gently and deeply, and continue lying down for three to four minutes to allow the oils to penetrate the cavities and perform their cleansing role.

- After a short time you will feel internal mucus secretions building up and searching for a way out. Proceed to release the secretions either via your nose or mouth.

. . . .

*In Ayurvedic terms, the nose is the door to consciousness
and the pathway to our inner pharmacy.*

. . . .

According to the classical Ayurvedic texts, brain congestion and headaches are associated with present and past emotional fears or anxieties, and nasal cleansing is a treatment for it. Nasal cleansing helped me recover normal mental activity and get rid of headaches caused by my accidents. Ever since my first *panchakarma* program, I have included *nasya* in my daily routine. I don't recall a single patient of mine who had a bad experience as a result of nasal cleansing, including people with septum deviation. It is effective for individuals who present symptoms of apnea. During sleep, when throat and tongue muscles are more relaxed, soft tissue or mucus can cause the airway to become blocked, causing apnea. Regular practice of nasal cleansing will support the evacuation of secretions building up via your nose or mouth. More details and references on nasal cleansing can be found in the references cited here.[6,7,8]

VITAL-POINT THERAPY: *MARMA*

Marma is a powerful therapy that originated in India around five thousand years ago. Its focus is the manipulation of the body's subtle energy *(prana)* to trigger healing processes. *Marma* is a highly precise application of touch and pressure on the vital points, which are energy points distributed throughout the body. According to Ayurveda, a vital point is an assemblage of muscle, blood vessel, ligament, bone, and joint, where *prana* inheres. The precise application of gentle pressure induces the flow of *prana* along a complex system of subtle channels called *nadis*. *Marma* was incorporated into a number of ancient Ayurvedic texts, which classify 107 or 108 therapeutic vital points and describe their impact on *prana*. Some of the benefits of *marma* are:

- Improvement in function of the digestive, respiratory, immune, and nervous systems by inducing release of neurotransmitters such as serotonin
- Increased production of melatonin, improving sleep quality and cognitive function
- Relief of chronic or acute pain, e.g., muscles, joints, headaches
- Balance of body temperature and *doshas*
- Body cleansing
- Healthy skin and a bright appearance

You can consider a vital points massage as a kind of Indian reflexology that focuses on strategic points in the body that act as energy centers.[9,10]

AROMATHERAPY/SCENT THERAPY

Aromatherapy is a holistic healing treatment that uses the scent of natural plant extracts to promote health and well-being. Sometimes it's called essential oil therapy, but it also includes the use of incense. Aromatherapy is used to support pain management, improve sleep quality, and reduce stress, agitation, and anxiety, enhancing both physical and emotional health. For many thousands of years, incenses and oil extracts have been used in religious and spiritual practices around the world. Now we understand why these practices extend far beyond purely ceremonial purposes, and scientists have shown that scent does remarkable things to the central nervous system by playing a therapeutic role. For instance, scents can alleviate psychiatric disorders and psychological symptoms among postmenopausal women.[11,12]

How does aromatherapy work? Let me give you one example. Through experimentation, scientists have identified the presence of an active molecule in incense known as incensole acetate. When mice were exposed to this molecule in olfactory form in a controlled setting, the researchers observed that the incense compound actually had a dual effect: it was an anti-inflammatory, and it boosted the mood of the mice significantly. Based on this information, they began to probe a little deeper. If it was true that incense had these positive effects on the brain and body, what was the actual mechanism causing this effect? They discovered that incense activates a part of the brain about which we still know very little. In the researchers' own words:

> There are opiate plants and there are plants that affect dopamine, serotonin, and similar substances that regulate the brain's activity. The substances in these plants work using special receptors. It turns out that the active component in frankincense acts via a receptor that is hardly known in brain science. What is known is that this receptor, known as TRPV3, is found in nerves located beneath the skin and responds to a sensation of warmth.

This receptor plays an important role in mood regulation and interacts with the active compounds in incense. In light of surprising study findings such as these, perhaps it is important to keep an open mind.[13,14]

PSYCHOACOUSTICS: *MANTRA*

Psychoacoustics is the scientific study of human perception of sound. Many cultures have used sounds or vocalizations as a tool for promoting physical, emotional, and spiritual healing since before the arrival of the written word. *Mantra* is a Sanskrit word that means sound healing: *man* refers to the mind, and *tra* signifies deliverance or projection. Indian culture has long given particularly deep significance to sound healing, as is shown by its long-standing use of mantras and sacred chants.

The ancient texts say chanted vocalizations in Sanskrit are designed to create sounds that vibrate in the body. According to Dr. David Frawley, studies of selected Vedic hymns or *mantras* show that they are not like our ordinary, artificial, rigid language; instead, they are composed of an "organic language in which sound and meaning correspond."[15] We also know that scientists generally agree that there was a Big Bang, a colossal sound wave critical to the creation of the universe. There is no greater example of the impact of sound. In 1973, physician and biophysicist Dr. Gerald Oster proved in his research article "Auditory Beats in the Brain" that sound affects the way the brain absorbs information and nearly all areas of our life, including healing.[16] Consequently, we can use certain frequencies of sound to change brain chemistry, affecting molecules such as serotonin.

Sound waves are a force that travels through particles, and sound and vibrations have the potential to influence matter. As Oster wrote in his article:

> *Our diverse states of consciousness are directly related to the continual electrical, chemical, and architectural environmental changes of the brain. Lifestyle with its daily habits of behavior and thought processes have the ability to modify the architecture of brain structure and*

connectivity, and per consequence, our neurochemistry and the electrical neural oscillations of your mind.

A series of experiments conducted by neuroelectric therapy engineers Dr. Meg Patterson and Dr. Ifor Capel revealed how alpha brainwaves boosted the production of serotonin, also known as the contentment or happiness molecule. Dr. Capel explained:

As far as we can tell, each brain center generates impulses at a specific frequency based on the predominant neurotransmitter it secretes. In other words, the brain's internal communication language is based on frequency. Presumably, when we send in waves of electrical energy at, say, 10 Hz, certain cells in the lower brain stem will respond because they normally fire within that frequency range.[17,18]

Sound as therapy can provide beneficial results for a range of conditions, such as depression, anxiety, stress, and stress-related issues such as posttraumatic stress disorder and pain management.

MUDRAS (HAND GESTURES)

Mudras are not only used in Ayurveda but also as symbolic or ritual gestures in Hinduism and Buddhism. The word *mudra* means "seal." These hand gestures are also used in yoga during various postures *(asanas)*, breathing exercises *(pranayama)*, and meditation. According to the ancient texts of Ayurveda, *mudras* direct the flow of energy into the body. Yoga scholars use *mudras* during their sessions to draw themselves inward. They believe that when hand gestures are used in conjunction with *pranayama*, they stimulate different body parts involved with breathing, affecting not only the flow of energy in the body but also one's mood. *Mudras* are generally practiced while seated in particular poses.

Ayurveda relates each finger of the hand to one of the five elements:

- The thumb represents fire and universal consciousness.
- The index finger represents air and individual consciousness.

- The middle finger represents space or connection.
- The ring finger represents earth.
- The little finger represents water.

Some yoga practitioners describe specific hand gestures for the mind and the brain that can help you to improve mental health and boost your intelligence.[19] For example, *mudras* like the *tse mudra, hakini mudra,* and *usahs mudra* are described as hand gestures that, when practiced along with yoga, can stop stress, anxiety, and depression, give you more energy, and lift your mood.[20] We do not yet have the technology to measure the energetic effects of these hand gestures, just as we could not really understand how meditation affected the brain before the development of EEGs and CAT scans.

AYURVEDIC HERBS

This book contains a full chapter addressing Ayurvedic herbal programs. However, I will describe here how the use of medicinal plants has long been a great source of biomolecules with therapeutic value for the treatment of depression, anxiety, and other conditions. Emerging clinical cases are attracting increasing interest in phytomedicine (plant medicine) among health practitioners and patients. The development of antidepressant and anxiolytic drugs from plant sources takes advantage of a multidisciplinary method that includes ethnopharmacology as well as phytochemical and pharmacological studies.

Mood disorders such as depression, with symptoms that vary from mild to debilitating to potentially life-threatening, are challenging to treat in both mainstream medicine and Ayurveda. Still, for centuries Ayurvedic herbs, spices, and other treatments have proved effective in helping to reduce the symptoms of depression. Your kitchen can become a very enjoyable home pharmacy. Just be ready to experiment and get better at the same time you are enjoying your food. Many of the most important, effective, and easy-to-use herbs and foods are included in the chapter on Ayurvedic herbal programs for your type of depression, which presents Ayurvedic herbs and herbal formulations along with some European plants.

Most people with depression complain of fatigue on a daily basis. If you are experiencing depression-related fatigue, I would like you to know about a group of rejuvenating or nootropic herbs known in Ayurveda under the name of *rasayanas*. The combination of *rasayanas*, made with a select group of rejuvenating herbs, with a balanced and wholesome diet will balance your *doshas* and stimulate your natural energy. From the thousands of medicinal plant species used in India, fewer than ten are considered *rasayanas*.[21]

According to their role, *rasayanas* can be divided into three categories:

- Promoting vitality and longevity
- Supporting body complexion
- Improving intellect, concentration, and memory

Rasayanas are classified as drug-based, dietary, or lifestyle. In today's busy world, the use of *rasayanas* is an excellent source of support and reinforcement, especially when considering the amount of stress with which we are bombarded and the low quality and selection of food that is sometimes on offer.

OIL PULLING

Oil pulling is a popular natural remedy from India that involves swishing a small amount of oil in your mouth, around your gums and teeth. It improves oral hygiene and is not only recognized by Ayurvedic practitioners but is also suggested and recommended by some Western dentists and doctors. Oil pulling has become increasingly popular for its purported health benefits.[22,23]

The health advantages of oil pulling extend beyond just mouth hygiene, in the following ways:

- Teeth and gums: helps maintain a normal mouth balance (pH acidity) and good oral flora, keeping microbes, plaque, and decay from building up within the mouth while strengthening the teeth and their enamel

- Promotes general sinus health, keeping them clear and free
- Regular practice refreshes the breath, diminishes dryness and wheezing, and eases breathing
- Reduces inflammation by preventing red, swollen, and inflamed or bleeding gums (gingivitis) by acting on the bacteria causing the formation of plaque
- Assists with joint comfort and flexibility
- Keeps the mandibles, jaw, and neck areas supple and mobile
- Supports the body's natural ability to detoxify

TONGUE SCRAPING

As your oral cavity is one of the main passages between your body and the environment, keeping proper oral hygiene helps create balance and overall general wellness. Your tongue is a favorable environment for bacteria to proliferate, especially toward the back of your mouth. In this practice you use a tongue scraper (usually made of stainless steel, and available online and in health stores) to gently scrape the tongue from the back forward, until you have scraped the whole surface. Afterward, rinse your mouth.[24]

Tongue scraping contributes to the balance between a healthy mouth and bodily well-being by performing these functions:

- Cleans the tongue of toxins and bacteria
- Removes coating on the tongue that leads to bad breath (halitosis)
- Helps eradicate undigested food particles from the tongue
- Cleans the taste buds, improving the sense of taste
- Improves the appearance of the tongue

EVACUATION: NONSUPPRESSION OF PHYSIOLOGICAL URGES

As you go about your daily life at home, work, or school, how often do you suppress the desire to urinate, defecate, sleep, or even cry? How often do you resist the impulse to pass gas, cough, or yawn? In our daily life quite frequently we find ourselves under circumstances where we are suppressing natural urges, sometimes without even being aware of it. Various studies of patients with psychological disorders show an association between chronic constipation and a shortage of serotonin.[25,26,27]

According to Ayurveda, we should not suppress our natural biological and emotional urges, particularly the following:

- Sleep
- Bowel movements
- Urination
- Flatus
- Thirst
- Hunger
- Tears
- Vomiting
- Coughing
- Sneezing
- Belching
- Yawning
- Heavy respiration
- Ejaculation

On the other hand, Ayurveda recommends that we suppress mental urges pertaining to:

- Greed

- Grief
- Fear
- Anger
- Vanity
- Shamelessness
- Jealousy
- Excessive desire
- Ill will, malice

The fundamental human need to express one's pain and try to find some way of ameliorating one's condition is at the heart of all this. We learn from the experience of undergoing pain, challenges, and difficulties; that is how we recognize who we really are. People transform through challenges.

We will end with the following quotation from Charaka:

Those [practitioners] who are accomplished in the administration of therapies, insight, and knowledge of therapeutics are endowed with infallible success and can bring happiness to the seeker. They are saviors of life.

—*Ca. Su. 9/4*

Disclaimer: The sole purpose of these descriptions is to provide information about the tradition and benefits of Ayurveda. This information is not intended for unsupervised use in the diagnosis, treatment, cure, or prevention of depression or any other disease. If you have any serious acute or chronic health concern, please consult a trained health professional who can fully assess your needs and address them effectively. If you are seeking the medical advice of a trained Ayurvedic expert, call or email a qualified Ayurvedic physician or practitioner in your area. Check with your doctor before taking herbs or using essential oils when pregnant or nursing.

Ayurvedic Mastery of Food, Diet, and Nutrition

FOOD AND THE BODY-MIND CONNECTION: HOW AYURVEDA CLASSIFIES FOOD

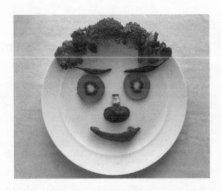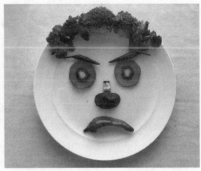

This chapter introduces basic practical information about food from an Ayurvedic perspective, including important concepts related to nutrition and diet that will help you restore balance and addressing depression in the most natural way.

According to Ayurvedic scholars, the pillars of proper body-mind health are:

- A balanced diet consisting of wholesome, nutritious food
- A strong digestive fire *(agni)* for the proper digestion and assimilation of food
- Surveillance of the absence or accumulation of *ama*

We start our discussion of food by describing the basic principles of wholesome food, based on the Ayurvedic concepts of constitution, taste, and quality. These descriptions allow us to integrate knowledge about wholesome food with modern nutritional concepts of diet and lifestyle.

Ayurveda evaluates foods according to the characteristics found in these three categories:

- The five elements—earth, water, fire, air, ether
- The twenty qualities of matter *(gunas)*—heavy, slow, cold, wet, sticky, dense, soft, firm, subtle, clear, and their opposites
- The six tastes—sweet, sour, salty, bitter, pungent, astringent

Before you think "This is becoming too complicated!" or "How am I going to follow all this information?" let me reassure you. Once you start to understand the basics of Ayurveda and how you can incorporate it into your life with appropriate adjustments to your diet and lifestyle, things begin to fall into place. It is not essential for you to know all the Ayurvedic terms. Some of them are presented here only because they help us to have a nomenclature. What is essential is to make the recommended adjustments in diet and lifestyle with an open mind and to welcome positive and productive changes in your life.

Be sure of one thing: our constant aim is to restore balance. For my part, I will illustrate the use of Ayurvedic terms with everyday examples to make clear what was beautifully, precisely, and systematically described by the Ayurvedic scholars so long ago and which is still highly relevant today.

The Five Elements

The concept of the five elements can be applied to your food intake. Nutritive elements are classified as earthy, watery, fiery, airy, and spacious. Ayurvedic doctors describe the elemental food categories in this way:

1. Earthy foods include all kind of vegetables, grains, and animal materials that are digestible. These give us the effect and sensation of solidity and heaviness.

2. Watery foods include liquid nutrients such as milk, buttermilk, fruit juices, soups, and ghee. These produce moistening and pleasantness, and they support tissular integration and body strength.

3. Fiery foods include spices such as red and green chilies, cayenne pepper, jalapeño pepper, and black pepper. These produce heat, spiciness, and warmth.

4. Airy foods produce lightness and cleansing. Importantly, Ayurveda considers air as food for metabolic processes in the body. This should not be a surprise: modern medicine tells us that because the digestive system breaks down food and uses muscular contractions to move food through the digestive tract, it needs oxygen to function properly.[1]

5. Spacious foods produce hollowness, softness, and lightness in the body tissues, allowing the blending and transformation of the previous four elements. Space needs to be created in the digestive system for the food to move through (*Ca. Su.* 25/5–50).

Ayurveda also classifies foods into these types of foods: cereals and grains; legumes, beans, and lentils; meat; vegetables; fruit; nuts; milk and dairy; water; wine and spirits; sugars; spices, minerals, fats, oils, and condiments; and cooked food preparations (e.g., soups, fruit juices, cooked milk).

Qualities of Matter: The Twenty *Gunas*

In addition to the five elements, in Ayurveda we use a simple but effective way to look at everything within and around us through the specific qualities of matter. In ancient Vedic times, the acknowledgment of the following ten fundamental qualities and their opposites were well incorporated into Ayurveda: heavy, slow, cold, wet, sticky, dense, soft, firm, subtle, and clear.[2]

One of the basic principles in Ayurveda is the concept that like increases like. This rule means that as the elemental qualities already present in our *prakruti* type are increased by similar qualities of the foods we consume and the environmental conditions we experience, we develop an imbalance, which is always due to an excess of one sort or another. By contrast, applying opposite qualities brings support and balance to your *prakruti*.[3]

The following table illustrates the relationship between the *gunas* and body.

Table 9.1. *Gunas* and the body

PROPERTY (GUNA)	SANSKRIT NAME	CONSTITUTION OF ELEMENTS (MAHABHUTAS)	EFFECTS ON THE BODY	V	P	K
Heaviness	*Guru*	Earth, water	↑ bulk. Heavy to digest.	↓		↑
Light	*Laghu*	Space, air	Bulk-reducing. Easy to digest.	↑		↓
Cold	*Shita*	Water, air	Cooling. Induces nourishment.	↑	↓	↑
Hot	*Ushna*	Fire	Sweating. Generates energy, appetite. ↑ *agni*.	↓	↑	↓
Unctuous	*Snigdha*	Water	Moistening. Supports body tissue nutrition.	↓		↑
Dryness	*Ruksha*	Air, fire	Dryness. Decreases fluids, fat, weight.	↑		↓
Dullness	*Manda*	Earth	Slowing. Decreases movement and digestion.	↓		↑

PROPERTY (GUNA)	SANSKRIT NAME	CONSTITUTION OF ELEMENTS (MAHABHUTAS)	EFFECTS ON THE BODY	V	P	K
Sharpness	*Tikshna*	Fire	Acuity. Appetite and *agni* ↑.	↓	↑	↓
Immobility	*Shira*	Earth	Stability, firm. → muscles, fat, bones.	↓	↓	↑
Mobility	*Chala*	Air, water	Motion, action.	↑	↑	↓
Softness	*Mrudu*	Space	Unstiffening.	↓	↑	↑
Hardness	*Kathina*	Earth	Rigidity, rough.	↑	↓	↓
Clear	*Vishada*	Space	Clearing. Disperses channels of circulation.	↓	↓	↓
Sticky	*Picchila*	Water	Adhering, coating. ↑ body bulk.	↓	↓	↑
Smooth	*Shlakshna*	Space	Softness.	↓	↓	↑
Coarse	*Khara*	Air, fire	Roughness.	↑		↓
Gross	*Sthula*	Earth	Obstructing. Induces bulking, obesity.	↓		↑
Subtle	*Sukshma*	Air, space	Piercing. Creates lightness.	↑	↑	↓
Dense	*Sandra*	Water, earth	Solidifying. → stability and strength.	↓		↑
Liquid	*Drava*	Water	Fluidity. Supports body exchanges.	↓	↑	↑

Key: ↑ = increases. ↓ = decreases. → = produces. *V* = *vata*. *P* = *pitta*. *K* = *kapha*. (*As. Hr. Su.* 1/18; *Ca. Su.* 26/65)

The Six Basic Tastes

Ayurveda distinguishes six basic tastes, flavors, or qualities of food, each of which has a specific influence on your mind-body physiology. The six tastes are sweet, sour, salty, bitter, pungent, and astringent. Each one affects our *doshas* differently. A well-balanced diet should include all six tastes in your food intake, attuned to your particular body-mind constitution, as each *dosha* requires nourishment. Are you one of those people who likes sweet and sour flavors, or maybe salty and spicy foods? Or perhaps you enjoy bitter and astringent tastes? Are you able to recognize those different tastes in the food you eat daily?

The taste of food originates from its own constitution or inner composition of elements. Everything we eat manifests distinctive proportions of the five elements, and many foods have a combination of two or three tastes. Ayurveda considers it essential to connect to our sensations through the six basic tastes. The list of twenty *gunas* as well as the description and understanding of the six tastes are valuable checklists to use in evaluating the wholesomeness of your food.

Let me give you examples of cases when your *prakruti* has too much of a particular element:

- *Pitta* constitution: foods that are preponderant in heat, such as hot peppers, will only be desirable in small amounts because they are going to increase your fire even more, as like increases like.

- *Kapha* constitution: foods that are preponderant in *kapha* elements, such as dairy products (constituted predominantly by earth and water), will induce production of mucus in your body, manifesting as congested sinuses among other symptoms. Once again we see that like increases like.

These concepts are very easy to understand, but regrettably, modern medicine rarely applies them. It is worth noting here that simply recognizing this concept—and doesn't it make sense?—is a step toward rebalancing without taking medications or making drastic changes in lifestyle or circumstances. It also costs nothing other than your time to take this first step. That is what I call a cost-effective health system!

Let me give you more examples of the direct impact that different types of foods or diet can have on your body-mind, according to their qualities:

- When the weather is hot and dry, you might find that your body, mind, or emotions become hot and dry as well. If you drink cooling coconut water or aloe vera juice, or you take a nap in the shade or a walk in cool, humid moonlight, you will start to address the conditions that give rise to this heat and dryness—all very much common sense.

- If you have a cold with a heavy mucus cough, what could be more helpful than drinking some channel-opening, warming, sharp, dry ginger tea to open your respiratory passages, or to rest for a while under a hot, dry, penetrating sun?

These examples are the flip side of the principle that like increases like. When we are aware of an excess, our natural instinct is to decrease the "like" around us. If you integrate the *guna* or quality concept with the concept of like increases like, you will realize that to correct diet and lifestyle imbalances you need to aim for the opposite qualities. In this way, those qualities present in you provide the intelligence needed to restore balance through diet and lifestyle.

Now, don't go to the other extreme and try to minimize the use or practice of the various tastes. According to Ayurveda, people whose diet predominates in only one taste are putting their health at risk. Why is this? If body tissues are not nourished properly, deficiencies will manifest sooner or later, gradually bringing about a poor immune response and making you more susceptible to physical or mental illness. Imagine somebody living on a food intake based on sugar; the result is an open invitation to diabetes. On the other hand, people whose diet includes the six tastes are likely to have well-nourished bodies and strong immune responses as a result of a well-rounded diet.

Note that for certain tastes, only a small quantity is necessary for it to satisfy and balance us; more is not always better. For most of us, the taste of bitter, spicy (pungent), and astringent foods is generally unpleasant, while sour, salty, or sweet foods generally provide a pleasurable sensation.

To encapsulate these points succinctly:

....

Ideal nutrition results from selecting foods with appropriate tastes matched to your prakruti, *prepared and eaten correctly in a health-promoting and soothing environment.*

....

Your *Prakruti* and the Six Tastes

- *Vata*-predominant people are inclined to enjoy food with tastes that are pungent, bitter, and astringent. However, the vigorous cooling and metabolic effect of pungent tastes (alkaline) can aggravate their body *prakruti.*

- *Pitta*-predominant people are influenced by food with the tastes sour, salty, and pungent. The vigorous heating and metabolic effect of sour (acidic) can aggravate their body *prakruti.*

- *Kapha*-predominant people are influenced by food with the tastes sweet, sour, and salty. The vigorous cooling and metabolic effect of sweet (neutral) can aggravate their body *prakruti.*

When you diversify your choices of foods and incorporate the six tastes into your daily meals, you will feel the difference. Then enjoyment of food will become a regular and welcome part of your daily life, gradually helping you reach and maintain balance. As you start listening to your body, you will start feeling the various tastes and will begin adjusting to them. Do not be surprised when you discover that, once you get to know which tastes are good for and resonate with your *dosha,* foods that once were familiar to your palate have been sending your *dosha* out of balance.

By using the Ayurvedic principle of "like increases and opposites decrease," the three *doshas* can be equalized either by increasing or decreasing their intrinsic qualities. Always take this important guidance into consideration:

- *Vata* is nourished by:
  - Sweet, sour, and salty tastes
  - Moist, smooth, warm, and strong qualities counteracting their dry, cold, bitter, and mobile *prakruti* nature
- *Pitta* is nourished by:
  - Sweet, bitter, and astringent tastes
  - Cool and fresh qualities counteracting their hot, pungent, sour, and forceful *prakruti* nature
- *Kapha* is nourished by:
  - Pungent, bitter, and astringent tastes
  - Warm and dry qualities counteracting their cool and sweetened *prakruti* nature

MODERN UNDERSTANDING OF NUTRIENTS

The modern understanding of a nutrient is a food substance that the body uses to support growth, maintenance, repair, and energy production. Your body contains thousands of different kinds of biological molecules, and for your well-being it needs to ingest foods containing certain crucial small compounds, such as essential amino acids, essential fatty acids, vitamins, minerals, and water.

It's important to note that most of the molecules in food, while metabolized or incorporated into the body, are not necessarily essential.[4] Let's consider carbohydrates as an example. If you decided to remove them from your daily food intake, their absence would not necessarily cause illness, if they were replaced by another type of food that provides the required calories for your normal bodily needs.

The basic nutrients considered essential for health are classified as follows:

- Macronutrients: carbohydrates (glucose), proteins (amino acids), and lipids or fats (triglycerides, cholesterol), which make up the bulk of our food intake and diet

- Micronutrients: vitamins and minerals, which, although essential for health, are required in minute quantities

- Water: the most essential of all. Your body loses water through breathing, sweating, elimination, and digestion. You need to rehydrate by drinking fluids and eating foods that contain water for all your cellular and tissular requirements.

All macronutrients require the presence of specific enzymes to become accessible for cellular absorption and perform their different functions. Fats or lipids consist of triglycerides that can be digested when they break down into fatty acids and glycerol; they are a very good source of calories. Another member of this group, which is also insoluble in water, is cholesterol, which plays essential roles from building healthy cells to acting as the precursor of many hormones.

Proteins are large molecules (macromolecules) composed of a variety of units called amino acids. A total of twenty different amino acids exist in proteins, and they play many vital roles, including building proteins and synthesizing hormones and neurotransmitters.

Carbohydrates are the sugars, starches, and fibers found in fruits, vegetables, grains, and milk products. In starches, they consist of very large chains of glucose molecules linked together, which eventually get broken down by enzymatic actions into smaller ones and ultimately into single molecules of glucose. Carbohydrates can also be small molecules like the lactose in milk or natural fructose in fruits. We get energy from carbohydrates by breaking them down into glucose, or blood sugar, which is absorbed into the bloodstream. Our brain accepts only glucose as fuel, despite the fact that we get different kinds of sugars from our diet.

While most nutrition labels group all carbohydrates into a single total carbohydrate count, the ratio of the sugar and fiber subgroups to the whole amount affects how the body and brain respond. Let me give you two examples to explain the importance of whole foods:

- White bread: this food's carbohydrates have a very rapid breakdown, intestinal absorption, and release of glucose, raising blood glucose levels higher and more quickly than most other foods (white bread is a high-glycemic food). Because carbohydrates from white bread are metabolized so quickly, blood sugar from this source is rapidly depleted, modifying your attention span and mood.

- Oats, grains, and legumes: due to their fiber content and more complex carbohydrates, they are broken down and absorbed more slowly, and glucose moves to the bloodstream over a longer period of time, keeping your attention span for longer with relatively less impact on your mood.

Something else to take into consideration here is that our bodies are able to convert the three major macronutrients into different substances, depending on our physical and mental needs. For example, glucose can be converted into nonessential amino acids and fats, and vice versa. These systems are metabolic interconversions of adaptation that involve several enzymatic reactions as part of well-known pathways and cycles.[5]

The amount of carbohydrates, proteins, and fat you should be consuming, and the combinations in which you should consume them, is a topic under continuous discussion by best-selling diet authors. However, their recommendations are striking in their divergence, from too much protein to too little, no meat versus a diet rich in meat, and so on. Some nutritional experts are big proponents of low-fat, low-protein, high-carbohydrate diets. Other nutritional gurus encourage just the opposite: foods high in protein and fat but low in carbohydrates. Others go for the minerals and vitamins. The question always remains, however: can these one-size-fits-all diets be sustained across a population of individual *prakrutis,* each of which has its own unique dietary and nutritional needs?

The clear answer Ayurveda gives is no. Perhaps the inability of these one-size-fits-all diets to distinguish among the needs of prospective dieters is one reason why they fall away as quickly as they rise in prominence.

The question of how to achieve an appropriate balance in our food intake is both exciting and confusing due to a variety of factors:

- The massive amount and diversity of general information and scientific literature available

- The disparity and complexity of scientific information concerning diets and nutrition

- Confusion generated due to the chemical composition of foods and their metabolic processes involving conversion and interaction of different kinds of food molecules

- Lack of understanding about when and how much food is required and in what combination

- Classification of natural foods combined with new, integrated, industrialized synthetic molecules and their potential toxicity

- Misunderstandings, predispositions, and biases coming from the agribusiness sector, the food industry, and nutritional gurus on social media

For these reasons I would like to set out here some basic information about how the different components of our food function and interact, alongside some digestive principles.

The ingested food traveling to our stomach passes through three processes—digestion, absorption, and assimilation—all executed by our *agni* (digestive fire). Nothing could happen at the digestive stage without the input of gastric acids and enzymatic action that break down our food. Their actions convert large particles of food into small molecules.

This process of digestive transformation allows them to be absorbed by the intestine and transported by the circulatory system, making them available at the level of the blood plasma. From there, processed and absorbed small nutrients can now be easily taken in by our cells and tissues and be assimilated structurally or functionally by our cells. Since body tissues are all made of cells communicating via minute channels receiving and distributing nutrients, this dynamic network will assimilate nutrients coming in the right quantity and quality. The elimination of metabolic waste products that are not required anymore or are present in abundance is also part of the same process, in order to maintain balance between inputs and outputs.

What is fascinating is that the description of digestion and cellular communication that was relayed through the classic Ayurvedic texts many centuries ago is consistent with the modern understanding of intercellular uptake and release of substrates and metabolites. These descriptions of the same processes are separated only by a few thousand years and different vocabularies.

The Ayurvedic texts summarize this process by saying what we take in is what we become, or you are what you eat. What we ingest and can digest becomes our strength, and what we cannot digest becomes our vulnerability. That vulnerability will manifest sooner or later in the form of imbalances and illnesses at a physical or mental level.

AGNI

The meaning of *agni* is "fire," an essential element for maintaining life. *Agni* is responsible for all metabolic functions, including digestion, absorption, and assimilation of ingested food. As this digestive fire is increased or depleted, our body-mind biological functions respond accordingly. Healthy *agni* supports a healthy body and mind. Depleted *agni* compromises physical and mental health. Thus, maintenance of healthy *agni* is fundamental to management of depression.

Fire is one of the five elements *(panchamahabhutas)*, and *agni* is one of its manifestations. Its qualities are described as hot, sharp, light, penetrating, spreading, luminous, subtle, and clear. Ayurvedic scholars describe up to forty types of *agni*, each defined by its specific physiological functions as well as its bodily location. Thousands of years ago, without the support of modern biomedical technology, Ayurveda described the digestive *agni* of the cell membrane *(pilu agni)* and of the *agni* inside the cell in the nuclear membrane *(pithara agni)*. Every single cell in our bodies requires fire (energy) to fuel all the many mechanisms of life, and their proper functions depend on the quality and quantity of *agni* available to them. In this section we will address *agni* in broad terms as the collective of digestive fires for the purpose of understanding body-mind imbalances.

> Agni *is said to be the root of our being, the root of our life, body, mind, and senses.*
>
> —*As. Hr. Ni.* 12/1

Functions of *Agni*

The mother of all *agni* is digestive or gastric fire, termed *jataragni*. It is said to be located in the stomach and small intestine and to be the central government of all the other types of "micro-*agni*" in our bodies. *Agni* has been divided into thirteen types (*Ca. Su.* 15/38):

- One *agni* in the stomach and duodenum *(jataragni)*
- Five *agni* representing each of the five elements *(bhutagni)*
- Seven *agni* in the seven body tissues, one per tissue *(dhatwagni)*

All types of *agni* depend directly on the quality and quantity of *jataragni*, since it provides energy from the intracellular components to all body tissues and through them to the entire body. We can see the different types of *agni* as various microfires controlling different micrometabolic processing in different cells and organs, with the aim of maintaining balance. So *jataragni* acts like a kind of distributor of energy from the main power station.

This *jataragni*, which we will call *agni* for simplification, governs cellular intelligence and cellular selectivity, and it is responsible for the processes of digestion, absorption, assimilation, and transformation. *Agni* processes include gastric mucus secretion, stimuli from the hunger center in the brain, peristalsis, opening of the pyloric valve, and secretion of the various gastric and intestinal enzymes.

Agni is equally in charge of the formation of urine, feces, and sweat, all of which neutralize potential toxins *(ama)*. When all these processes are working in harmony, they keep us in a state of balance, guaranteeing continual nutritional restoration and good cellular communication. All of these functions allow us to have strength and vitality and to maintain body temperature. At a mental level, *agni* supports our mental clarity, intelligence, discrimination, sensory perception, and enthusiasm for life (affection, contentment, courage, confidence, joy, and laughter), providing strength, tolerance, and longevity.

Imbalances of *Agni*

When *agni* is disturbed, the digestive fire does not burn or metabolize our food intake adequately, so those substances remain as undigested material that eventually becomes toxic in the body if it is not eliminated. This undigested material, either physical or mental, is what we call *ama*. If these foodstuffs or mental thoughts are not well digested, the unprocessed particles create dysfunction in our cellular metabolism. For example, they can affect the space between cells (intracellular fluid), impairing cellular communication by settling in and around the cell, resulting in a process of cellular shutdown known as apoptosis.

If more *ama* keeps recirculating in our body, it will eventually end up lodged in our vessels or arteries, which are really designed to transport wholesome food to the body instead of housing *ama* deposits. This will cause conditions such as arterial blockages at all levels, including the heart and brain. These unmetabolized accumulations also give rise to toxicity in blockages of the channels and tissues of the brain, creating mental imbalances and individual distress manifesting as heaviness, dullness, stagnation, and cloudiness of emotions and perception.

It is not just a poor-quality diet that gives rise to depleted *agni* and *ama* accumulation; even high-quality foodstuffs, if not digested properly, could make you sick. Here is a list of signs and symptoms of *ama* production and accumulation in our body-mind systems:

- Coated tongue
- Indigestion or poor appetite

- Congestion of body channels

- Stagnation of energy flow

- Fatigue

- Taste scarcity or spoiled taste in the mouth

- Heaviness

- Sexual weakness

- Abnormal *vata* flow

- Mental confusion

- Sickness

- A feeling of filthiness

Ayurveda also describes three other related metabolic processes known as *virya, vipaka,* and *prabhava.* I am going to describe them briefly because they are very important concepts in Ayurveda. We are not going to directly integrate them for the purpose of rebalancing, but they will be part of your own research if you would like to go deeper into these subjects.

- *Virya:* potency or energy of a substance, e.g., of a food or curative herb. It is the secondary action of an ingested substance experienced after taste. Cold and hot are considered the chief potencies.

- *Vipaka:* the final postdigestive effect of food that happens in the colon, having an effect on our eliminations (sweat, urine, and feces). It is described as sweet, sour, and pungent.

- *Prabhava:* the special dynamic efficacy of a substance that cannot be explained based on its energy, taste, and postdigestive effects.

Table 9.2 describes four metabolic conditions based on the type of inner fire *(agni),* its connection with your associated preponderant *dosha,* and their physiological potential consequences.

Table 9.2. Four metabolic conditions

Balanced metabolism *(sama agni)*	Balanced inner fire; balanced *doshas*	State of perfect health: normal appetite, digestion, elimination, stable health/immunity, calm/quiet mind, clarity
Fluctuating or irregular metabolism *(vishama agni)*	Irregular inner fire; associated with *vata;* an on/off digestive fire that cannot digest food completely	Irregular: erratic appetite/digestion, indigestion, gut distension, gases, constipation, abdominal pain, diarrhea (seldom), heaviness after eating, guts gurgling, desires for fried/hot-spicy food; dry mouth/skin, receding gums, cracking joints, sciatica, low back pain, muscle spasm, restlessness, anxiety, insecurity, neurological/mental troubles
Excessive or hypermetabolism *(tikshna agni)*	Sharp inner fire; associated with *pitta;* an overly intense digestive fire that can burn food, preventing complete digestion	Intense: strong appetite. Following digestion: dry lips/throat/palate, heartburn, hot flashes, strong desires for sweets; hyperacidity, gastritis, hypoglycemia, colitis, diarrhea, dysentery, liver pain, nausea, vomiting, inflammatory states; anger, hate, envy, judgmental
Diminished or slow metabolism *(manda agni)*	Dull inner fire; associated with *kapha;* a digestive fire that burns often at low temperature, giving partial digestion	Dull/heavy: fast to gain weight, sluggish digestion, gut heaviness, cold, congestion, cough, oversalivation, low appetite, craving hot/sharp/dry/spicy food; allergies, nausea, mucus, edema, obesity, diabetes, hypertension, lethargy, extreme sleep, clammy skin, generalized body weakness, attachment, greed, possessiveness

Perhaps you can see a correlation or association between the *doshas* and *agni,* and you are asking yourself: is *agni* the same as *pitta*? Well, that was and still is a subject of discussion, and theories have their own importance.[6,7] According to Sushruta, there is no existence of any other *agni* in the body without *pitta* (*Su. Sū.* 21/9).[8]

In any case, try to see how you relate to one of these four types of *agni*. Most of us feel inclined to identify with one or more of them. Regrettably, today's lifestyle pressures from processed foods, social media, and other factors make it quite rare to keep up a balanced metabolism.

Reasons for *Agni* Imbalance

Now let's consider the most common causes of imbalanced *agni*, which often generates physical or mental *ama* in our body-mind system. Most probably we can recognize ourselves in more than one of the following factors that cause *agni* imbalance:

DIET:

- Overeating
- Eating at the wrong time
- Extremely dry/cold food
- Leftover food
- Incompatible food combinations
- Inappropriate fasting
- Excessive water intake

PSYCHOPHYSIOLOGICAL:

- Emotional stress (worries, anxiety, fear, nervousness, grief, sadness, frustration, anger)
- Suppression of natural urges
- Smoking, drinking, and drug addiction

ENVIRONMENTAL:

- Unseasonable weather (rainy or extremely cold)
- Social media

Recommendations for Managing *Agni*

By learning how to use our body's interior fire and manage it skillfully, we are walking on the right path toward the development of good body-mind health. Eating food in a conscious way in terms of quality and quantity is the secret for a proper inner fire. An unwholesome diet, an unsupportive lifestyle, and unresolved emotions can easily impede *agni* by diminishing its qualities. You need to fuel this fire regularly, and especially when the fire gives you signs of hunger. Provide suitable food at a proper time to keep *agni* healthy and secure your health based on good digestive processes and the resultant immunity.

> *Strength, health, longevity, and vital breath are dependent upon the power of digestion, including metabolism. When supplied with fuel in the form of food and drink, this power of digestion is sustained; it dwindles when deprived of it.*
>
> —*Ca. Su.* 28/342

Bad digestion and lack of interest in food are manifestations showing that your emotional state, and with it your *agni*, are moving in a wrong direction. This is especially the case if these symptoms keep manifesting in a stubborn way and their duration is for longer periods of time. These are the symptoms that your body-mind is in a state of disorder and requires some balancing actions. It is important to point out here that the physical manifestations of disturbed *agni* may be readily observable, such as fainting spells, gastric ulcers, or obesity, but the mental impact is harder to observe and may therefore deteriorate undetected for some time. An example of a general Ayurvedic approach is to eliminate *ama* first by increasing the power of *agni* to a normal functional level; then treatment is implemented to reduce the increased quantity of the affected *dosha*.

When studying Ayurveda in greater detail, one grasps that *agni* is something far more than just a simple digestive fire; it is more like a higher intelligence giving us the chance to live free of the suffering caused by imbalances. *Agni* is the principle that functions through the metabolic processes to transform food and sensations into consciousness.

Ayurveda states that low or depleted *agni* (low internal fire) is the root cause of our many physical and mental diseases.

I see this daily, both personally and in my patients, and for that reason I advise you to perform this key task for the improvement of your mental and physical condition: secure your inner fire. Don't neglect the language of your guts, despite all the external pressure around you. *Agni!*

UNDIGESTED FOOD (AMA)

Ama translates to "undigested," "uncooked," "unripe," "raw," or "immature." Essentially *ama* is a form of unmetabolized waste that the body cannot use. In all our cellular metabolic processes, including digestion, molecules and compounds are formed that our body cannot process and that we need to have removed. This is especially true for people who overeat. The formation of small amounts of *ama* is a normal part of the digestive process, and under normal conditions of a strong *agni* or metabolic fire, *ama* will be efficiently eliminated. However, when our body systems cannot clear these components for one reason or another, such as a weak *agni*, then we risk entering into a vicious and self-perpetuating cycle. The etiology or causes of *ama* formation were very well studied by the Ayurvedic scholars, for example in pathologies such as obesity.

Ayurvedic scholars recognize various types of *ama*, as described in the table 9.3:

Table 9.3. Descriptions of *ama*

TYPE OF *AMA*	DESCRIPTION
Heavy and sticky	Produced through bad dietary habits and low *agni;* these undigested, unassimilated foodstuffs gradually accumulate in body systems, blocking channels and instigating disorders
Reacting	Mixing with body tissues or its accumulated waste products (urine, feces, sweat, and *dhatu malas*), initiating chronic issues

TYPE OF *AMA*	DESCRIPTION
Environmental	Associated with bioaccumulation of environmental pollutants
Aggravated *dosha*	Attacking *dhatus*
Mental	The result of unresolved, repressed emotions

The human body has hundreds of different tissues and cell types. Under balanced circumstances, every single cell of your body recognizes itself as being part of you and knows where it has to be integrated in order to communicate to neighboring cells via complex carbohydrates coating the surfaces of the cells.[9] This is a part of the continual process of maintaining equilibrium that we call inner intelligence. In the dynamic realm of cells, intelligent communication must flow. *Ama* blocks that flow of intelligent communication at the level of our circulatory systems, a topic I explored as a medical scientist for many years.[10]

When *ama* is located in the digestive tract, it is fairly easy to clear, but once it extends into the deeper tissues, it becomes far more difficult to eradicate. Once *ama* accumulates in other tissues it inevitably obstructs the channels of the body and disturbs tissular nutrition. A simple example of *ama* blocking communication at the level of body channels is the arterial accumulation of molecules of oxidized LDL (also known as "bad cholesterol"). This prevents nutrients from being delivered efficiently to the cells and waste from being discharged efficiently from the body. Accumulated waste in abnormal tissues inhibits arterial flow and cellular communication, and it even weakens the immune response.[11]

Removing the *ama* generated in our daily life by the constant attack of environmental pollutants, either by combining with our natural bodily molecules or by bioaccumulation in our tissues, is a big challenge today. Ayurvedic protocols can play a valuable role in achieving environmental *ama* removal. This type of *ama* leads to a loss of intelligence at a cellular level and is strongly associated with a wide variety of body-mind imbalances that can lead to chronic illness if not properly addressed.

How *Ama* Forms

Ama can manifest in two different ways: by accumulation in your body tissues, disturbing physiological processes, and by accumulation or interference at the level of your mind via your thinking, causing mental imbalances such as anxiety and depression.

Ayurveda says *ama* results when there is more deviation than can be tolerated between the individual and nature. When that harmony is lost, a physical or mental disease can arise. The human being is a combination of *sattva* (mind), *atma* (soul), and *sharira* (body). The universe and the individual interact through the eternally shifting interplay of three factors that exist in both realms and form a bridge between the universe and the human being: intellect *(buddhi)*, sense objects *(indriyartha)*, and natural rhythms *(kala)*.

Ayurveda gives special value to these three fundamental causes of disease:

1. *Asatmyendriyartha samyoga* means an "inappropriate correlation of the sense organs with certain sense objects." Excessive indulgence, underuse, or distorted or perverse use of the sense organs all cause disease. An excessive visual stimulus produces a distorted effect in the mind, which in turn causes stress and a vulnerability to disease. Examples are continuous exposure to bright lights, objects observed for long periods of time (either closely or at a distance), and overexposure to cell phones or TV screens. These activities can aggravate the *doshas*, transforming an initially mental phenomenon into a somatic manifestation.[12] Overindulgence in a bad diet,[13] hyperactivity, or any other extreme indulgence in any physical or mental activity results in an increase of *vata*, causing the release of neurotransmitters and endocrine regulators that will start all the metabolic and transformational actions of *pitta*, causing structural changes at the cellular level that represent the involvement of *kapha*. The three *doshas* are affected, resulting in imbalance and potential disease.

2. *Prajnaparadha* means "improper behavior due to incorrect knowledge." This is a failure of the natural knowledge of the body

due to the loss of wisdom or discrimination *(dhi)*, patience or conviction *(dhrti)*, or remembrance or memory *(smrti)*. From the allopathic point of view, this can be understood as various emotional stress conditions causing different biochemical reactions in the body, with the subsequent release of certain neurotransmitters, e.g., catecholamines increasing the uptake of endogenous and exogenous lipids such as LDL, affecting the physiological balance of *dosha* homeostasis.[14]

3. *Parinama* means "being out of harmony with the rhythms and cycles of nature." *Parinama* has to do with two types of time: seasonal variations of the *doshas* and predominance of *doshas* according to a person's age. Seasonal and age-related variations cause vitiation of the *doshas: vata* accumulating during the summer and vitiating in the rainy season, *pitta* accumulating in the rainy season and vitiating in fall, and *kapha* accumulating in the cold season and vitiating in spring.[15] With regard to age, *kapha* is predominant in childhood, *pitta* in middle age, and *vata* in old age.

You should become aware of these cycles and modify your lifestyle accordingly to avoid discordance through *tridosha* imbalance. Our chronobiological rhythms were well known to the classical Ayurvedic scholars. Here I cite scientific studies illustrating the mental disturbances caused by perennial disrespect of our biorhythms.[16,17]

Signs and Symptoms of *Ama*

If you do not change the oil in your car for a prolonged period of time, the engine is going to give you trouble, and the whole system will not function well. The same happens in your body when channels are blocked. That is the case when plaque formation at an arterial level causes strength deficiency, a lethargic feeling, or heaviness. Cases of indigestion when your body manifests gas, bloating, constipation, or diarrhea, or even cases of mental confusion and physical exhaustion are also particular cases where *vata*—the *dosha* of motion—feels disturbed, and its fluidity is not normal.

Five Methods for Reducing *Ama*

1. Avoid the formation of *ama* by refraining from:

   • Overeating heavy, fried, processed foods, rich desserts, or incompatible foods

   • Eating again before the preceding meal is digested

   • Irregular eating routines, not having lunch (main meal), skipping breakfast, eating a heavy dinner

   • Drinking ice-cold water and cold drinks when eating your meal; eating cold-food meals

   • Eating food that is not fresh, uncontaminated, and organic, e.g., stale, packaged, or long-frozen foods

   • Eating without paying full attention to the meal (using your phone, watching TV, or reading) or eating very quickly

   • Eating under intense emotional tension or without a supportive state of mind

   • Avoidance of exercise

2. Digest the *ama* by sipping hot water or using specific spices or herbal preparations.

3. Cleanse the digestive tract based on your *prakruti*, since certain spices may be too heating. Basically, a simple application of this is to drink hot water and lemon in the morning and could include the use of particular spices such as ginger and black pepper.

4. Increase or ignite the digestive fire by implementing a strict diet, starting with liquid meals, moving gradually to semiliquid ones, then to more consistent soups, and finally moving to solid food. The process involves the use of specific spices and herbal preparations taken at specific times during the day.

5. Eliminate *ama* via Ayurvedic herbal formulas; or, for a more rigorous *ama* reduction, use a supervised detox program or *panchakarma*. Ayurveda's cleanse is fully planned around loosening *ama*,

toxins, and excess *vata, pitta,* and *kapha* from the deep tissues and cells, and moving them toward the digestive tract and then out of the body.

A gentle way to detoxify your body on a daily basis is to use *triphala*, a well-known and highly effective polyherbal Ayurvedic medicine consisting of fruits of the plant species *Emblica officinalis* (amalaki), *Terminalia bellerica* (bibhitaki), and *Terminalia chebula* (haritaki). Triphala is a foundation of gastrointestinal and rejuvenative treatment, and it is rich in antioxidants.[18,19,20]

Remember, our bodies were not designed or destined to become toxic dumps. However, inadequate food ingestion, overstress, and chemical contaminants present in the air we breathe, the water we drink or wash with, and the foods we eat are endlessly creating metabolic byproducts that can create a toxic scenario in our bodies. You need to flush them out of your system on a regular basis. Ayurveda offers you the above protocols to use before this potential toxic buildup manifests as a strong imbalance. The older we become, the less capable our body's mechanisms for eliminating impurities tend to be, so I stress the need for periodic cleansing therapy. As always, I recommend that you discuss these matters with your doctor or a qualified Ayurvedic practitioner before taking any steps.

OPTIMIZING YOUR NUTRIENTS

The Intrinsic Quality of Food (Food *Prakruti*)

Everything that exists has a *prakruti*, and that includes food. The quality of food is the first factor to take into consideration when tailoring a diet to assist in managing the imbalances that manifest as depression.

The most important quality to remember in food is its taste *(rasa)*. The taste of food is the result of the predominance of some basic molecular particles (qualities) that are part of the food's composition. The combinations of these particles manifest in the many types of food substances we find in nature, creating the different tastes. Since most of us have the ability to recognize different tastes, you can explore them by training your tongue to recognize and differentiate the great variety of combinations of tastes present in food.

Ayurvedic scholars have devised tables of foods to eat according to your body *prakruti,* the qualities that each taste holds, and the influence it will have on your *doshas.*[21] To discover which diet is more suitable for you, remember the results of your individual *prakruti* constitution test from earlier in this book.

If you prefer to have a diet tailored for your depression by consulting with a recognized Ayurvedic practitioner or diet consultant, do not be surprised if the prescribed diet does not look like the one you need to support your main body-mind constitution. Perhaps this initial prescribed diet is designed to reduce a particular symptom or *dosha* related to your condition and the type of medications you are taking. You will follow that diet until the symptoms of your disorder abate, and then you will return to the diet tailored for your body-mind constitution.

Methods of Preparation (*Karana*)

Certain methods of cooking harm the inner qualities of food. Preferably, food should be eaten soon after it is cooked. For vegetables an enhanced option is to steam them rather than boiling them. We have to learn to prepare our food in a way that prevents the intrinsic adverse effects for a particular body-mind constitution. For example, to control the flatulence that most beans tend to cause, supplementation with such spices as cumin, ajwain, asafetida, and turmeric are very supportive, especially for *vata* constitutions. Another combination that can reduce flatulence is when cumin and parsley are combined with potatoes.

Another beneficial supplementation we can use during food preparation is to add garlic and onions when cooking rice or any food in general, due to the antibacterial properties of their components, i.e., allicin in garlic.[22]

Additionally, I think we can agree that food cooked with pleasure and awareness is of a higher quality than food cooked in an indifferent or unfriendly manner, with scant regard for our taste buds and digestive impact. The notion that the healthiest diet is the one with copious amounts of salads is incorrect, especially if you eat them at night. Eating industrially precooked food stored in freezers and then reheated in microwave ovens can be very practical, but in the long term your body will be affected by all the processing and artificial components present in those foods that are there simply to maintain their cosmetic appearance and to prevent very old food from going bad.

Avoid buying prechopped vegetables from grocery stores. They are not as healthy as you think. They can save you cooking time but also can build up endotoxins by sitting there, which undermines some of their benefits. The golden rule here: chop your own.

Food Combinations (*Samyoga*)

Ayurveda teaches us that unwholesome combinations of foods of opposing qualities have to be avoided, such as cooking fish with milk or curds, or cooking sour fruits, such as apples, with milk.

Quantity (*Rashi*)

Ayurveda indicates that we should consume a good mixture of solid foods and liquid, in these proportions: one-third of the stomach's volume should be filled with food, and the other two-thirds should be filled with water and air, respectively. That advice is very logical, since our gastric juices and enzymes need to properly mix with food for good digestion. Per the concept of the five elements, space is required for free movement of the food/gastric secretion mixture, allowing for proper performance of the digestive fire *(agni)*.

Foods Grown Locally (*Desha*)

Ayurveda recommends eating foods grown near our place of residence, since they are exposed to the same climate and nourished by the same conditions as you. We should not consume exotic foods on a regular basis. Local food should be fresher and higher in nutritional value, as it has not had to travel long distances or be stored (often frozen) for long periods of time before being consumed.

Time of Food Intake *(Kala)*

Ayurveda says digesting food requires a strong *agni,* so you should eat your largest meal at midday, when the digestive fire is strongest.

Ayurvedic texts also say breakfast should be light and rather stimulating. Dinner should not be too ample, and it should be eaten before seven p.m.

Mental and Physiological State of the Eater *(Upayogasamastha)*

Do not eat when you are tense, anxious, or under any other kind of emotional stress. Before eating, try to calm your mind and collect your senses, and then proceed to eat.

Season *(Ruta)*

Ayurveda recommends adjusting your food intake according to the season. During spring, increase the intake of *kapha*-decreasing foods; during the summer, increase the intake of fresh foods, and be careful to avoid heat-producing foods. Eat more salads and fruits in the summer, even if you have a *kapha* constitution. During the cold season, eat more *vata*-reducing foods.[23]

FOOD FOR THE BODY: WHEN AND WHERE?

Regardless of your predominant body-mind constitution, eat only after full digestion of the previous meal. Please do not eat because it is "mealtime"; eat when you are really hungry (except for late at night).

Western society has developed in us a very strong tendency to eat far too much. If you eat before the previous meal has been fully digested, you are forcing the body to simultaneously deal with the arrival of fresh food while still handling the half-digested food from the previous intake. If you had a late breakfast, how can you expect that your body will be able to digest and assimilate a full lunch at midday? Eating when the previous meal is half-digested invites the production and secretion of enzymes and other factors present in the digestive juices. In the long run this situation alters the normal balance of your internal organs that support your digestion.

The result is that you are inviting the *doshas* to become vitiated (impaired), which ultimately means you are creating bodily and mental imbalances.

Typical examples of what happens in the physical body as the result of such imbalances include fermentation of food substances, decrease of enzymatic secretions, and flatulence. With regard to mental processes, such imbalances will cause bad moods, weariness, fatigue, and a deeper descent into depression.

Similarly, if you are stressed, anxious, or depressed and haven't eaten for a while, if hunger comes, eat well—but not too much, to avoid exhausting the body by giving it a large load of food to digest. Build your determination to respect your three meals per day in terms of proper time and right quantities. In order to achieve that real state of hunger, make the effort to avoid having unnecessary snacks (or only a very small snack, if unavoidable) between meals.

EATING WITH AWARENESS

How often do you eat in front of screens, at your desk while managing documents or emails, or even standing up or walking along the streets in a hurry? Do you think that is the way your body will appreciate food and get a sense of being nourished? Are you surprised if later on your body struggles to assimilate hurriedly ingested food?

Realize how important it is to take time before each meal to really appreciate the food you are going to eat. Aroma, flavor, color, and a relaxing atmosphere add another dimension to the nutritional value of your meal. Take the time to chew your food. All these factors send signals to the brain and will induce the release of secretions from the salivary level to gastric juices and enzymes, ensuring they play their proper role in breaking down your food and allowing proper absorption and assimilation.

FOOD AND DIET ACCORDING TO YOUR PREDOMINANT *DOSHA*

The tables presenting food for your preponderant *dosha*, included in an appendix in this book, describe in great detail the different types of foods each person should eat. These recommended foods will keep you in a state of balance or rebalance your *doshas* based on your predominant *dosha*, if it is not under a very strong imbalance.

I am not inviting you to follow a particular type of diet, such as eating or avoiding meat or becoming vegan. I am very respectful of those issues, since I deeply agree with the Ayurvedic principle that your diet has to be tailored to your individual constitution. It took me a while to abandon my belief that I had a deep understanding of diets after three intense years researching vegetarian diets as part of my master's degree in biochemistry at medical school.[24,25]

AYURVEDA AND DIET

Ayurveda believes that understanding the individual is the key to finding a truly balanced diet. It teaches that the digestive/gastric fire or *agni* in the stomach and digestive tract is the main gateway through which nutrients enter the tissues and then pass into individual cells to maintain life functions.

Our suffering society could benefit greatly from a clear, scientific Ayurvedic exposition on how body, mind, and food interrelate and function, in order to clarify and raise awareness of the nutritional and metabolic aspects of disease for conditions such as depression. Integration of Ayurvedic knowledge with today's modern medical tools is the way to get a proper vision of the physiological, biochemical, and psychological aspects of depression.

Ayurvedic literature describes five types of nutritional disorders:

1. Quantitative dietary deficiency: insufficient food causing undernutrition and even starvation

2. Qualitative dietary deficiency: malnutrition through lack of essential nutrients or certain food combinations upsetting the normal functioning of the gastric secretions, interfering with the state of our *doshas* and creating *ama*

3. Qualitative and quantitative overnutrition: emotional overeating, as well as other factors creating conditions such as obesity, high cholesterol, hypertension, heart attack, or paralysis

4. Toxins in food: certain nutrients causing toxemia, leading to digestive disorders

5. Foods unsuitable to one's constitution: these may affect natural resistance and cause disease

Food Combining

According to Ayurveda, every food has its own taste *(rasa)*, a heating or cooling energy *(virya)*, and a postdigestive effect *(vipaka)*. Some also possess *prabhava*, an effect that cannot be explained in terms of the prior three effects. Therefore, while it is true that an individual's *agni* largely determines how well or poorly food is digested, food combinations are also of great importance. When two or more foods having different tastes, energies, and postdigestive effects are combined, *agni* can become overloaded, inhibiting the enzyme system and resulting in the production of toxins. Yet if these same foods are eaten separately, they might well stimulate *agni*, be digested more quickly, and even help to burn *ama*.

Poor food combining can produce indigestion, fermentation, putrefaction, and gas formation, and if prolonged, can lead to toxemia and disease. For example, eating bananas with cold milk can diminish *agni*, change the intestinal flora, produce toxins, and cause sinus congestion, cold, cough, and allergies. Although both of these foods have a sweet taste *(rasa)*, their digestive energies *(virya)* are very different. Bananas are heating, while milk is cooling. Their postdigestive effects *(vipaka)* are also different. Bananas are sour, while milk is sweet. This confuses our digestive system and may result in toxins, allergies, and other imbalances.

Similarly, milk and melons should not be eaten together. Both are cooling, but milk is laxative, whereas melon is diuretic. Milk requires more time for digestion. Moreover, the stomach acid required to digest the melon causes the milk to curdle, so Ayurveda advises against taking milk with sour foods.

You might want to introduce yourself to food combining by eating fruit by itself, because many fruits create a sour and indigestible "wine" in the stomach when mixed with other food. Once you have adopted this change into your eating habits, try other suggestions from the list below.

. . . .

Always remember that whatever you eat,
eat it with moderation and awareness.

. . . .

Factors That Can Decrease the Consequences of Bad Food Combinations

- A strong digestive fire (if we are so blessed) can be the most powerful tool of all to deal with "bad" food combinations.

- Different quantities of each food involved in a combination can sometimes help significantly. For instance, equal quantities by weight of ghee and honey are a bad combination—ghee is cooling, but honey is heating—whereas mixing a 2:1 ratio of ghee to honey is not toxic.

- Ayurvedic cooking often adds spices and herbs to help make foods compatible or to ease a powerful effect, e.g., cooling cilantro is added to very spicy food.

- If our bodies have become accustomed to a certain food combination through many years of use, such as eating cheese with apples, then it is likely that our body has made some adaptation or become accustomed to this. This is not to say we should continue this practice, but this explains why the newcomer to apples and cheese may experience a strong case of indigestion, while the "old-timer" digests it adequately.

- Correctives, like cardamom in coffee or ghee and black pepper with potatoes, often can help alleviate some of a food's negative effects. (Coffee is stimulating and ultimately depressing to the system, and potatoes cause gas.)

- If foods with different and possibly aggravating qualities, such as a mixture of vegetables, are cooked together in the same pot, the foods tend to learn how to get along. Using appropriate spices and herbs helps with this too.

- Occasionally eating a "bad" combination usually does not upset the digestion too much.

It is difficult to understand Ayurvedic nutrition from the Western point of view, in which quantity is determined by portion size or caloric intake. In Ayurveda, nutritional advice is based on each individual rather than on seeing the population as a unitary group to which one solution is to be applied. Since the 1990s, various governmental bodies have been providing nutritional and dietetic guidance on food classifications and components based on rigid concepts such as the "four-food-group" approach to daily meal planning, which was then superseded by the "food pyramid." Health care providers routinely used the pyramid, which was adapted on the basis of cardiovascular and cancer risk factors known at the time. The pyramid guide recommended the reduction of total fat intake and promoted servings of complex carbohydrates, fruits, and meat or animal products at different ratios. Over the years and after more research, it was concluded that the food pyramid provided an unsuitable model for a balanced diet, because obesity was increasing. Today the pyramid concept is considered obsolete, and in 2005 it was replaced by the "my plate" model.[26,27]

Some nutritionists are working hard to bring about healthful change by encouraging diets centered on whole grains, beans and other legumes, fresh fruits, and vegetables and by sharing their concern with regard to salt, fats, and refined sugar. One example is a 2018 systematic review of many studies showing that adhering to a healthy diet (in particular a traditional diet common throughout the Mediterranean countries) and avoiding an inflammatory diet is associated with reduced risk of several pathological conditions, including depression.

The Mediterranean diet primarily consists of plant-based foods, such as fruits, vegetables, whole grains, legumes, and nuts. Fats such as olive oil and canola oil are used instead of butter. Herbs and spices are used to flavor foods instead of salt. Large portions of red meat are limited to no more than a few times a month, and fish and other seafood are eaten about two times per week and in small quantities. In other words, people who eat the Mediterranean diet are consuming many different types of foods, giving more importance to those with the most health benefits.[28,29]

In contrast, inflammatory diets have been associated with conditions such as depression. These diets include processed meat, red meat, fish other than dark-meat fish, high- and low-energy carbonated beverages, and vegetables other than green leafy and dark yellow vegetables.[30,31,32]

These two Western diets represent two different types of food intake—one based on intake of natural foods like the diet described in the scholarly Ayurveda texts, sourced in a cultural climate of living in contact with nature, and the other strongly affected by the impact of mass food production and industrialization.

Since scientific studies have explained how proteins and enzymes participate in digestive processes, many people—qualified and unqualified—have been promoting models of the best diet. For instance, not long ago it was recommended to limit intake of eggs and butter because they were considered unhealthy, and parts of the scientific community instead recommended the consumption of margarine, due to its perceived benefits. We now know that margarine is not recommended, due to the large amount of damaging fats within it. Now eggs and butter are considered valid components of a healthy diet, and today's new debate is over olive oil versus coconut oil. Who knows what's coming next?

We do know there has long been a continuous rise and fall of trendy diets, each new one better for you than the last. One thing these new diets have in common is how they are marketed to a mass audience. One size fits all! Ayurveda, on the other hand, asks you: what food combinations are best for you as an individual?

We also have to consider that when people reduce dietary fat intake, they tend to replace it with high-calorie snacks overloaded with sugar or other simple carbohydrates, causing other metabolic issues. The idea that we need to drastically reduce fat in our diet has been circulating for many years. This concept is a survivor of the deep-rooted hypothesis that dietary fat is the cause of cardiovascular disease, coronary heart disease, and obesity. The vilification of dietary fat originated in the late 1950s, for example in the work of U.S. scientist Ancel Keys's "Seven Countries" study. The findings of his work, followed by the publication of the first American dietary goals to reverse the increase in heart disease in 1977, have resulted in what is now known as the standard American diet.[33,34] Unfortunately, the vilification of fat has taken little note of the fact that essential fatty acids are required for the good functioning of our bodies.

In another example, during the 1980s American dietary associations recommended low-fat diets as the best way to control body weight.[35] When a food product is marked "low in fat," that often means the removed fat has been replaced with something else, such as sugar. This is not a beneficial replacement. It is not unreasonable to ask that our food be healthy for us. Unfortunately, this is not the most important goal of industrialized processing, where cosmetic longevity is a prime component of mass food production.

Another challenge we face is the lack of awareness of true nutritional integrity and of the potential of food to be used for healing instead of becoming a cause of chronic diseases, such as depression.

We are facing daily doses of food misinformation based on questionable science or simple business motives. We do not need to dwell here on the financial links and collaborations among scientific groups, multinational food manufacturers, and agrochemical producers, because our focus is on more pressing matters. Still, I am always reminded of the phrase "you get what you pay for."

Let's now "pay" attention to our next chapter, which will discuss how you can use herbs for your type of depression.

Ayurvedic Herbal Programs for Your Type of Depression

THE HERBAL CONCEPT

Humans have used plants as medicine for as long as we have existed. Archeological excavations of artifacts dated from sixty thousand years ago have found remains of medicinal plants, such as cannabis, opium poppies, and ephedra. The earliest records of herbs are from the Sumerian civilization, where hundreds of medicinal plants, including opium, are listed on clay tablets. The Ebers Papyrus from ancient Egypt, circa 1550 BCE, describes about 850 medicinal plants.[1]

Ayurveda as a "prescribed" practice dates back to the period of the Indus Valley civilization (about 3000 to 5000 BCE, based on recent archeological findings), and its system is mentioned even in the ancient Vedas and other scriptures. Its concept, as previously described, appeared and developed between 2500 and 500 BCE in India, with Charaka's compendium of 120 chapters describing more than two thousand medicines. The Indian subcontinent is a vast source of medicinal plants that are used in traditional medical treatments. Today about 70 percent of India's rural population depends on the traditional Ayurvedic system.[2] In essence, humans have been involved for thousands of years in a vast "clinical trial" of medicinal plants.

Perhaps you have wondered how herbal medicines work and why we don't use them more often. The WHO reports that 75 to 85 percent of the world's population continues to rely on botanical medicines dispensed by traditional healers for primary health care, as has been their tradition for centuries.[3] In the United States and other developed countries, we have gone down the path of synthetic replacements.

Herbal medicines are plant-based medicines made from combinations of plant parts such as leaves, flowers, bark, or roots. Each part of the plant can have different medicinal uses according to its chemical constituents. Both fresh and dried plant materials can be used after following specified methods of extracting the active components, depending on the plant. The methods of extraction vary; the most common preparations are water-based preparations (infusions, decoction syrups, poultices, lotions, and compresses), alcohol-based preparations, and oil-based preparations.

Ayurveda deeply understands the complex interactions of substances, compounds, and plants that occur naturally. Concepts such as incompatibility (creating toxic reactions or side effects), antagonism (reducing the desired effect of one substance by combining it with another substance), detoxification (one substance reduces the toxicity or side effects of another), enhancement (one enhances the effects of the other), and synergism (two substances of similar nature reinforce each other's effects) were evidently part of the Ayurvedic scientific understanding of plant interactions. Ayurvedic practitioners applied these concepts for healing purposes.

In nature, all members of the vegetal kingdom live in a perpetual dance of synergism in order to maintain biological balance. Indeed, this is how our ecosystems grow, despite the regular presence of incompatibilities or antagonisms. This energetic exchange was, is, and always will be there, and it is the basis of adaptability and sustainability. It is a healthy sign—although it's coming late in the day—that we are taking more action to protect plants and green life more widely by reducing the toxic emissions of our everyday lives.

Ayurvedic formulations, in the form of combinations of parts of plants, are the embodiment of a deep understanding of nature and of how to put that understanding at the service of people who are mentally or physically imbalanced. But life has its own plans, and when in the 1940s scientists started studying drugs and medicines at a cellular level with the aim of producing useful (and sometimes harmful) effects, modern Western pharmacology took an expansionary path toward single synthetic chemicals for treatment of disease. That is where we are now.

Ultimately researchers believed there was no need to use plants in drugs because chemists could synthesize single molecules that could be more potent (and often more toxic) than natural products. Currently, most pharmaceuticals are single synthetic compounds. One argument for synthetic production is that it avoids the depletion of plant life that may result from overharvesting and exploiting the natural occurrence of these plants. However, synthetic production has its own impact on the environment.

AYURVEDIC HERBS FOR DEPRESSION

We know well that depression is not just a question of feeling sad or blue. Depression is a mood disorder with symptoms that range from mild to debilitating, and it can even be life-threatening. The mainstream modality of treatment for depression is antidepressant drugs. The chemical substances used in the treatment of disease such as depression generally come from synthetic sources. Western health care has an excellent biomedical technology for the diagnosis of disease; unfortunately, the Western treatment approach is often focused on treating the symptoms, not the root cause. For this reason, the use of some drugs can be literally lethal, and even when properly prescribed and administered they typically treat symptoms ("managing" rather than curing) while harming the patient's health or contributing to their deterioration.

The use of herbal medicinal products and supplements (adaptogens, phytonutrients, or nutraceuticals) has increased tremendously over the past three decades, with at least 80 percent of people worldwide relying on them for treatment of various health challenges. Some plant-based natural medicines are as effective as pharmaceuticals—and some are even more effective than pharmaceuticals. A few plant-based natural medicines can be unsafe, but overall this type of medicine causes fewer toxic side effects than prescription drugs, and it costs much less.[4]

As patients have become more active in learning about their conditions and more participatory in their treatments, more and more of them are searching for relief from depression by exploring the use of natural plants and herbal formulations, instead of taking mainstream drugs to repress the manifestation of symptoms. There are many factors involved in this decision process, but perhaps the main ones are the fear of drug dependency, the limited efficacy of mainstream drugs, the high costs of mainstream therapies, and the occasional severe side effects.

Ayurvedic scholars described a vast variety of plants and herbal-mineral formulas as a natural approach to the prevention and treatment of mental disorders. The classical Ayurvedic texts describe numerous herbs acting in a safe and effective way for thousands of years. Herbs can address specific needs and support your condition of depression if taken in the proper way and under the recommendation and supervision of a qualified Ayurvedic health practitioner.

To better understand Ayurvedic herbal programs, it is important to define or differentiate natural, medicinal herbs from adaptogens and nutraceuticals, which are recent innovations developed and marketed by the food and pharmaceutical industry. For many centuries, Ayurvedic medicinal traditions have used herbs, roots, bark, and other parts of plants, as well as minerals, as single or combined herbal formulas. Preparations like these are having something of a renaissance today. As a result it has become easier to spread the message and meaningfulness of Ayurveda in the West.

The companies that make adaptogens describe them as molecules from nontoxic plants that help the body resist stressors of all kinds by "hacking" the body's stress response at a molecular level, regulating a stable balance in the hypothalamic, pituitary, and adrenal glands. The nutraceutical industry defines its product as a food or fortified food product that not only supplements the diet but also assists in treating or preventing disease, thus providing health benefits. Nutraceuticals are not tested and regulated to the extent of pharmaceutical drugs. They can come from plant, animal, and mineral origin, and they are generally referred to as health products. They try to emulate the pharmaceutical model by focusing on identifying a single chemical and standardizing the delivery of each alleged "active ingredient" as if it were a pharmaceutical drug.

Certainly there is no singular magic bullet among the foods and herbs responsible for reproducing a whole plant's healing power. Scientific studies suggest that the potential benefits of medicinal plants come from the interaction or cooperation of two or more molecules or active principles to produce a combined effect greater than the sum of their separate effects, an effect called synergism. What we have in most medicinal plants and foods are hundreds of compounds orchestrated by the unseen, intelligent, synergistic hand of nature, which could never be reduced to the activity of an exclusively quantifiable phytocompound or molecule.

New research is demonstrating a growing level of interest in Ayurvedic medicinal plants among Western health practitioners. Ayurveda has the advantage of centuries of clinical observation and patient experience in the treatment of depression via medicinal herbs, diet, and lifestyle rebalancing. There is little that stands in the way of integrating this modality into the Western medical model, other than knowledge of and professional expertise in diagnosis and tailoring solutions. Such an integration would bring a breath of fresh air and natural solutions to the realm of treating depression.

I believe that in the particular case of depression, the patient has to participate more actively in taking control of their health. Your body has an innate ability to heal. We may let our minds get in the way of that by thinking we are weak, lost, or confused, but it's useful to always try to come back to this simple, powerful rule: your body, despite your perceptions, is designed to move toward health and away from disease, provided you give it the basic support it needs in terms of mental enthusiasm, nutrition, physical activity, and other lifestyle factors and natural health strategies that Ayurveda offers.

I invite anyone with depression who feels skeptical about herbal protocols to sincerely evaluate the available evidence and put some of the following herbal health principles to the test. At the end of the day, your own experience is all the proof you need. Go ahead and discuss the use of herbal treatments with your specialist. I am not asking you to drop your antidepressants. Instead perhaps you can discuss options relative to your current medication, which may include implementing some Ayurvedic herbal protocols in parallel with your medication. If you try these protocols, they will either work or they won't, but at least you will be giving yourself the opportunity to find out. Remember that when adopting a rebalancing program in Ayurveda, you are addressing your depression in a fundamentally different way. Ayurveda is not a symptomatic health system; instead it addresses the root causes.

Disclaimer: All the information concerning herbal programs in this chapter is only for the purpose of education. This information is not intended to be used to diagnose, prevent, treat, or cure any disease. Always consult your doctor for any health issues. Self-medication is dangerous. Some of the health claims indicated here are not necessarily approved by the U.S. Food and Drug Administration. Always pay attention to an herbal preparation's organic origin and absence of heavy metal contents.

AYURVEDIC HERBS AND HERBAL FORMULAS

There are thousands of herbs with a variety of medicinal purposes. I am presenting here single herbs or herbal combinations that will support you in your effort to conquer depression.

Ayurvedic tradition calls this category of herbs *medhya rasayana* in Sanskrit because they are beneficial for the intellect *(medha)*, and *rasayana* means renewal or rejuvenation. In Ayurveda herbs are considered to be foods that contain health-giving properties and have medicinal benefits. These herbs can nourish the nervous system, enhancing memory and other cognitive functions along with antistress effects.[5]

Some Key Ayurvedic Spices

Your kitchen can and should be your own personal pharmacy. Integrating the right herbs and spices into your daily cooking will not only provide flavor but will also improve your digestion by stimulating enzymatic secretion to support absorption of food and maintain a balanced gut microbiome.

In addition to exciting your taste buds, spices are also composed of a remarkable list of phytonutrients, essential oils, antioxidants, minerals, and vitamins that are essential for your general well-being. Spices have been an integral part of our diet for centuries, and they have become even more relevant for us today as food for health. Thanks to the fusion of Eastern and European cultures, as well as technological advances, some of the spices described here are no longer confined to the people of India or just for Ayurvedic purposes. These spices are going to help you address your depression, directly or indirectly acting at the level of your gastrointestinal system or other body systems.

I only have one specific request for you: whether you are going to use single herbs or an herbal combination, make your very best efforts to obtain certified organic products. There is always room for the possibility of contamination with heavy metals or other chemicals when using nonorganic herbs.

In general, when shopping for herbs, quality matters—and quality varies widely. Choosing the least expensive product can be a big mistake if you want a high-quality product. When purchasing herbs, try to meet the following criteria as much as possible:

- 100 percent organic components
- Includes the entire part of the most potent part of the plant, i.e., leaves, bark, root, flowers, etc.

- Free of fillers, additives, and excipients
- Manufactured by an organic company knowledgeable in traditional Ayurvedic practice and with a track record of Ayurvedic medical plant production

The list below contains spices that may be in your kitchen and that have a direct or indirect effect on depression, since they play a role in rebalancing various body systems.

- **Asafetida:** flatulence easing (carminative), antispasmodic, anthelmintic
- **Bay leaf:** warming, digestion (stimulate bile flow), pain relief
- **Black mustard seeds:** increases appetite, digestive, reduces edema and joint pain
- **Black pepper:** antioxidant, carminative, warming, digestive, antibacterial
- **Cardamom:** antioxidant, diuretic, stimulates digestion (boosts metabolism)
- **Cilantro:** cooling, comforting, carminative, digestive
- **Cinnamon:** antioxidant, anti-inflammatory, improves sensitivity to insulin
- **Cloves:** antioxidant, antibacterial, digestive stimulant
- **Cumin:** antioxidant, promotes digestion, carminative, balances *doshas*
- **Fennel:** supports digestion, heart health; reduces water retention, constipation
- **Fenugreek:** lowers blood sugar, inflammation; increases milk production, testosterone
- **Garlic:** antioxidant, antibacterial, antifungal; reduces cholesterol, blood pressure
- **Ginger:** potent digestive stimulant (antioxidant), anti-inflammatory
- **Neem:** detoxification, immune function and liver and skin health

- **Saffron:** cooling, antidepressant, tonifying, digestively balances all *doshas*

- **Triphala:** supports colon cleanse and detox; antioxidant and anti-inflammatory

- **Turmeric:** supports all organ systems, facilitates digestion, anti-inflammatory

Single Herbs

Ayurvedic herbs are usually available in the West in powdered form or tablets, and they can be taken on an ongoing basis after discussing the proper dosage with a qualified Ayurvedic doctor. The following herbs are not described in great detail here, but they are part of the array of Ayurvedic herbs used for the management of stress, anxiety, and depression:

- Sankhapuspi *(Convolvulus pluricaulis):* neurodegenerative ailments, anxiety, hypertension, memory

- Mandukaparni *(Centella asiatica):* nervine tonic (depression, anxiety and tension) as tranquilizer

- Sarpagandha *(Rauwolfia serpentina):* tranquilizer, antipsychotic, reduces anxiety and insomnia

- Jyotishmati *(Celastrus paniculatus):* neuroprotective, antioxidant, improves digestion, carminative

- Yastimadhu *(Glycyrrhiza glabra):* stress/depression management, soothes gut, lung cleanser

Below we will discuss some Ayurvedic herbs in more detail, specifically a few that relate directly to depression.

Single Ayurvedic Herbs

Ashwagandha *(Withania somnifera)* helps the body adapt to stress (i.e., it acts as an adaptogen). Ashwagandha belongs to the same family as the tomato and is a plump shrub with oval leaves and yellow flowers. It bears red fruits about the size of a raisin. It is sometimes known as Indian ginseng, even though ginseng and ashwagandha are not related botanically.

In Sanskrit, ashwagandha means "the smell of a horse," signifying that the herb has the potential to impart the vigor and strength of a horse. The root of the plant is also described as having a smell evocative of horse sweat. It has been used since time immemorial in the traditional Ayurvedic medical system because of its rejuvenating properties (*rasayana* in the Ayurveda tradition). It is considered a *vata*-fortifying herb and hence is used in patients with an imbalance in *vata dosha*. Scientific studies show that the active steroidal compounds present in ashwagandha (alkaloids, steroidal lactones, saponins, withanolides, and essential oils) can reduce stress caused by emotional and physical fatigue, balance mood swings, and increase mental alertness, focus, and concentration. Several studies provide scientific validation that ashwagandha works as well as or even better than antidepressant drugs used for the relief of anxiety and the treatment of depression and inflammation.[6,7]

A recent randomized, double-blinded study of ashwagandha compared a treatment group to a group receiving a placebo. This study suggests that cortisol, the primary biological marker of stress reaction, can show a marked decrease after the patient takes one 300 mg capsule of ashwagandha per day for sixty days with minimal side effects, establishing ashwagandha as a suitable support against stress and anxiety.[8] Ashwagandha has also been shown to be effective in ameliorating the effects of other mental disorders, such as bipolar conditions, by improving auditory-verbal working memory, which is a measure of both reaction time and social cognition.[9]

Brahmi *(Centella asiatica)* is also known as gotu kola. It is a small perennial creeping herb that has an age-old reputation for curing stress. Gotu kola is also used for fatigue, anxiety, depression, psychiatric disorders, Alzheimer's disease, and improving memory and intelligence. Sometimes it gets confused with the cooling herb bacopa *(Bacopa monnieri)*, which has a traditional use in both neurological and psychiatric disorders, since neurology is also considered part of Ayurvedic psychiatry. This adaptogen herb is so highly esteemed in Ayurvedic medicine that it's also known as brahmi, a derivation of the word *Brahman*, which means "the energy of universal consciousness." Brahmi and bacopa are not related, and they do not look similar, but in the East they are both known as brahmi, which causes confusion. Both of these herbs act as adaptogens, supporting cognitive function and improving memory and learning skills.

Brahmi also has antidepressant effects. It is believed to increase levels of serotonin in the brain, which helps the mind keep calm and gives relief from anxiety and nervousness.[10,11,12]

Guduchi *(Tinospora cordifolia)*, also known as amrit, is a highly valued herb in folk and Ayurvedic systems of medicine due to its versatile effects, including those beneficial to patients with depression. According to myth, when the ancient gods churned the primordial ocean, an ambrosial nectar was created that would grant immortality to any who drank it. The nectar was named *amrit*, a Sanskrit word that means "imperishable." Guduchi contains the bitter, pungent, and astringent tastes. Although it's traditionally used to remove accumulated *pitta*, guduchi can balance all the *doshas*. Its chemical constituents are reported to be antistress, antidiabetic, antiperiodic, antispasmodic, anti-inflammatory, antiarthritic, and antioxidant, among other medicinal properties.[19,20]

Jatamansi *(Nardostachys jatamansi)* is a perennial herb known for its antidepressant, antistress, and antifatigue properties, as well as for providing relief from insomnia and other sleeping disorders. The root of jatamansi is used for medicinal purposes in Ayurveda. It is known to provide a therapeutic effect for mood swings and stress disorders.[21,22]

Kapikacchu *(Mucuna pruriens)* is a creeping vine that grows in the tropical areas of India and is also found in tropical regions of Africa and the Caribbean. The name kapikacchu means "one starts itching like a monkey," in reference to the velvety coating of hairs on its seedpods that, if touched, can indeed cause severe itching and skin irritation. The herb's other common name is atmagupta, which means "secret self." In English, the common name for this plant is cowhage. There are traditional uses for the seed of *Mucuna pruriens*, the root, and the irritating hairs themselves (trichomes). They provide a natural source of levodopa, support the body's ability to handle stress, and promote a healthy central and peripheral nervous system, supporting healthy motor skills and coordination.[38]

Punarnava *(Boerhaavia diffusa)* removes excess *kapha* from the system and supports proper function of the heart, liver, and kidneys. It also promotes balanced fluid levels in the tissues and the healthy flow of urine, and it supports optimal weight management. Its alkaloid, punarnavine, exhibits antidepressant-like activity, possibly by initiating a decrease in plasma corticosterone levels.[23]

Saffron *(Crocus sativus)* is best known for producing the spice saffron from the filaments that grow inside the flower. It is a sterile plant that requires human assistance to proliferate. Saffron contains bioactive components (picrocrocin, crocin, and safranal) that have demonstrated a wide range of therapeutic applications for healing. There is a rather extensive body of clinical literature on its role in treating depression. One example studied its function as an antidepressant among other potential therapeutic applications.[24] A meta-analysis of the literature found saffron to be as effective as fluoxetine (Prozac) in the treatment of mild to moderate depression.[25,26]

Shatavari *(Asparagus racemosus)* is a powerful rejuvenating plant that is native to India and is in the same family as the common asparagus. Shatavari has small, uniform pine needles and produces white flowers and blackish-purple berries. The plant has been shown to aid in the treatment of neurodegenerative disorders and in alcohol abstinence-induced withdrawal symptoms. In Ayurveda, shatavari has been described as a *rasayana* herb and has been used extensively as an adaptogen to increase the nonspecific resistance of organisms to a variety of stresses, such as mood swings and mental irritation.[27,28]

Tagar *(Valeriana officinalis L.)*, also known as valerian, is a member of the Valerianaceae family. This plant and its related species are used in traditional medicine in many other parts of the world, including India. Recent research shows that tagar exhibits properties including anxiolytic activity, antidepressant activity, antispasmodic activity, a hypotensive effect, sleep-inducing activity, liver cleansing, and antistress activity.

Stress may lower your body's levels of a powerful neurotransmitter in gamma-amino butyric acid and may trigger anxiety and poor-quality sleep.[33,34,35]

Tulsi *(Ocimum tenuiflorum)*, also known as holy basil, has been recognized as a sacred plant in India and many other parts of the world. The Vedic sages knew the benefits of tulsi, which means "the incomparable one," and it was personified as a goddess that needed to be taken care of by all people. Tulsi leaves, stems, and seeds have great medicinal properties. Holy basil is commonly used to help with anxiety and as a stress stabilizer. Early research suggests that taking holy basil leaf extract twice daily after meals reduces anxiety and associated stress and depression in people with anxiety.[29,30] Studies also show that tulsi supports the immune system, protects the liver, eases pain, and assists with management of diabetes symptoms. It is a remarkable antibiotic, anti-inflammatory, and antioxidant, and it increases immunity and helps to prevent diseases.

Turmeric *(Curcuma longa)* is an Indian spice that gives yellow coloring to foods like curry and that has long been a pillar of Ayurvedic medicine as a treatment for various ailments. Turmeric is widely known for its edible roots containing curcumin. Turmeric is the most versatile healing spice in the world, with more than eight hundred experimentally confirmed health benefits, and a long-standing history of its power to alleviate human suffering. It may also represent the pharmaceutical industry's single biggest existential threat because the preliminary science shows that turmeric is at least as effective as many drugs, and it is much safer with regard to toxicological risk. The database MedlinePlus, for example, contains more than ten thousand abstracts of studies on turmeric or its components, called curcuminoids.

The main health benefits of curcumin compound are to:

- Help maintain a healthy digestive system by facilitating proper digestion

- Moderate some of your genes

- Regulate several physiological pathways

- Make your cells' membranes more organized

- Apparently switch back on the self-destruct mechanism within cancer cells

- Affect signaling molecules, since curcumin can directly network with inflammatory molecules, cell survival proteins, DNA, carrier proteins, and metal ions

Several studies show curcumin to be as effective as fourteen conventional pharmaceuticals with more than 160 potentially therapeutic activities, including antioxidant, anti-inflammatory, and anticancer effects. The natural substance curcumin "appears to be safe, well-tolerated, and efficacious among depressed patients" and can function as a "novel antidepressant," the literature says. Three trials also reported significant antianxiety effects. Researchers are finding increasing evidence that an anti-inflammatory compound in this common kitchen spice might help reduce symptoms of major depressive disorder.[13,14,15]

A randomized, controlled study of curcumin and depression that compared the efficacy of 1,000 mg curcumin to 20 mg fluoxetine (generic Prozac) in sixty patients diagnosed with major depressive disorder provided clinical evidence that curcumin may be used as a safe, effective treatment for patients with this disorder who do not have coexisting suicidal thinking or other psychotic disorders.[16] One of the mechanisms behind curcumin's beneficial impact on depression appears to be its ability to pacify the fires of inflammation, which is now thought to be a foundational cause of depression.[17,18]

Vacha *(Acorus calamus)* is a flowering herbaceous perennial plant native to India. It is called sweet flag in English. For ages, the rhizomes of vacha have been useful for sedation, behavior modification, and antidepressant effects.[36] The main mechanism of vacha activity involves a potent interaction with gamma-amino butyric acid receptors.[37]

Valerian *(Valeriana officinalis)* is a perennial flowering plant native to Europe and Asia. It is used for conditions such as insomnia, stress, anxiety, menopausal syndrome, painful menstruations, obsessive-compulsive disorder, and premenstrual syndrome. When researchers compared valerian to benzodiazepines for insomnia, they found valerian obtained equally effective results with fewer side effects.[31,32]

Herbal Formulas (Compounds) for Depression

In addition to the single herbs listed above, Ayurveda uses a variety of herbal compounds to treat depression, including the following:

Mamsyadi kashaya: antidepressant activity[39]

Jyotishmati taila: improves microcirculation and increases memory and concentration[40]

Anu taila: nasal treatment (*nasya*) effective in generalized anxiety disorder[41]

Ashwagandharishta: used in treatment of depression, mental disorders, and dementia[42]

Brahmi ghee: clarified butter with brahmi is helpful in improving intelligence, learning skills, and speech. Other ghee preparations such as siddharthaka ghee, dhanwantari ghee, and mahapaishachika ghee are equally useful in conditions of psychosis and depression.[43]

Other herbal formulas described in Ayurvedic texts are:

- Saraswatarista
- Smriti sagar rasa
- Krisna chaturmukha rasa
- Unmada gajankusa rasa
- Unmada gajakeshri rasa

Non-Ayurvedic Beneficial Herbs

Maca *(Lepidium meyenii)* is also known as Peruvian ginseng and is an adaptogenic herb that increases stamina and decreases excessive anxiety. Maca has been traditionally used in Peru to treat depression and to stimulate libido. Several international studies show the effectiveness of maca for diminishing anxiety and the symptoms of depression in women with menopause.[44,45]

St. John's wort *(Hypericum perforatum)* is widely used to treat mild to moderate depression and mood disorders. It has been used for hundreds of years to promote mental health, and it is currently prescribed for depression in Europe. Its effects have been validated in clinical research.[46] People with bipolar disorder should not take St. John's wort, as it could trigger mania.

Ginseng *(Panax quinquefolius)* has been used in Chinese medicine for thousands of years. Ginseng effectively regulates immune response and hormonal changes due to stress, thus maintaining homeostasis. In addition to suppressing the occurrence of psychological diseases such as anxiety and depression, ginseng also prevents stress-associated physiological diseases. Ginseng also has effects on stress-related depression, anxiety, and the hypothalamic-pituitary-adrenal axis.[47,48] Like St. John's wort, ginseng has been found to trigger mania in people with bipolar disorder.

Chamomile *(Matricaria recutita)* has been shown to provide greater relief from depressive symptoms than a placebo. Studies have shown that chamomile is particularly beneficial for those dealing with both depression and anxiety.[49,50] A randomized, double-blinded study comparing chamomile extract with a placebo for treatment of generalized anxiety disorder showed that chamomile was associated with a statistically significant reduction in anxiety after eight weeks of use.[51]

Lavender *(Lavandula angustifolia)* is a popular essential oil, traditionally used for relaxation and to reduce anxiety and mood disturbances. A review of various studies in 2013 suggested that lavender may have significant potential for reducing anxiety and improving sleep. Lavender cream decreases postpartum stress, anxiety, and depression.[52]

Peppermint *(Mentha piperita)* has been used for centuries to cure nervous system disorders due to the presence of menthol, which helps calm frazzled nerves and has a cooling effect. Menthol assists in the curing of insomnia by keeping your mind calm and allowing you to sleep in peace.[53]

Rosemary *(Rosmarinus officinalis)* is a woody plant. Its leaves are useful for seasoning purposes, making it a great addition to the spice medicine cabinet. Its active ingredients—rosmanol, circimaritin, and salvigenin—show good antidepressant and anxiolytic effects.[54]

The two scientific reviews cited here will give you an idea of the enormous potential of natural compounds present in plants.[55,56]

Ayurveda and Cannabis for Depression

The desperate need for safer alternatives to manage pain relief, in light of the horrors of the opioid crisis in the United States and around the world (killing an estimated 47,600 Americans annually), makes us reflect on the possible use of medical cannabis as a substitute.

Cannabis is a term increasingly used to refer to "weed" or marijuana. There is legalized mass production of cannabis now in parts of the United States, but my intent here is to discuss its role in Ayurveda. Cannabis has grown wild in the Himalayas and in India from Kashmir in the west to beyond Assam in the east, as well as in Iran and all through central and west Asia. The Latin names *Cannabis indica* and *Cannabis sativa* indicate that cannabis was traditionally grown and used in India. The Atharvaveda, an ancient Vedic text, mentioned cannabis more than two thousand years ago. The earliest known cultivation in India dates from 900 BCE. Archives of Ayurvedic traditional texts describing cannabis date from the Middle Ages. The most common Ayurvedic names of cannabis are *vijaya*, "the one who conquers," and *siddhi*, "subtle power," "achievement." Ayurvedic texts describe the plant as having three therapeutic parts that have rather different actions on the body and are given separate names.

Today the cannabis plant is cultivated mainly in the tropical and subtropical parts of India. In certain regions of India, the leaves of male and female plants are called *bhang;* other regions use the same name for flowers of the male plant. The flowering top of the female plant is called *ganja.* The name for the plant's resin, which naturally exudes from leaves, stems, and fruits of plants that grow in the mountains, is *charas.* Do note that some confusion exists between south and west India regarding the names for this plant and its parts.

The Indian pharmacopeia describes all parts of cannabis as narcotic, designating the resin or *charas* as the most powerful narcotic part. Different parts of the plant are described as having actions such as analgesic, nervous system stimulant, sedative, digestion stimulating, diuretic, spasmolytic, and aphrodisiac. According to the Ayurvedic concept of *virya* (basic energy), cannabis potency is considered warming. Its continuing use dries up the body, and its moderate use works initially as a nervous system stimulant and powerful aphrodisiac, and later as a sedative. Ayurvedic texts say that the habitual, continued use of cannabis drives the body to a state of imbalance of all three *doshas*, manifesting as a persistent poor digestion, melancholy, sexual impotence, and body wasting.

Ayurvedic texts describe many uses of the different parts of the plant. *Bhang* is used for short-term stimulation of the nervous system as well as in aroused psychiatric states, manic states, chronic pain, and chronic insomnia for short-term use. Ayurvedic treatises say doctors recommended the use of cannabis over opium, because cannabis did not produce nausea, loss of appetite, headache, or constipation. They also describe more than eighty different traditional herbal formulas in which the actions of parts of the cannabis plant are modified according to the other herbs present in the formula.[57]

Here are some examples of how Ayurvedic doctors *(vaidyas)* have used the cannabis plant through many centuries to heal different medical conditions.

Use of Leaves or Their Extracts

- Nervine medicine: as a tonic to stimulate the nervous system, and to regain power following conditions of severe exertion or fatigue
- Digestive complaints: cannabis leaves as an appetizer
- Anti-inflammatory and analgesic: compress of the fresh, bruised leaves for ocular problems associated with photophobia; also applied in orchitis (testicular inflammation) conditions to relieve pain and inflammation

- Disinfectant: leaf extract or paste applied on the scalp to remove dandruff and vermin; when dropped into the ear, it alleviates pain and destroys worms; also used to control the discharge in diarrhea and gonorrhea conditions

Use of Resin or Oil

- The concentrated resin exudate (resinous matter) extracted from the leaves and flowering tops or agglutinated spikes of *C. sativa*, known as *nasha* or *charas* (which forms the active principle when collected separately), is used to induce sleep in cases of insomnia in which opium is contraindicated. The resin is also used for prevention and cure of neuralgia, headache, migraine (malarial and periodical), acute mania, cough, asthma, dysuria, menses, and pain of the last stages of pulmonary tuberculosis.

- Oil extracted from the seeds is used for rubbing in cases of rheumatism.

- There are many descriptions of uses of different parts of the plant in combination with herbs and other compounds, such as ghee, sugar, black pepper powder, poppy seeds, asafetida, and belladonna.

- Several "sweets of *bhang*" are described in Ayurvedic texts. As the phrase implies, they are considered aphrodisiac and are also used in nervous debility and chronic bowel disorders. Most of them are prepared by using equal amounts of tonic and aphrodisiac substances in small quantities, with an equal quantity of *bhang* by weight. Then the ingredients are mixed with sugar, honey, and the usual aromatics.[58]

Some medicinal practitioners consider that the uplifting qualities of marijuana facilitate conversation, encourage social relationships, support physical awareness, highlight a deep enjoyment of life, and elevate social contact. These features suggest that cannabis could be effective where depression and isolation are primary concerns. Cannabis is made up of more than 120 components known as cannabinoids. Experts still aren't sure what each cannabinoid does, but they are getting a much better understanding of two of them, cannabidiol (CBD) and tetrahydrocannabinol (THC), which have particular effects:

- CBD is a nonpsychoactive cannabinoid, meaning it will not get you "high." It is often used as a support to reduce inflammation and ease pain, and it helps with nausea, migraines, seizures, and anxiety.

- THC is the main psychoactive compound in cannabis. THC is responsible for the "high" that most people associate with cannabis.

Research is being conducted to understand the mechanisms and effectiveness of these compounds for medical use. Much of this research is being financed by Big Pharma, who are looking to capitalize on many states' increasingly relaxed attitudes toward cannabis. The profit hole left by the falling rate of opioid prescriptions will not fill itself.

Recent studies on cannabis do not offer a very clear definition of its role when used as the whole plant. Let me give you some examples from a mixed bag of research:

- The association between cannabis use and depression was studied in 6,900 Australian people. Cannabis use was associated with modest increases in rates of depressive symptoms. The association was stronger in adolescence and declined thereafter. However, it was not possible from the available data to draw a definitive conclusion as to the likely direction of causality between cannabis use and depression.[59]

- Cannabis use was both phenotypically and genetically associated with depression and self-harm in a study of 126,291 British adults aged forty to seventy. Future work dissecting the causal mechanism linking these traits may have implications for cannabis users.[60]

- Another study of 8,598 Swedish men and women, aged twenty to sixty-four, with a three-year follow-up found no associations between depression/anxiety and cannabis use onset.[61]

- A cannabis use disorder medication trial in 302 adults showed that reductions in cannabis use were associated with improvements in anxiety, depression, and sleep quality, but not quality of life.[62]

Other recent studies show that cannabis is becoming a more viable option as legalization makes it possible for users to obtain a more reliable dosage. A newly characterized cannabinoid molecule—tetrahydrocannabivarin (THCV), which is very similar to tetrahydrocannabinol (THC)—is under study. THCV is not psychoactive but can nevertheless create a sense of focused euphoria. For those reasons, THCV seems to be effective for depression, anxiety, and pain. That particular feeling could be very beneficial for individuals with depression and anxiety. Ongoing studies will tell us whether it can reestablish balance for people experiencing symptoms of depression, anxiety, and neuropathic pain.

Ayurveda has been using different parts of the cannabis plants for many medical conditions for centuries. Nevertheless, I do not recommend its open use as an Ayurvedic medicinal herb. The main reasons are that everything depends on your individual constitution, your type and degree of depression, the proper source and purity of the plant or its compounds, and the legal ramifications of where you live. Remember also that cannabis is usually detectable in your bodily fluids for up to thirty days after use; for daily users it can be detectable for several months after use. Even in places where cannabis is legal, if you are considering using it I advise you to discuss it with your specialist or at least a qualified pharmacist beforehand, to make sure it will not interact with any medications or supplements you are taking. You really need to weigh the potential benefits and risks to your health.

General recommendation and disclaimer: Before you consider using herbal remedies, it is important to discuss the protocols with your doctor to avoid contraindications. It is also important to discuss dosage and the forms in which herbal remedies will be taken with your qualified Ayurvedic practitioner.

Applying the Ayurvedic Mastery of Food, Diet, and Nutrition for Your Depression

EXPLORING YOUR DEPRESSION ACCORDING TO YOUR *MANAS PRAKRUTI*

There is one constant that continually crops up in my professional practice: a large proportion of my clients with depression and anxiety conditions have bad dietary habits and a high intake of unwholesome foods. If you are dealing with depression, anxiety, or other mental health issues, the material in this chapter will explain which foods may be contributing to your symptoms and stopping you from making progress in freeing yourself of your depressive state.[1]

Ayurveda offers this very simple and straightforward advice: eat the right food, in the right quantity, at the right time, at the right place, and with the right attitude. Nature will take care of everything else. If you follow this simple advice, you may take a giant leap forward in addressing your depression. It sounds easy to say this, but perhaps you feel it is hard to put into practice and hard to change habits. Well, habits are what got us here, and we need to change direction to restore balance. In reality, addressing depression through diet is just like many things in life: it's more achievable when done step by step.

It is appropriate here to describe the Ayurvedic understanding of nourishment and digestion:

> *The world around us is digested by our five senses; ideas are digested by the mind and intellect; the body digests feelings and wholesome foods. Nourishment—the process of extracting information and energy from our environment to make it available to our mind-body physiology—is received and perceived via our five senses, as well as through our minds and emotions.*
>
> —*Ca. Su.* 8/13, 8/15; *Ca. Su.* 11/11, 11/25, 7/60

You can appreciate that Ayurvedic perception goes further than just biochemical characterization of digestive metabolic processes, to address the concept of other subtle energies via the science of energetics. The Ayurvedic perspective involves our feelings as well as our environment, conditions that all of us experience when ingesting food, even though we are often oblivious to these factors. There is just too much going on elsewhere!

Manas prakruti (our mental constitution) is based on the three constituents *sattva, rajas,* and *tamas.* Ayurveda uses these constituents to explain different types of depression and allow us to better understand our own condition. Vedic scholars categorized human personalities one step further by examining the individual differences in psychological and moral temperaments as well as people's reactions to sociocultural and physical environments. The scholars couched these descriptions in terms of the previously discussed basic qualities *(triguna).* Let me give you my basic interpretation of this concept:

- The "truth—what is" mental constitution *(sattvic)*
- The action/movement mental constitution *(rajasic)*
- The inertia/heaviness mental constitution *(tamasic)*

The three *gunas* of these mental components and constitutions can be seen in everyday life. They are in constant interplay within us. The relative prevalence of their expressions that are responsible for individual psychological constitutions are described as follows:

SATTVIC PRAKRUTI = KNOWLEDGE/PURITY

- Physical/mental: active, very strong body-mind relation in all aspects of life
- Intellect: creative, intelligent, humble, respectful
- Emotional: happy, joyful, aware, alert and fresh, doesn't get angry or upset easily
- Spiritual: intuitive, humanitarian, caring for all kinds of life

RAJASIC PRAKRUTI = MOVEMENT/ACTIVITY

- Physical/mental: perfectionist; enjoy power and control, prestige, position; egoistic, proud; tendencies are toward having a life of sensual enjoyment, seeking pleasure, avoiding pain
- Intellect: hardworking, active, restless, competitive, scarce proper planning and direction
- Emotional: jealous, ambitious, angry, stressful, fear of failure, loses mental energy quickly
- Spiritual: loving, friendly, faithful, calm, doubtful of inner awareness, patient when mutually supported

TAMASIC PRAKRUTI = INERTIA/HEAVINESS

- Physical/mental: thoughts tend to focus on themselves and their possessions
- Intellect: short attention span, enjoy work with low responsibility, feel tired quickly
- Emotional: greedy, possessive, attached, irritable; loves to eat, drink, sleep, and have sex

- Spiritual: careless, able to harm others in self-interest
- Tendencies toward laziness, lethargy, oversleeping, even during the day

After completing the three tests from previous chapters, you should now have a clear idea of the way your body-mind functions.

- You evaluated your constitution type in the body *prakruti* evaluation, which gave you your predominant *dosha*.

- You also evaluated your potential *dosha* imbalances by the use of the *vikruti* evaluation, which allowed you to see the potential causes of your modified (and unbalanced) *dosha* state.

- Finally, you did the third test, evaluating your mental constitution through the *manas prakruti* evaluation, helping you to perceive some temporary mental threads that could be associated with depression, such as feelings of lack of pleasure or hopelessness in your activities.

With this accumulated information and understanding of yourself, we should now seek to discern the areas in your activities that prompt feelings of sadness, guilt, failure, or hurt, and how your state of depression has been manifesting. As a result of the Ayurvedic analysis of your body-mind processes, you now have substantial data on the way you function and the way you interact with others. Having considered this data, you may well now have a clearer idea of the subtle causes and effects and how these manifest in your approach to daily life. This new state is where Ayurveda invites you to live: in search of awareness. Try not to give any color to that awareness; just be a witness of your observations.

Enjoy trying this homework, and enjoy accepting the process. Let me tell you, though, it is not easy to complete this task, and it takes practice not to let feelings interfere with and color the process of observation.

We will be discussing in more detail current scientific work regarding how the condition of depression has a direct connection to our biology. We are starting to understand that our state of body-mind-consciousness balance is directly related to our biochemistry and physiology. These processes occur under the control of certain amino acids that can convert into neurotransmitters, and they may generate feelings and dispositions toward processes such as satiation, hunger, pleasure, or even happiness.

But for now, let's come back to food. First I will summarize the ways in which mainstream medicine's understanding of food corresponds closely with the Ayurvedic understanding. Then I will take you one step forward, showing you examples of tailored food and diet recommendations based on your *manas prakruti* to complement the food and diet recommendations you already have based on your body *prakruti.*

YOUR BRAIN ON FOOD: UNDERSTANDING DEPRESSION

Food Components

If you extracted all the liquid out of your brain and then broke the remaining tissue down to its constituent nutritional contents, what would it look like? Most of the weight of your dried brain would be constituted by fats (lipids, including cholesterol), proteins (amino acids), traces of micronutrients, and glucose. Of course, your brain is more than just the sum of its nutritional parts, but each component has a unique impact on functioning, development, mood, and energy.

Fats: your diet requires the essential fatty acids, omega-3 and omega-6, which have been linked to preventing degenerative brain conditions. Eating omega-rich foods, like nuts, seeds, and fatty fish, is vital to the creation and maintenance of cell membranes. Although omegas are good fats for your brain, long-term intake of other fats, like trans and saturated fats, could compromise brain health as well as body health.

Amino acids: these building-block nutrients of growth and development influence how we feel and behave. However, reaching your brain cells is tricky, and amino acids have to compete for limited access. They are precursors of neurotransmitters—chemical messengers carrying signals between neurons and affecting things like mood, sleep, attentiveness, and weight. They are part of the reason why you feel more alert after a protein-rich meal or feel calm after eating a large plate of pasta. The intricate combinations of food can stimulate brain cells to release mood-altering norepinephrine, dopamine, and serotonin. A proper diet with a range of food supports that maintains a balanced combination of brain messengers will help keep your mood from being tilted in one direction or the other. A detailed description of the role of amino acids will be presented later.

Micronutrients: like all the other organs in your body, the brain requires a steady supply of micronutrients. For example, antioxidants in fruits and vegetables support the brain in fighting off free radicals that destroy brain cells, enabling your brain to work well for a longer period of time. Vitamins B6, B12, and folic acid protect your brain from susceptibility to brain disease and mental decline. Trace amounts of the minerals iron, copper, zinc, and sodium are also essential for a healthy brain and early cognitive development.

Glucose: this is the fuel required for the brain to efficiently transform and synthesize the above valuable nutrients. It is interesting to consider that although the brain represents only about 2 percent of our body weight, it uses up to 20 percent of our energy resources.

Selecting a varied diet of wholesome foods is an essential tenet of Ayurveda. The choice of good-quality foods has a direct and long-lasting effect on our brain and body.

Food and the Body-Mind Connection for Depression

Food intake based on wholesome foods is vital in nourishing and treating your physical health, preventing significant imbalances of your body-mind-consciousness trilogy, and safeguarding you from depressive patterns. The foods that maintain your body tissues in equilibrium are the ones considered natural or wholesome, causing the growth of living beings. Unnatural or unwholesome foods cause diseases through accumulation of *ama*. Earlier, we addressed in detail how wholesome or unwholesome food constituents bring about opposite effects depending on variations in quality, quantity, process of preparation, time of ingestion, body constitution, age of the individual, potential disease stage, and environment.

To protect your physical and mental health, the above factors need to be studied to create diets tailored according to your unique *prakruti*, *manas prakruti*, and personal conditions, without creating too many restrictions or making your life too challenging.

Unfortunately, if we are honest, whether under a condition of depression or not we mostly eat without actually being hungry, simply because it is that time of the day or due to our senses' attraction (taste, looks, or a good smell), our family and educational habits, or based on how much we understand about nutrition.

As a result of not necessarily knowing the right way of eating, we potentially contribute to the decline of our mental health, increasing the struggle with depression and collateral manifestations such as anxiety, loss of focus, sleeplessness, fatigue, brain fog, or even more severe mental issues. If you are also taking a mixture of antidepressants or other drugs, they are also affecting your body-mind-consciousness trilogy, causing the formation of more *ama* (undigested particles), the underlying cause of many health issues.

Agni and Depression

Agni, your digestive fire, is affected when confronted by unwholesome food, when eating at the wrong time of the day, or under stressful or inappropriate circumstances, such as eating while watching a TV or computer screen, driving a car, or taking public transport. In such instances, there is very little connection with the food you are eating. What is the result of this loss of connection? It is a cycle of formation of more and more *ama* (undigested particles or metabolic byproducts).

Ama and Depression

What you eat absolutely does matter, and the choices of the foods you are eating at every meal or snack are either promoting imbalance and disease in your body or promoting improved health, depending on your digestive fire *(agni)* at the time you decided to eat, as well as the quality and quantity of what you are eating. These are all potential factors leading to the accumulation of *ama* (unassimilated metabolic byproducts).

Ask yourself: are the foods I am eating day in and day out associated with my condition of depression, anxiety, or brain fog? Let's be realistic; you are already aware that certain foods contribute to the incidence of diabetes, heart disease, high blood pressure, irritable bowel syndrome, celiac disease, and autoimmune diseases. The list goes on and on concerning the connection between the type and quality of food we eat and the diseases this behavior contributes to. The common denominator is the formation and accumulation of *ama,* undigested or unmetabolized products in your body. It is important to point out how the wrong foods, medications, and impressions can cause alterations of your mental health. I believe this area has not been explored sufficiently in the modern treatment of depression.

Consider your digestive fire *(agni)* as your bank account, and the type of food you eat (potential *ama*) as a kind of savings. Now let's look at your options: you can accumulate a wealth of robust health by depositing wholesome foods, since your *agni* will be functioning efficiently; or you can make continual withdrawals through consumption of unwholesome foods, which will drain your healthy bank balance. The consumption of unwholesome foods will end up depleting your *agni,* building *ama,* and causing body-mind imbalances. As you can see, building *ama* is a very bad investment because it drains your savings account—or even worse, it can leave you in debt.

Of course, there is always an underlying cause or reason why we feel the way we do. Every effect has a cause. We have to remember that *ama* can alter our body-mind system in two different ways: *ama* has a material manifestation by accumulating in your bodily tissues, but it is equally able to manifest through accumulation or interference at the level of your mind, causing mental imbalances such as anxiety and depression. Ayurveda refers to the process of accumulating mental *ama* as mistakes of the intellect, senses, and time. Mistakes of the intellect begin when a person sees what is harmful as useful, or they do not eat according to their level of hunger or digestive power. Mistakes of the senses arise through sensory desire, which is often seen in cases of overeating. Mistakes of time include not eating according to the seasons. These mistakes lead to poor diet, wrong eating habits, overeating, unnecessary cravings, and wrong routine. These manifestations in turn lead to aggravation of the *vata, pitta,* and *kapha doshas,* imbalance within the channels of the body, and weak or dull digestive fire *(agni),* which can lead to accumulation of more *ama.*

TAILORING FOOD FOR YOUR BODY-MIND CONNECTION

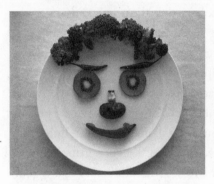 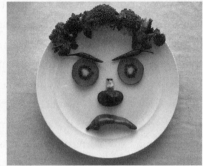

Food, though necessary for our existence, is also one of the major pleasures in our life. It is important to recognize that when we eat food, we acquire energy and materials from nature that we then convert into cellular-intelligent energy that we integrate into our body. In Ayurvedic terms, imbalance arises from incorrect food intake. This is the main physical factor in the causes of imbalance and development of diseases such as depression. Ideally, your food intake should build, provide energy to, and repair the cells in your mind-body organism. Thanks to the subtle dynamism of your tissues, the food you eat also influences your emotions. We frequently overlook the fact that just as food influences your digestive processes, it also plays an influential role in your mental processes.

Food and Mind: Foods for Truth *(Sattva)*, Action *(Rajas)*, and Inertia *(Tamas)*

. . . .

Qualities of the mind = qualities of the body.

. . . .

Conventionally, food is an often-ignored factor when considering our mental health. To me, that is quite strange because we all can reflect on the role food has played in our lives in relation to our moods. Think of the times in your life when you've been unable to eat a meal because you were feeling angry, sad, or upset. What better example is there than to see how your emotions are informing your physical body that now is not the time to eat? Your body very cleverly decided to tell you not to eat under these circumstances, because your *agni* will not be at its best. We know from psychoneuroimmunology that the stress and anger you feel in these moments is also going to decrease your immune system, disturbing your body-mind balancing processes. By the same token, how many times do we celebrate our happiness with a very good meal?

Ayurvedic texts state that all disease processes start from the subtle, psychic level, and from there they influence the physiology of a person. If an imbalanced mental state continues, it will manifest as an imbalance or disease at the somatic (bodily health) level. Balance in our food is paramount for the balance of our *prakruti*. Ayurveda holds that a good appetite indicates a well-functioning *agni* (digestive fire), so for that reason the quantity of food you eat should be determined accordingly. However, it is important to establish the difference between hunger and appetite. The feeling of hunger is an authorization to eat, while appetite must be delimited according to your real needs.

Ayurveda describes foods according to their *guna* characteristics: foods are light *(sattva)*, rich or passionate *(rajas)*, or sluggish or dull *(tamas)*.

Foods with a Light Quality *(Sattva)*

A *sattvic* diet generally consists of wholesome foods, such as:

- Fresh, organic fruit and vegetables
- Whole grains, nuts
- Dairy products, i.e., milk and ghee
- Pulses (beans, lentils, etc.)
- Plant-based oils

- Mildly sweet foods (natural, unrefined sugars), i.e., honey and molasses

- Spices such as cinnamon, basil, coriander, ginger, and turmeric

Food constituents of this group are agricultural products grown and processed in an organic way. When eaten in proper amounts they will not cause body-mind imbalances. As an example, practitioners who administer the Ayurvedic detoxification protocols *(panchakarma)*, which require a *sattvic* diet, generally observe quick recovery and improvement in their clients due to the combination of treatments and the digestibility of wholesome foods, improving the intellect and sense organs of the individual, evoking conscious awareness and bringing the psyche to a state of harmony.

Foods with a Rich or Passionate Quality *(Rajas)*

Below are some common *rajasic* foods:

- Fruit: sour apples, apples, banana, guava, tamarind

- Grains: millet, corn, buckwheat

- Vegetables: potato, cauliflower, broccoli, spinach, winter squash

- Beans: red beans, yellow dal, mung beans

- Dairy: old, sour milk, sour cream

- Meat: fish, shrimp, chicken

- Highly spicy food; sour, salty, hot, and dry foods

The word *rajasic* originates from the word *raja*, a Hindi word of Sanskrit origin meaning "king" or "prince." *Rajasic* food's effect on the mind is to stimulate the individual beyond normal capacity and capability, energizing virtually all the body systems and especially the nervous system. For these reasons, *rajasic* food in moderate quantities stimulates creativity and activity by providing energy and drive. However, if eaten in excess or when imbalanced, it can also leave the individual feeling restless, busy, overwhelmed, and tense, encouraging aggressive and domineering tendencies that disrupt the body-mind balance.

We are all under continual demands from the external world. In order to handle those pressures we require sensible support from these passionate energies. The main point here is to eat according to your daily life activities. For example, an individual who does heavy physical labor every day cannot afford to eat like a monk or a nun living in a monastery or convent. Our passionate potential has to be kept up to a certain level. However, in order to maintain balance, our diet cannot consist of only passionate foods; it also requires foods of a *sattvic* quality.

Foods with a Sluggish or Dull Quality *(Tamas)*

Common *tamasic* foods include the following:

- Meat: lamb, beef
- Fruit: avocado, watermelon, plums, apricots
- Grains: wheat, brown rice
- Vegetables: mushrooms, garlic, onion, pumpkin
- Beans: black, pinto, pink, black gram, black lentil
- Dairy: cheese

Ayurveda says what we eat affects who we are and how we think and act. The *tamasic* food category must be included in the diet with caution. The concept of *tamasic* food also varies according to the food you've been eating since your childhood, i.e., foods that your body is familiar with and recognizes well, and that you will metabolize well too. From this consideration arises the importance of being careful when eating exotic foods.

Tamasic food lowers the body's ability to fight disease and disrupts the proper functioning of the immune system. Under certain conditions, such as overeating, reheating food, or eating leftover or stale food, what was once *sattvic* food can turn *tamasic*. Eating *tamasic* food solely or in large amounts is considered inappropriate and unwholesome because it makes people lazy, inefficient, slow, and resistant to change, because these foods require so much energy to digest. *Tamasic* tendencies often lead to disease and distress.

Since the natural state of the mind is creative and productive, *tamasic* food brings about stagnation in thinking, leading to body-mind imbalances. Gradually this sluggish *tamasic* food brings about strong mood swings, insecurity, pessimism, irritability, cravings, and lethargy. As a result, the *tamasic* individual is quickly exhausted, may be unable to deal with others in a peaceful way, and often needs long hours of sleep.

In today's lifestyle *tamasic* foods include such unwholesome foods as heavy pastries and cakes, canned and frozen foods, meat products that have been stored or treated, dry milk, grains that cause dryness, leftovers, overcooked food, processed food, stale food, strong alcoholic drinks, and strong medicines. Some of these foods are part of this *tamasic* group despite the fact they have high nutritional value. Remember also that much of the meat we buy over the counter or pull from the store freezer is packed with hormones and antibiotics that you probably would not even touch—let alone ingest—if they were presented to you separately in a cup. Most of these products can even taste and look as fresh as if they were wholly natural foods, as a result of chemical additives introduced during the manufacturing process.

The light at the end of this dark tunnel of *tamasic* food is that, as with everything, when consumed in moderation *tamasic* foods can bring stability. We know from experience that *tamasic* qualities come in handy during phases of strong physical pain and stress, such as bitter cold or physically strenuous work. In such situations *tamasic* food helps to temporarily dull the senses, giving your body the space to repair itself, thus providing stability and restoring your drive. Nevertheless, under normal conditions, keep *tamasic* foods at bay.

It is important to remember that the most general body *prakruti* traits for the three body constitutions are:

- *Vata*-type people are anxious and have a tendency to lose weight.

- *Pitta*-type people will manifest anger and preoccupation.

- *Kapha*-type people will manifest a tendency to sleep excessively and gain weight.

Describing the body *prakruti* traits in such a succinct way can be misleading because we are a combination of the three *doshas* in different proportions according to our parents' *prakruti*, i.e., the combination of our parents' DNA. In the same way, when Ayurveda considers *manas prakruti*, you can see that people are not only *sattvic* or only *rajasic* or only *tamasic*. Our nature and behavior are a complex interplay among all of the three qualities *(triguna)* in varying degrees. As described previously, for some people their conduct is *rajasic* with a significant influence of *sattvic guna;* in others it is *rajasic* with a significant influence of *tamasic guna.*

What Ayurveda conceptualized so long ago, and what I recommend to you here, is that for your best body-mind functioning, you need to eat primarily *sattvic* foods, with just enough *rajasic* and *tamasic* qualities to complement strength, energy, and stability to support your life activities and keep you motivated and purpose oriented. Note that the trend in modern nutritional guidance is to recommend more *sattvic* diets. This is happening irrespective of any Ayurvedic influences on nutritionists, so perhaps we are relearning the ancient wisdom of Ayurveda subconsciously.

Optimizing Your Nutrients: Quality and Quantity *(Gunas)* = Digestion, Assimilation

Imbalance arises from an inappropriate diet. Ayurveda advises us to follow a tailored diet to balance your *prakruti* based on enjoyment and benefit, taking into consideration the breaking down of natural food either under regular or depressive conditions in order to maintain your acid/alkaline balance. Showing the importance of natural food, Charaka says:

> *Food sustains the life of all living beings; and complexion, clarity, good voice, longevity, genius, happiness, satisfaction, nourishment, strength, and intellect are all conditioned by food.*
>
> —*Ca. Su.* 27/349–51

The amount of food that gets digested and metabolized in the proper time is to be regarded as the proper quantity.

An important Ayurvedic recommendation for those under pressure or suffering from depression is to eat warm and unctuous foods, because these foods stimulate the digestive fire. Under these conditions, food is also quick to digest, reducing gas and mucus formation.

For example, the traditional European practice of making a salad dressing with oil and vinegar makes lots of sense because you are adding other complementary tastes and providing some essential fatty acids and vitamins present in the oil, which will aid digestion and assimilation. More pertinent Ayurvedic advice for all body types is to avoid eating raw salads at night, particularly during winter or if you live in cold areas or countries.

....

Depressed? Please, optimize your cooking.

....

Bringing Joy and Diminishing Depression by Food Combining

We have talked a lot about food and diet without any mention of calories in tailored Ayurvedic diets. That is as it should be. The Ayurvedic take on eating food is not at all about counting calories or having a mechanical approach to food. It is more about learning how to prepare the right amount of a variety of healthy meals that are wholesome and easy to digest, thus preventing the accumulation of *ama*. The proper quantity of food to eat depends on the properties of the food as well as your constitution. For instance, foods that are difficult to digest should be eaten in small quantities, and foods with lighter properties can be taken in larger quantities.

....

Heavy substances, when taken in small quantities, become
light, while light substances taken in large quantities become heavy.

....

Researchers from Macquarie University in Australia studied 76 university students aged seventeen to thirty-five years who exhibited moderate to severe depression symptoms and followed an unhealthy diet (high in processed foods, sugar, and saturated fats). After only three weeks of moving to a healthier diet, they showed significant improvements in mood, and their depression scores went into the normal range. What you eat affects your mood; beyond that, your diet is powerful enough to influence symptoms of depression, for better or for worse.[2]

Let me emphasize that the people in this study are not my clients, this is not my own research or data, and this is not even a research paper trying to convince the scientific and nonscientific community of the virtues of Ayurveda. It is a controlled study conducted by researchers who may or may not know of Ayurveda. Still, in their protocols they applied a dietary framework—the most fundamental of Ayurvedic principles. The study participants were probably people similar to many of you, going through experiences of depression and searching for the right door that will allow them to leave behind this challenging condition of imbalance. They decided to take a step forward by changing just one aspect of their lifestyle: a clear diet change, just one of the principles of Ayurvedic rebalancing. And through that one small change in their lifestyle, they discovered that it is possible to be an active participant in getting better.

Pleasing the Palate, Eyes, and Other Senses

What we in the West call Ayurvedic or Indian food is plentiful and accessible, and it will offer you many options of great varieties, flavors, combinations, and recipes. Also, consider traditional cuisines such as Thai, Singaporean, Mexican, and many others that offer many combinations of spices.

Because food is essential and it is all about joy and pleasure, we have to treat our palate well. Therefore, eat slowly, and chew properly. A new relationship with food doesn't mean eating insipid or bland food. On the contrary, your palate is so essential to your life that food should always be satisfying to the palate, in addition to being nourishing.

Even if you are feeling unwell, not very positive, or in a depressive state, make the effort to ensure your food presentation is appealing to the eye. The visual impression your food makes is always important for the digestive processes. That is why so much time and effort is put into cookbook photography; it's all about healthy seduction!

When you eat, always make sure you are sitting in a restful posture. Do not eat standing. Create a pleasant atmosphere at your dinner table or the space where you are eating by including suitable light adapted to your eyes. Relaxing music will be a plus for your digestive fire. Refrain as much as you can from listening to the news or eating in front of screens, because this divides your attention, making you unaware of the process of eating and what you are ingesting. Also, give yourself a rest from your mobile phone. After all, you are eating.

. . . .

If you eat and process food in a conscious way, then you can connect to deeper and calmer places within yourself. When you honor the food you are eating, you will change your state of mind by removing internal considerations that may be feeding your depressive state.

. . . .

FOODS TO EXCLUDE IF YOU HAVE DEPRESSION:

- **Coffee:** caffeine can make you feel jumpy and nervous, and it can disturb your sleep. Withdrawal of caffeine can also disturb you. Verify whether caffeine is having a negative effect on you. If it is, cut caffeine out of your diet gradually. If it is too difficult to completely remove it, then drink decaf coffee.

- **Energy drinks:** these can cause anxiety and depression because they are mostly sugar and artificial sweeteners. They cause altered heart rhythms and sleep issues.

- **Alcohol:** follow the daily or weekly recommendations for the consumption of alcoholic units.

- **Fruit juices:** avoid them. They don't contain fiber, and they only provide quickly absorbed sugar water, giving you a high and bringing you down very quickly. In that condition of hunger, anxiety and depression will rapidly manifest. Instead, eating a whole fruit and its fiber satiates you, supports your microbiome, and slows down the way your blood integrates the calories.

- **Diet soda:** these beverages can provide an overload of caffeine. Perhaps you don't feel the energy crash that comes with having too much sugar, but diet soda could make you feel down and depressed.

- **Sugar-sweetened drinks:** colas and other sugar-sweetened drinks have a direct link to depression. All they do is cause your blood sugar to spike, without providing any nutrition.

- **Packaged dressings and marinades:** these are loaded with sugar, generally listed as "high-fructose corn syrup." Alternatively, they may be sweetened with the artificial ingredient aspartame, which is associated with anxiety and depression. Try to make your own dressing, or at least check the composition of the packaged ones.

- **Ketchup:** this condiment contains more sugar per tablespoon than you think. The "light" version may include artificial sweeteners that could be connected to anxiety and depression.

- **Soy sauce:** this can cause anxiety and depression, making you feel lethargic if you have a gluten sensitivity.

- **Toasted bread:** have the wholesome version. White bread, doughnuts, and pastries are made of highly processed white flour, which quickly increases your blood sugar after you eat it. Afterward you experience energy spikes and crashes that can be bad for anxiety and depression. Remember, products made with white flour contain little fiber and in general lots of added sugar and unnatural types of fats, and they are considered depression inducers.

OPTIMIZING YOUR DIGESTION

The Role of Food

The clear outcomes of the various findings discussed above correspond exactly to what Ayurveda has recommended as a balanced diet for thousands of years. The value of a healthy, balanced, wholesome diet *(pathya)*, as opposed to an unhealthy or unwholesome diet *(apathya)*, is well described by Charaka when he says, "The body is made up of diet."[3] He also says, "A patient who follows a healthy diet *(pathya)* doesn't need medicine as much as a patient who doesn't follow a wholesome diet" (*Su. Sū.* 1/25).

In other words, Ayurveda says a person who eats a healthy diet doesn't need medicine because their body is in a state of equilibrium. On the other hand, the patient who doesn't follow a wholesome diet doesn't need medicine either, because medicine will be ineffective in an unhealthy body. This concept has usually been attributed to Hippocrates, traditionally seen as the father of medicine, even though Ayurvedic scholars came up with it long before. Hippocrates is often quoted as saying, "Let food be thy medicine and medicine be thy food."

Ayurveda is unique in its clarity about how food, environment, lifestyle, and habits influence not only your physical health but also the way you think and feel. The perpetuation of an imbalanced diet creates imbalances of the mind that gradually manifest in the form of depression. Balance can be achieved when mental and spiritual qualities are organized according to the principles of balance and dynamism instead of imbalance or inertia. However, balance has to come from within yourself.

The following recommendations concern how to optimize the benefits of a healthy diet to prevent mood changes or exacerbations of depressive conditions. They apply to all body constitutions and need to be considered carefully when selecting and preparing your food.

Connecting with Your Food

If you would like to have a proper relation with the food accessible where you live, this advice is important:

- Identify your *prakruti*.
- Learn to recognize the qualities of a diverse variety of foods.
- Evaluate your environmental conditions and seasonal changes.

- Organize the foods' *doshic* qualities relative to your *prakruti*, based on the seasons.

Making Your Meal Pleasurable

When eating your food, remember the following:

- Eat only when you are hungry.
- Stop eating when you are satisfied; do not keep eating until you are full.
- Be aware of your inner signals telling you when you are satisfied.
- Do not get involved in other activities while you are eating.
- Do not eat if you are upset or stressed.
- Pay full attention to the process of eating.
- Create an enjoyable environment around your eating space.
- Understand that food should really have only a nutritional role.
- To carry on eating after reaching satiety is lavish.
- Eating to gratify other desires will not fulfill those desires.

Proportioning Your Meal

Remember the general principle that you should never eat up to your saturation level. Ayurveda offers the following advice for your stomach's contents:

- One-third should contain solid food.
- One-third should contain liquids.
- One-third of the stomach should be left empty to give the digestive processes room to take place.

Like everything else, the effectiveness of Ayurvedic constitution-based diets for treating depression requires further study. Still, it is clear that a tailored diet based on your Ayurvedic constitution using the basic principles described above will be helpful in supporting and creating a more balanced mental state.

Digesting Your Food

The four main stages of digestion are: ingestion, digestion, absorption or assimilation, and elimination. To guarantee that all four stages of digestion will function well to generate a healthy physiology, be sure to do the following:

- Include all six tastes at every main meal.
- Select tastes that are appropriate to your body-mind constitution.
- Choose the right spices and herbs for your body-mind constitution.
- Appreciate the process of eating.
- Become confident of your inner feelings.

FOOD AND TASTE FOR BODY BALANCE

Above we have considered general recommendations for all three types of constitutions. Let's now consider the way to optimize your digestion according to your specific constitution, based on your preponderant *dosha* according to the results of your *prakruti* evaluation. At the beginning of chapter 9 we described food and tastes. It is time to put those concepts together in a practical way to achieve a balanced metabolic condition that will prevent or reduce depressive episodes.

- *Vata:* If your *prakruti* evaluation described you as a *vata*-dominant person, your constitution is influenced by the cooling and alkaline effects of pungent, bitter, and astringent tastes. For those reasons, you need to compensate for those *vata* characteristics with foods that are sweet, sour, and salty. Those types of energetic foods are going to nourish your predominantly *vata* body by keeping it moist, smooth, and warm.

- *Pitta:* If your *prakruti* evaluation described you as a *pitta*-dominant person, your body constitution is influenced by the energetic of heating and the metabolic effect of sour tastes of acidic character. For those reasons, you need to compensate for those *pitta* characteristics with foods that have sweet, bitter, and astringent tastes. Those types of foods are going to nourish your predominantly *pitta* body by keeping it cool and fresh. That is the best way to balance your hot, pungent, sour, and forceful nature.

- *Kapha:* If your *prakruti* evaluation described you as a *kapha*-dominant person, your body constitution is influenced by the energetic of cooling and the metabolic effect of tastes of sweet or neutral character. For those reasons, you need to compensate for those characteristics with foods that have pungent, bitter, astringent tastes to counteract their cool and sugary sweetness. In that way you can balance the sweet, sour, and salty *kapha* tendency by integrating warm and dry qualities into your food intake.

Ayurveda clearly states that people whose diet predominates in only one taste are risking their health. Why? Because if their body tissues are not nourished properly, deficiencies will manifest sooner or later, gradually leading to a poor immune response and making the body-mind more susceptible to illness. The Ayurvedic approach to selecting food based on its taste is not to stick only to the recommended three types of tastes. The real intention is to make you aware of your food choices and keep you away from your natural tendency to overeat certain types of food that are going to feed imbalances again.

We are using the Ayurvedic principle of "like increases and opposites decrease" to balance the predominance of each of the three types of *doshas* by either increasing or decreasing their intrinsic qualities. Start increasing your choice of foods by including all of the six tastes, and you will feel the positive changes and the gratification of wholesome food in a balanced body. Food is to be enjoyed!

FOOD AND TASTE FOR MIND BALANCE

According to several studies, selective serotonin reuptake inhibitors and other antidepressants have been shown to distort or diminish tastes. Researchers from the University of Bristol believe a reduction in serotonin or noradrenaline in our brains and bodies might also affect our taste buds and how they respond to different tastes.[4]

Perhaps when you are in a phase of depression, as a result of a lack of energy or a low mood you are not motivated to cook. In this situation you may end up eating mainly one food product, such as rice or pasta. In those cases you will probably be feeding only two or maybe three different tastes, instead of feeding five or six tastes with a proper multicomponent meal. I understand if you feel you do not have the energy to cook or eat, but your choices are going to play a role in your general digestion. When you make a wrong food choice you will end up disturbing your systems even more while feeding emptiness and imbalances, both mental and physical.

It is extremely important to note that for certain tastes, only a small quantity is required for it to satisfy and balance us; more is not necessarily better. For most people, the taste of bitter, spicy (pungent), and astringent foods is generally unpleasant, while sour, salty, and sweet-tasting foods mostly provide a pleasurable sensation. Perhaps we can try to get out of the box and explore these "unpleasant" tastes in more detail. Spices, for example, are very important because in small quantities they provide "extra" tastes that are often missing from our diets, such as pungent, astringent, and bitter. At the same time, they provide an easy approach for exploration.

Below is a series of short questions that are intended to stimulate your inquisitive mind. Try to engage with them and visualize how your own condition of depression could be related to your daily food intake and your pattern of food intake over an extended period.

- Are you taking medication? Are medications or antidepressants affecting your taste?
- Which tastes do you prefer when you are or are not taking medication?
- How many of the six tastes are in your daily intake of food? Do you eat them all together or throughout the day?
- Perhaps due to a depressive phase without eating, do you decide to eat something one or two days later?

- Do you eat the same food type habitually?
- Do you know how to cook, or do you dislike cooking?

DIGESTION STAGES OF FOOD INTAKE FOR BODY *PRAKRUTI* AND MIND *PRAKRUTI*

All body systems are necessarily interconnected for proper function, but you can sense which ones feel more disturbed under conditions of depression.

- *Vata:* As previously described, life exists thanks to the independent movement of *vata* controlling all body functions, including all sensory and motor functions of the nervous system, i.e., enthusiasm, inspiration, and expiration, and all voluntary and involuntary actions of the body, such as circulation of blood, plasma, and lymph throughout the body, as well as bodily excretions. A *vata*-type physiology achieves proper digestion thanks to the main *vata* organ, the large intestine, as well as the kidneys and bladder, all under regulation of the brain, the *vata* organ with the main function of providing communication and organization of the bodily functions. In depression, the principal *vata* manifestation is dryness. In terms of digestion, dry colon leading to constipation is a clear manifestation of wrong function turning into body debility, emaciation, and loss of physical activity and consciousness.

- *Pitta:* The role of *pitta* is digesting or metabolizing ingested food for correct biological transformation and generation of body heat, metabolic energy, and inducing impressions. The small intestine, the main *pitta* organ, is the primary site for digestion, breaking food down into particles to form the various constituents of the human body. This organ also regulates assimilation, hunger, and thirst. At the same time, another *pitta* organ, the heart, responsible for the circulation of blood throughout the body, is affected. As a result, the liver and gallbladder, both involved in digestion and circulation, are affected, causing alteration of bile production and digestion of fats. Because circulation is affected, the spleen, a *pitta* organ involved in blood formation and destruction, is also affected.

- *Kapha:* According to Ayurveda the structure of the body, including the muscles, fascia, ligaments, tendons, and skeleton, manifests the stable physical organization and cohesion of the body as well as providing nourishment to the whole body and mental balance, all qualities of *kapha.* The *kapha*-type physiology is responsible for digestion of proteins, carbohydrates, and fats via its main organs of stomach and pancreas. The other *kapha* organs, the lungs and respiratory system, provide oxygen for all cellular metabolic processes and elimination of carbon dioxide as a waste product. Abnormal ingestion of food manifests clearly in terms of the digestive *kapha* functions. Since *kapha* is the slowest and steadiest of all three *doshas,* an imbalanced diet, wrong food practices, changes of natural tendencies, food intake disconnected to the seasons, and hereditary traits instigate a visible imbalance manifesting as obesity, with collateral physical and mental implications.

Even before reflecting on the role of food, Ayurveda teaches us that poor digestion (low *agni*) is the primary cause of most diseases and that imbalance affects our body and mind. *Ama,* generated from undigested food in the digestive tract, is the source of gastrointestinal disorders. An inefficient digestive tract is unable to process food intake, generating *ama.*

Ama subsequently leaks from the gastrointestinal tract into other body systems and settles in vulnerable or fragile places, including our nervous system. The ancient Ayurvedic scholars called those defective tissular or organ spaces *khavaigunya:* places where *doshas* begin to settle and initiate subsequent pathologies. We all have an Achilles' heel or vulnerable area in our bodies susceptible to emotional or physical lesions. Inherited disorders or unhealthful lifestyle choices can also be the cause of *khavaigunya*. This Ayurvedic conception of weakness is analogous to the concept of a weak immune system in mainstream medicine. It is well known that everyone has an immune system that is sensitive to conditions such as weather and food, as well as emotions.

The strength of *agni*—digestive fire, playing the role of biochemical energy to break down, metabolize, absorb, and assimilate nutrients without creating much waste—determines a person's appetite. *Agni* regulates digestion, absorption, and metabolism of nutrients to transform them into part of our functional cellular structures.

Agni transforms food molecules into energetic molecules at the service of the whole organism. If your *agni* is inadequate, the processes of digestion, absorption, and metabolism of nutrients will be improper, leading to poor nourishment and *ama* generation. Under these circumstances, your *ama* will eventually start disturbing your cellular functions, creating all kind of tissue alterations and dysfunctions that are going to affect your metabolic processes on various levels, from the digestive system up through the nervous system. Those dysfunctions will manifest in your moods, mental imbalances, and strongly depressive manifestations.

Let me be crystal clear: What you eat absolutely does matter. The kind of food you eat each time you have a meal or a snack is either causing disease, building disease in your body, or reversing disease and improving health, depending on your individual constitution, digestive power, and factors such as what, when, and how much you eat. From now on, please try to see the kind of food you eat as a sort of savings account of bodily strength—although it could become a savings account of sickness if you deplete *agni* as a result of *ama* accumulation. Nothing could be better than depositing noble savings in your body. Are you the kind of person who becomes sick as a result of making continuous deposits into the illness account by accumulating toxins and withdrawing from the well-being savings account? If that's the case, then it's time to change!

NURTURING YOUR BODY AND MIND ACCORDING TO YOUR TYPE OF DEPRESSION

Vata Dosha Depression

BODY NURTURING (FOOD INTAKE/DIET):

- Good, rich, heavy, wholesome, nutritive food to avoid weight loss and ground the mind
- Dairy products (fresh milk and cheese, homemade yogurt, ghee)
- Sweet potato, lentils, rice, tapioca, zucchini, squash, nuts, seeds, whole grains
- Mangoes, figs, raisins, peaches, pears
- Nervine brain tonic *(rasayana):* brahmiprash
- Avoid spicy foods; warm, spiced teas with honey or natural sugar are good

MIND NURTURING (EMOTIONS):

- To be promoted: truth, harmony, fearlessness, patience, courage, self-acceptance
- To be discouraged: confusion, lack of direction, blues, grief, unhappiness

Pitta Dosha Depression

BODY NURTURING (FOOD INTAKE/DIET):

- Appropriate *dosha*-pacifying diet
- Milk, yogurt, rice, beans (kidney beans, lentils), sprouts, zucchini, squash
- Keep the body hydrated with cooling drinks and sweet fruits
- Pomegranate, coconut water, aloe vera juice

- Nervine brain tonic *(rasayana):* brahmiprash
- Avoid spices, salt, acidic foods (sour), oily/fried foods
- Avoid eating late at night (this is one of the most harmful food activities you can engage in)

MIND NURTURING (EMOTIONS):

- To be promoted: forgiveness, serenity, friendship, kindness, devotion
- To be discouraged: attachment, possessiveness, greed

Kapha Dosha Depression

BODY NURTURING (FOOD INTAKE/DIET):

- Reduce food intake, and eat between ten a.m. and five to six p.m.
- *Dosha*-pacifying light diet: salads, hot spices, yellow squash, beans (mung dal, kidney beans, yellow/brown lentils), and grains (brown rice); pomegranate; hot water and teas
- Avoid *kapha* products such as dairy; oily, salty food; and sweets (cookies, candy)
- Attention to eating disorder/overeating to avoid obesity
- Avoid ice, cold water, ice cream, and soft drinks

MIND NURTURING (EMOTIONS):

- To be promoted: courage, flexibility, independence, disengagement
- To be discouraged: deep confusion, nothingness

GENERAL RECOMMENDATIONS FOR YOUR SPECIFIC PREDOMINANT *DOSHA*

General Recommendations for *Vata Dosha* Depression

These recommendations mainly address feelings of fear, anxiety, and terror, which can manifest into insomnia.

DAILY NURTURING (LIFESTYLE):

- Regular daily routine with regular times for eating, working, sleeping, etc.
- Good, deep sleep, rest, and relaxation; relaxing, slow evening activities
- Avoid stress, overwork, and personal conflicts; develop a hobby to divert your depression
- Avoid exposure to cold, wind, or dryness
- Nasal drops: vacha oil (sweet flag) *nasya*
- *Bhringaraja* oil on scalp and soles of the feet at bedtime
- Triphala (½ teaspoon) at bedtime (to support elimination or in case of constipation)
- Don't suppress your natural urges

FRAME NURTURING (EXERCISE):

- Full body self-massage *(abhyanga)* with sesame oil, followed by a hot shower
- Light exercise, yoga postures, qigong, tai chi

BODY NURTURING (FOOD INTAKE/DIET):

- Eat good, rich, heavy, nutritive food to avoid weight loss and ground the mind
- Avoid spicy foods; warm, spiced teas with honey or natural sugar are good
- Dairy products (fresh milk and cheese, homemade yogurt, ghee)
- Sweet potato, lentils, rice, tapioca, zucchini, squash, nuts, seeds, whole grains
- Mangoes, figs, raisins, peaches, pears
- Nervine brain tonic *(rasayana):* brahmiprash

MIND NURTURING (EMOTIONS):

- To promote: fearlessness, patience, courage, self-acceptance, harmony
- To discourage: confusion, lack of direction, blues, grief, unhappiness

HERBAL NURTURING (KITCHEN PHARMACY):

- Ashwagandha (addresses neuronal exhaustion and supports healthy weight), jatamansi (Indian variety of valerian/tranquilizer and nervine boost), tagar/*Valeriana* (for sleeping disorders), vidari (improves communication between neurons), dhattura/belladonna (analgesic and tranquilizer)

BREATH NURTURING *(PRANAYAMA)*:

- Calming, slow, deep *pranayama*
- Right-nostril-breathing *pranayama (surya bhedana)*

SPIRITUAL NURTURING (MEDITATION):

- Meditation on light and fire, focusing on a candle or a light that is not bright
- Meditation to calm emotions and develop devotion to protective deities

SCENT NURTURING (FRAGRANCES):

- Quieting incenses and fragrances such as frankincense, rose, sandalwood, champak

General Recommendations for *Pitta Dosha* Depression

These recommendations mainly address anger, irritability, and a sense of failure.

DAILY NURTURING (LIFESTYLE):

- Full body self-massage *(abhyanga)* with sunflower oil, followed by a warm shower

- Nasal drops: brahmi ghee *nasya*
- Avoid bright light, sun, heat, and fire
- Avoid competitive activities, disputes, or personal conflicts
- Relaxation of strength; searching from introspection instead of condemning others
- Bhumi amalaki (½ teaspoon) at bedtime (if constipated)
- Don't suppress your natural urges

FRAME NURTURING (EXERCISE):

- Mild exercise, noncompetitive swimming, relaxing yoga postures addressing the abdominal area
- Walking in cooling natural places (forests, gardens)

BODY NURTURING (FOOD INTAKE/DIET):

- Appropriate *dosha*-pacifying diet
- Milk, yogurt, rice, beans (kidney beans, lentils), sprouts, zucchini, squash
- Avoid spices, salt, acidic food (sour); avoid oily/fried food
- Avoid eating at night
- Keep the body hydrated with cooling drinks and sweet fruits
- Pomegranate, coconut water, aloe vera juice
- Nervine brain tonic *(rasayana):* brahmiprash

MIND NURTURING (EMOTIONS):

- To promote: forgiveness, serenity, friendship, kindness, devotion
- To discourage: attachment, possessiveness, greed

HERBAL NURTURING (KITCHEN PHARMACY):

- Nervine and cooling products such as brahmi, jatamansi, shatavari, licorice, gotu kola, mint
- Liver cleansing with aloe vera, turmeric

- Blood cooling and cleansing with red clover or manjista
- Purgation with bitter products *(virecana):* rhubarb root, aloe vera

BREATH NURTURING *(PRANAYAMA):*

- Cooling and pacifying *pranayamas: anuloma viloma* (alternate nostril breathing), *shitali, siktari*

SPIRITUAL NURTURING (MEDITATION):

- Meditation on special expansion/outer awareness with compassion
- Meditation on peaceful deities

SCENT NURTURING (FRAGRANCES):

- Cooling fragrances such as sandalwood, vetiver; sweet flower aromas such as rose, jasmine, gardenia, champak
- Apply sandalwood to the forehead and brahmi oil to the head

General Recommendations for *Kapha Dosha* Depression

These recommendations mainly address excessive sleep.

DAILY NURTURING (LIFESTYLE):

- Avoid extreme sleep and daytime sleep
- Avoid sedentary activities
- Full body self-massage *(abhyanga)* with sesame oil, followed by a warm shower
- Nasal drops *(nasya)* with warm ghee or medicated ghee to lubricate and clean the nose passages
- Emetic therapy *(vamana)* for expectoration: ginger, pippali, shilajit, cinnamon, cardamom
- Bibhitaki (½ teaspoon) at bedtime
- Don't suppress your natural urges

FRAME NURTURING (EXERCISE):

- Strong daily exercise: walking, aerobic exercise, swimming to activate physical and mental circulation
- Vigorous yoga postures
- Sweating therapies: saunas and hot tubs *(svedana)*

BODY NURTURING (FOOD INTAKE/DIET):

- Reduce food intake, and eat between ten a.m. and five to six p.m.
- *Dosha*-pacifying light diet: salads, hot spices, yellow squash, beans (mung dal, kidney beans, yellow/brown lentils), and grains (brown rice); pomegranate; hot water and teas
- Avoid *kapha* products such as dairy; oily, salty food; and sweets (cookies, candy)
- Avoid ice, cold water, ice cream, and soft drinks
- Attention to eating disorder/overeating to avoid obesity

MIND NURTURING (EMOTIONS):

- To promote: courage, flexibility, independence, disengagement
- To discourage: deep confusion, vacuity

HERBAL NURTURING (KITCHEN PHARMACY):

- Ayurvedic herbs and spices for cooking: hot spices, i.e., long pepper (pippali), ginger, parsley, basil (tulsi), garlic, hing (asafoetida)
- Brahmi, punarnava, valerian, sage, bayberry, St. John's wort, ginkgo
- Nighttime: haritaki

BREATH NURTURING *(PRANAYAMA):*

- *Anuloma viloma:* alternate nostril breathing on the right side *(surya bhedana)*
- Strong, deep breathing/fast breaths *(kapalabhati, bhastrika)*

SPIRITUAL NURTURING (MEDITATION):

- Meditation on the limitless, the shapeless, pure grace
- Meditation on formless divinities or presences

SCENT NURTURING (FRAGRANCES):

- All kinds of stimulating aromas (eucalyptus, mint, ginger, heena, camphor)

SUMMARY

The big picture presented here is just a fraction of what Ayurveda has to offer you. I hope we have covered enough to whet your appetite and stimulate a desire to understand yourself better. Put these recommendations into practice, and read more about this subject. This information represents just the beginning of a personal invitation to you to take a challenging path to correct your imbalances. Enjoy learning about food and diet, even cooking more or learning to cook.

There is always a cause or reason for why you feel the way you do. As we've said before, every effect has a cause. Like many other organs and tissues of the body, your brain is very sensitive to conditions such as inflammation caused by contaminants or metabolic byproducts *(ama)*.

If you would like to support your body-mind health regardless of the diagnosis your doctor has given you, you need to ask yourself: What are the true driving factors of my mental state? What are the causes? What role does food play in all this? By exploring the causes of your imbalance, you will discover the path back to balance.

Depression, Food Contamination, and Social Media

INESCAPABLE CONTACT
WITH HAZARDOUS CHEMICALS

We are surrounded in our inner and outer lives by contamination and toxicity. How can we get rid of these toxins and contaminants around and inside us? Your natural detoxification organs are the liver and kidneys, with the gut and urinary tract as extensions of these organs acting to eliminate waste products from your body. The skin (via sweat) and the lungs (via expelling CO_2) are also considered detoxification organs.

If we go back to our great-grandparents and try to visualize their lifestyle—connected to all the elements of nature, independent of continent, country, racial group, or economic background—we understand that they faced natural pressures. Our modern lifestyle, on the other hand, is largely detached from nature, so it exposes us to many kinds of contaminants that simply didn't exist when our ancestors lived or when Ayurvedic medicine was created. The conditions we face are fundamentally different from theirs, starting with the air we breathe and the food we eat, and extending to the innumerable new kinds of impressions we receive, be they physical, digital, or emotional, overcharging our detoxification organs and affecting our minds. A holistic approach to our mental and physical well-being cannot ignore our direct connection to all types of nourishment.

Despite the readily available tools offered by Ayurveda, we in the West are not familiar with them as an option for addressing the physical and mental contamination we face. Every aspect of Ayurvedic lifestyle teaching provides a foundation for handling change. This principle was fundamental to the essence of Ayurveda as first practiced and recorded centuries ago, and it has stood the test of time ever since. The foundations of Ayurveda apply to our modern situation more or less unchanged because, despite the many damaging changes of diet and environment humanity has endured, the role of Ayurveda remains constant through time: restoring balance against the changing backdrop of our lives. Ayurveda holistically addresses the factors disturbing what this system calls our *prakruti* and *manas.*

FOOD FOR THOUGHT

Research in the field of nutritional psychiatry supports the scientific assertion that what you eat and how you feel about it are connected by your brain-gut axis, especially when it comes to managing anxiety and depression. This fact is of great interest to us because we need to view these conditions in light of how to limit our exposure to harmful chemicals and other types of contamination, especially in cases of depression-related imbalances, where people could be more susceptible to the impact of contaminants.

It is not news that the very influential food, agrochemical, pharmaceutical, and media industries play a significant role in affecting our normal biological functions, both physical and mental. Along these lines, I would like to share several examples of the ongoing risks we are exposed to. Please understand that my intention is not to alarm. On the contrary, as you read this information, try to analyze it, and perhaps verify it if you feel the need to. Because of your new awareness of our situation, the important thing is for you to move to a place of participation within yourself, from where you can take proper action. At the end of the day, we are addressing the environmental risks to your health before it is too late.

Our world is filled with more environmental contaminants than at any other time in recorded human history. For example, pesticides are so widely used in our food system that most people assume they must be safe. Unfortunately, that's not always true. For that reason, I am focusing on a variety of chemicals to which you are exposed in daily life, either knowingly or not. We are exposed to innumerable chemicals every day that affect the nervous system, such as medications for attention deficit disorder, attention deficit hyperactivity disorder, hormonal regulation, weight gain, infertility, and immune disorders, as well as bisphenols, phthalates, perfluoroalkyl chemicals, nitrates, and nitrites, to name only a few.

For now, let's not worry about the names of these chemicals. Instead, try to perceive how your body attempts to cope with them. For example, when your body is exposed to a toxic chemical such as a pesticide, your detoxification organs have to generate a biological transformation of these toxic molecules to remove them from your system. Let us not forget, pesticides shouldn't be there in the first place. But if your body cannot handle the toxic load, then you absorb the toxic chemical more quickly than it is being removed by elimination. The term for this process is bioaccumulation. We can accumulate dioxins, heavy metals, pesticides, PCBs, and other toxic chemicals in our bodies in the same way that mercury can accumulate in fish before we eat it.

Research conducted by the Environmental Working Group found that on average there are two hundred industrial chemicals and pollutants in the umbilical cords of newborn babies in the United States. The chemicals identified included pesticides; perfluorochemicals used as stain and oil repellents in fast-food packaging, clothing, and textiles; Teflon; flame retardants; and other pollutants present in consumer goods.[1]

A joint report on several studies, released by the WHO with the United Nations Environment Programme, suggested a ban on chemicals that disrupt our hormonal systems needed to protect the health of future generations. The comprehensive report highlights a wide variety of complications stemming from contamination with these chemicals, such as nervous system deficiencies; the development of attention deficit disorder and attention deficit hyperactivity disorder in children; undescended testicles; and breast, prostate, and thyroid cancers associated with exposure to chemicals commonly found in plastics and food additives.[2] An example of those compounds is the phthalates widely used to make plastics more durable and flexible, which are present in food packaging, vinyl gloves, household cleaners, cosmetics, and personal care products. Although they are used to strengthen a product's durability, they are not strongly bound to it, and they tend to leak out over time.

There is a groundswell of activism from environmental and consumer groups demanding accountability from the food, agrochemical, pharmaceutical, and media industries for their actions. Concentrated animal feeding operations, as well as the farms that grow the corn and genetically modified soybeans that feed them, are the number one source of water pollution in the United States and a main cause of air pollution. Bayer/Monsanto's genetically modified soybeans and animal feed are the top destroyer of grasslands and forest in the Amazon and other regions.[3,4,5]

Your condition of depression or anxiety is not only centered in your feeling of being unable to break out of the cycle of depression by yourself. Your condition is also influenced by your life context and your larger environment. Again I emphasize that eating in a natural way, in the right amounts and at the right time, is one way to improve your mental health.

Your nervous system is affected by contamination, so below we will discuss the most relevant contaminants, both physical and mental. At the end of this chapter I will offer Ayurvedic lifestyle recommendations aimed at reducing your exposure to toxic substances affecting your neural, immune, and metabolic systems.

THE FOOD INDUSTRY AND THE CREATION
OF ADDICTION AND DEPRESSION

For years, many of us have been aware that the large and influential food corporations have been blending "pleasure" with "happiness" so we cannot differentiate them any longer, all for the commercial purpose of selling us unwholesome food. Pleasure has a short life span. Physiological and biochemical studies and neuroscience imaging reports show how the food industry has altered our food supply with the clear intention of creating desirable and addictive foods. As a result of nutritional deficiency, many people have become obese. Yes, this is not a contradiction; it is the result of our bodies searching for nourishment, and since food has been nutritionally depleted, we have to eat more and more. The results leave many people concerned and depressed. Even neuroscientists are hired by large food corporations to collaborate in achieving the goal of creating those desirable and addictive foods.[6]

You are at risk. We are all at risk. We are all seduced by clever, psychologically adept marketing about food. However, recall what we discussed earlier: *you are more than habits.* By now you have an understanding of various Ayurvedic tools. What's the first thing to do? Let me help you: look at the quality and quantity of nutrients in your diet. What to do next? Evaluate your diet, and be honest about the types of foods you eat. How much junk food is part of your daily intake? How respectful are you of your food intake schedules? Please keep asking yourself these questions in an open and honest way. Deep inside you have all the proper answers. Trust yourself. It is time to engage and take the right actions.

Different "Sugars" and Their Effects

Sugar is the common name for sweet-tasting, soluble carbohydrates, many of which are used in food. Simple sugars include glucose, fructose, and galactose. The combination of glucose and fructose is referred to as sucrose, regular sugar, table sugar, or granulated sugar. In the body, sugar is broken down into fructose and glucose. We all require a certain level of circulating glucose in our bodies (generally known as blood sugar), mainly because glucose is the only fuel naturally used by our brain cells. Since our neurons cannot store glucose, they literally depend on the constant bloodstream supply of this fuel. There are other molecules, such as the fatty acids in food, that are rich energetic fuel. Unfortunately, fatty acids do not serve as fuel for the brain, because they journey through the bloodstream bound to a protein called albumin, so they become a very big molecule that is unable to cross the selective blood-brain barrier.

If the levels of glucose in the brain are very high or very low, your body-mind consciousness will be affected. Spikes or alterations of sugar levels could be the cause of your irritability, lack of motivation and energy, and depression. It is important to quickly find a remedy for this situation, because long-term imbalances could cause chronic cycles of hypoglycemia or could affect insulin levels, eventually causing insulin resistance. The role of the hormone insulin is to regulate how the body uses and stores glucose and fat. If you are in a prediabetic state because your blood sugar is too high as a result of wrong or irregular eating habits, that could stimulate depression. Ayurvedic lifestyle recommendations set out by the ancient scholars are based on the importance of respecting the proper times for food intake and proper balance of quality and quantity of natural foods, including carbohydrates. These recommendations protected people's health for centuries. Because natural carbohydrates break down into sugar and then into glucose and fructose, and natural carbohydrates were the only ones available when the foundations of Ayurveda were being developed and recorded, the risk of being exposed to artificial sugars was nonexistent.

Our love for sweetness goes back to the beginning of civilization. Today the food industry works hard to exploit that love, employing scientists and manufacturers to produce synthetic artificial sweeteners for commercial reasons. On average a U.S. citizen eats 150 pounds of added sugar a year. Approximately half of the added sugar we consume today comes from soft drinks, sports drinks, energy drinks, fruit drinks, and the like.[7] We cannot be surprised that the consumption of artificial sweeteners in these drinks correlates with the increased risk of developing obesity, metabolic syndrome, type 2 diabetes, and mental imbalances.

We can all choose whether to eat natural sweeteners or artificial ones. Natural sweeteners are slightly processed and offer certain nutritional value to the body. These include cane sugar, coconut sugar, blackstrap molasses, raw honey, maple syrup, and molecules from plant leaves such as stevia. Artificial sweeteners are molecules synthetically produced in a laboratory. These can also include sugars that have been chemically processed to fulfill the craving for sugar without providing the additional calories. These artificial sweeteners can deplete the body of essential nutrients, as well as being converted into potentially toxic compounds. They have the harmful effects of increasing triglycerides and insulin response, boosting health risks that instigate metabolic disorders, cancer, and neurotoxicity. Examples of these compounds are monosodium glutamate, acesulfame potassium, sucralose, aspartame, and sodium benzoate.

Let's discuss in more detail the artificial sugars created by the food industry and their potential toxic effects, such as altering our metabolism, affecting our body systems, and creating mental imbalances.

Sucralose

In 1998 the U.S. Food and Drug Administration approved Splenda as a biologically inert compound sweetener for use in many food products, such as baked goods, nonalcoholic beverages, chewing gum, frozen dairy desserts, fruit juices, and gelatins. Splenda is the brand name for sucralose, a chlorinated sugar marketed under the claim that as an inert molecule, it is unable to be metabolized or bioaccumulated in the human body—although this may not be the case. Animal studies have revealed that sucralose is, in fact, metabolized in the body and accumulates in fat tissue, so it doesn't pass as an inert substance.[8]

Other studies show that this chlorinated sugar causes renal and hepatic inflammation and damages the thymus gland and the gut, creating microbial imbalances that cause chronic inflammation and weakened immunity. It is also associated with disorders such as irritable bowel syndrome, obesity, Crohn's disease, and ulcerative colitis.

Researchers tested saccharin, sucralose, and aspartame, the artificial sweeteners in Sweet'n Low, Splenda, and NutraSweet respectively, and found that noncaloric artificial sweeteners induce glucose intolerance by altering the microbiome. They found that after just one week of using saccharin, some participants experienced exaggerated blood-sugar responses related to changes in their gut bacteria.[9,10] Further studies showed that sucralose is particularly able to harm the gut because it is metabolized and stored in our fat cells, and it could cause liver damage when used regularly.[11,12] Sucralose has a detrimental effect on your microbiome by reducing gut bacteria by as much as 50 percent, preferentially targeting bacteria known to play important roles in human health.[13]

Artificial sweeteners like sucralose and aspartame have zero calories, but they fool your body into thinking they're sweet like caloric sugar. It's this biological deception that triggers the various disorders discovered in the studies cited above. How does it work? When your tongue gustatory receptors get hit by a sweet taste, your body will anticipate calories to follow; that is the natural way our bodies behave. Unfortunately, when the sweet taste comes without the calories, your body begins to store whatever kind of calories come to it. Consider what human life looked like many thousands of years ago, when we all were nomads dealing with how seasonal changes made it difficult to obtain food. Our bodies learned to store food in the form of calories to be used in case of an unexpected situation, e.g., inability to hunt animals or grow crops due to climatic, seasonal, or other conditions. Your body's storage of calories, stimulated by artificial sweeteners, can result in weight increase, metabolic disorders, and additional health complications.

Aspartame

Aspartame, a widely used artificial sweetener, is one of the most popular sugar substitutes in low-calorie food and drinks, including diet sodas. It is also a component of some medications. In the United States it is available under the brand names NutraSweet and Equal. It is made with a combination of the amino acid phenylalanine (50 percent), aspartic acid (40 percent), and methanol (10 percent), and it is two hundred times sweeter than sugar.

High concentrations of phenylalanine produce abnormal serotonin levels in the nervous system, causing depression and emotional and psychotic disorders. People who regularly consume aspartame have excess phenylalanine in their systems. Phenylketonuria is a disorder in which a person cannot metabolize phenylalanine. Consequently, aspartame must never be consumed by infants or pregnant or nursing women. The chemical aspartic acid functions as an excitotoxin, stimulating neurons and destroying nerve cells, with potential neurophysiological indicators such as learning problems, headaches, seizures, migraines, insomnia, irritable moods, anxiety, and depression.[14,15]

Processed Fructose

Fructose, which makes up half of table sugar, was our natural source of energy for many decades. High-fructose corn syrup (HFCS), or processed fructose, is not the same as fructose. HFCS was first introduced by the food and beverage industry in the 1970s as a cheap alternative to sugar to be used for sweetening foods and beverages. In 1980, Coca-Cola began using HFCS in its beverages, and within a few years most other soft drink companies had followed suit. The average American consumes 5.4 ounces of sugar per day, half of which is processed fructose. If you would like to avoid the collateral consequences of depression, such as obesity and diabetes, the best way is to reduce the amount of processed and treated food in your diet. It is a simple step to take; there are no mysteries here.

Let's analyze this processed fructose in more detail. Recent studies confirm that processed fructose is more harmful than table sugar because it aggravates insulin levels and reduces glucose tolerance.[16] Other research confirms that sugar intake from sweet foods and beverages has an adverse effect on long-term psychological health and suggests that lower intake of sugar may be associated with better psychological health. Intake of sweet foods, beverages, and added sugars has been linked to depressive symptoms and an increased chance of mood disorders in several populations.[17]

Studies confirm that all calories are not created equal. Enhanced sugars and processed fructose are more harmful than other carbohydrates. In the U.S., adults consume three times the recommended level of added sugar (5 percent of energy intake), with sweet foods and drinks contributing three-quarters of the intake.[18]

The preponderance of the evidence clearly shows that processed fructose, primarily in the form of corn syrup, has become a major health issue in the United States. Studies show an association between sugar ingestion and the promotion of synthesis of lipids, a disorder correlated with fat accumulation in the liver. This accumulation causes harmful levels of fat storage, encouraging inflammation that triggers insulin resistance, hyperinsulinemia, metabolic syndrome, and associated diseases, including type 2 diabetes, hypertension, lipid disorders, circulatory disease, cancer, and dementia. These kinds of metabolic disorders are the cause of metabolic syndrome. Among children who have metabolic syndrome, these disorders can be reversed in a short period of time if you take sugar out of their diet and substitute starch in an equal calorie-for-calorie exchange. In the same way, it is possible to reverse insulin resistance, fat accumulation in the liver, and the pancreatic load of increased insulin production. Essentially, all of the metabolic perturbations caused by sugar intake can be reversed.[19]

Consider the following facts as reasons to reduce or avoid foods with HFCS: they add unnatural sugars to your food; increase your risk of fatty liver disease, obesity, and weight gain; and are linked to diabetes and other serious conditions. Above all, like other added sugars, HFCS is "full" of empty calories, offering no essential nutrients. Today, even in India, mother of Ayurveda, obesity has reached epidemic proportions. India is also considered the diabetes capital of the world as a result of drastic changes in lifestyle, partly promoted by the modern food industry.

Food Additives

Here are some examples of food additives that may pose dangers to your mental health and physical functions.

Acesulfame Potassium

This artificial sweetener is two hundred times sweeter than sugar. It does not increase blood-sugar levels, but it does stimulate insulin secretion and is associated with chronic respiratory disease, increased risk of leukemia, thymus cancer, changes in gut bacteria, and breast cancer.[20]

Monosodium Glutamate (MSG)

MSG is a flavor enhancer and preservative added to many packaged and canned goods. Its intake is associated with symptoms of headaches, brain lesions, heart palpitations, and Parkinson's disease. Research has found that MSG is associated with chronic inflammation, liver damage, weight loss resistance, and chronic pain. MSG is hidden on food labels under different deceptive names such as autolyzed yeast extract, textured protein, soy protein, and whey protein isolate. Scientific literature shows that increased consumption of MSG could be associated with harmful health effects.[21]

Sodium Benzoate (E211)

E211 food preservative is present in soft drinks, such as energy drinks and sodas. Neurodevelopmental conditions such as ADHD, asthma, and other inflammatory disorders have been linked to sodium benzoate exposure.[22] Vitamin C is also added to many popular beverages. When E211 is combined with vitamin C, they form a highly carcinogenic compound called benzene.[23,24]

Trans Fats

Trans fats are liquid oils that have been chemically treated through a process called "hydrogenation" so they will be solid at room temperature. They are used to give food a certain taste and texture, and trans fats can increase shelf life. However, the body is not well equipped to break down, use, or eliminate this artificial substance. According to the FDA, here are some foods that commonly contain trans fats: baked goods (crackers, cookies, cakes, and frozen pies), snack foods (microwave popcorn, potato chips, and corn chips), coffee creamers, refrigerated dough products, ready-to-use frostings, margarine, and shortening.

Our bodies need natural fats to function properly, but trans fats do more harm than good. Studies have shown that high levels of trans fats may reduce serotonin production in the brain, leading to depression and adversely affecting memory. Remove trans fats from your diet by inquiring, checking labels, and avoiding processed and fried foods you do not prepare yourself. Also avoid foods whose ingredient lists include partially hydrogenated vegetable oil or esterified fats. Instead, consume healthy natural fats such as olive oil, coconut oil, and butter, which are better for your body and brain health.[25] Studies have observed a relationship between trans fat intake and depression risk.[26,27]

Endocrine-Disrupting Chemicals (EDCs)

Most EDCs are artificial substances (pesticides, metals, additives, or contaminants in food or personal care products) that interfere with hormone biosynthesis or metabolism, or otherwise cause a deviation from normal homeostatic control or reproduction. EDCs increase incidence of breast cancer, abnormal growth patterns, and neurodevelopmental delays in children, as well as changes in immune function.[28,29]

Many EDCs take the form of pesticides, which can be grouped according to the types of pests they kill: insecticides (insects), herbicides (plants), rodenticides (rats and mice), bactericides (bacteria), fungicides (fungi), and larvicides (larvae). Agricultural use accounts for 80 percent of pesticide use in the United States. The FDA's pesticide residue monitoring program has disclosed that pesticide residues are extensive in popular foods, including strawberries, apples, and grapes. Altogether, 84 percent of domestic fruits—along with 53 percent of vegetables, 42 percent of grains, and 73 percent of "other" foods, such as nuts, seeds, candy, and beverages—were recently found to carry pesticide residues.[30,31]

A 2019 review listed a number of physiological functions affected by EDCs, including cancer, reproductive impairment, cognitive deficit, and obesity.[32]

Human exposure to EDCs occurs via ingestion of food, dust, and water, inhalation of gases and particles in the air, and through the skin.

A pregnant or nursing mother can also transfer EDCs to the developing fetus or infant child through the placenta or breast milk. Pregnant mothers and children are the most vulnerable populations to be affected by developmental exposures, and the effect of exposures to EDCs may not become evident until later in life. Research also shows that such exposure may increase susceptibility to noncommunicable diseases.[33,34]

The reality is that EDCs are on our daily menu, and food is a major vector of exposure to these artificial chemicals. For instance, studies have shown that the plastic containers made for roasting chickens convey EDCs into the blood. The Future Generations Association reported in September 2018 that more than six out of ten pesticide residues identified in the European diet are suspected to be EDCs[35]. Although concentrations are low, populations remain vulnerable because it is not so much a question of dosage; it's a question of the length of exposure and the vulnerability of the individual. A dietary dose of an endocrine-disrupting pesticide might be harmless for a fifty-year-old but catastrophic for a fetus. Fetal formation, early childhood, and puberty are periods of increased vulnerability to EDCs, and the effects of these agents can be transmitted between generations. A 2020 study showed that fungicides can have toxic effects in humans by causing stress and inducing changes in neurons.[36]

Scientists are still assessing how much EDCs can damage our body-mind health. In the meantime, learn more about the risks of EDCs by reading food labels warning you of their presence in the products you use and consume. Based on the research, we should be most concerned about the EDCs discussed below.

Bisphenol A (BPA)

Did you know that it is estimated that about 42.6 billion bottles of water per year are purchased in the United States alone? What you might not know is that each of these bottles contains toxins that have been scientifically proven to have a negative effect on our health.

BPA is the chemical compound used to shape and harden plastic. It is also used to line food and beverage cans, in particular soup and tuna cans. This toxin has been trivialized into our daily lives; it has been part of our "daily toxins" since the 1960s, and by now we don't give it a second thought. It has become one of the highest-volume chemicals produced in the world, with billions of pounds produced each year. This EDC was first developed about a century ago as a synthetic estrogen, but it wasn't until the 1950s that manufacturers realized it could be used to make polycarbonate plastic. After that, BPA quickly became one of the most fabricated and used chemicals worldwide, despite its known hormonal effects. In fact, BPA is known to change the timing of puberty, reduce fertility, affect the immune system, increase body fat, and affect the nervous system by interfering with neurotransmitters. Although BPA is banned in baby bottles and sippy cups, it continues to be used in a variety of readily available products.[37,38]

Bisphenol S (BPS) and bisphenol F (BPF) are chemicals similar to BPA. A recent study showed that 97.5 percent of children and adolescents had detectable levels of BPA in their urine, 87.8 percent had BPS, and 55.2 percent had BPF. All three chemicals correlated with an increased risk for obesity, even after the researchers controlled for caloric intake. Following the rising concern associated with BPA, some companies are substituting similar chemicals that have not been so well tested and whose structure is chemically similar to BPA, including BPS and BPF.[39,40]

Phthalates

This is a group of hormone-disrupting chemicals used in the making of PVC plastics and in industrial food production to make plastics more flexible. Phthalates are also used as a fragrance carrier in personal care products, soaps, and cosmetics to make them more liquid, and it's used in children's and adults' toys. Phthalates are associated with changes in male genital development, increased risk of childhood obesity, contributions to cardiovascular disease, and induction of oxidative stress and depression.[41,42] In 2017, the U.S. Consumer Product Safety Commission banned the use of some phthalates in child care products. To identify them, look for items listed as DBP, DEP, and BBP.

Perfluoroalkyl Chemicals (PFCs)

These chemicals are used to grease-proof paper and cardboard food packaging. PFCs may affect brain development, thyroid function, digestion, and bone strength, and they may reduce fertility, immunity, and birth weight. Recent studies show that hormonal disturbance from PFCs starts before birth, significantly affecting development of sexual organs. Exposure to PFCs in cookware, fabrics, microwave popcorn, and fast-food packaging also affects liver and kidney health, lipid metabolism, hypothyroidism, obesity, and ulcerative colitis. Perfluorooctanoic acid (PFOA), also known as C8, is a PFC used in the production of Teflon by DuPont. In 2017, DuPont agreed to pay $670 million to settle 3,500 lawsuits in the United States brought by people who claimed they were poisoned by drinking water contaminated with PFOAs that the company knowingly released into surface water.[43,44,45,46]

Perchlorate

Perchlorate is a manufactured chemical free radical; it also occurs naturally. It is generally used as an oxidizer in rocket propellants, munitions, fireworks, matches, and signal flares. It is also added to some dry food packaging to control static electricity. Perchlorate reduces hormonal production in the thyroid gland, which is of particular concern to the developing fetus and infant.[47]

Other Artificial Chemicals in Our Food

Nitrates and Nitrites

Cured and processed meats such as beef jerky, salami, hot dogs, and other processed meat snacks are treated with nitrates and nitrites to extend shelf life and enhance color. An analysis of more than one thousand people with and without psychiatric disorders showed that nitrates and nitrites may contribute to mania, an abnormal mood state characterized by hyperactivity, euphoria, and insomnia.[48]

Artificial Food Colors

Artificial food colors are often added to foods to make them more visually appealing. Tartrazine, also known as yellow 5, has been associated with behavioral changes including irritability, restlessness, depression, and difficulty sleeping. Artificial food colors are linked with aggravation of the symptoms of attention deficit disorder and ADHD.[49]

In addition, recent studies have confirmed that many hair products contain EDCs and carcinogens potentially relevant to breast cancer, which indirectly affects one's mental condition.[50,51]

Baby Food

The organization Healthy Babies Bright Futures recently discovered that 95 percent of baby foods they tested contained the heavy metals lead, arsenic, cadmium, and mercury. The food items tested included 61 brands and 13 types of food, including infant formula, fruit juices, teething biscuits, and cereals. Lead was discovered in 94 percent of the foods, cadmium and arsenic in nearly 75 percent, and mercury in about 30 percent. Fifteen of the foods accounted for 55 percent of the heavy metal contaminants.[52]

Cow's milk from conventionally raised cattle contains dozens of reproductive hormones, allergenic proteins, antibiotics, artificial chemicals, inflammatory compounds, and growth factors, some of which are known to promote cancer. The dairy industry has somehow convinced us that drinking milk is the only way to ensure healthy, strong bones, but in reality there are other foods that have more bone-boosting nutrients than milk, such as sardines, arugula, and tahini. These foods contain more calcium than milk and are rich in other nutrients necessary to build strong bones, such as magnesium, vitamin K, and vitamin D.

Microplastics Found in Food

When larger plastic items are tossed out as litter or wash out of landfills, wear and tear from the elements can break them down, contributing to massive amounts of tiny plastic pieces in the environment. Pieces that are five millimeters in size or smaller are called "microplastics." Animals that accidentally ingest these microplastics can suffer toxic effects. If microplastics enter the human food cycle via meat consumption, the toxic and carcinogenic chemicals used to make these plastics become part of our bodies, and our detoxifying organs have to try to eliminate them to keep our body balanced.[53]

Skin Care Products with Potentially Dangerous Ingredients

Perhaps it would be a good idea for you to check the ingredients of your daily skin care products. You may not be happy to discover that they contain one or more of the following common ingredients:

Mineral oil, paraffin, and petrolatum: These petroleum products coat the skin and clog pores, resulting in a buildup of toxins. When they accumulate they can cause dermatological issues, such as slowing cellular development or altering hormonal activities.[54]

Toluene: Made from petroleum or coal tar, toluene is present in most synthetic fragrances. It is harmful if absorbed through the skin or inhaled. Chronic toluene exposure is associated with anemia, decreased blood cell count, and liver or kidney impairment.

Parabens: Extensively used as preservatives in moisturizers and other industrial cosmetics, parabens are present in more than ten thousand skin care and cosmetic products. Studies associate their use with cancer because of how they mimic estrogen's effect on the endocrine system.[55]

Microbeads: These can be of two types: either tiny plastic particles that easily pass through water filtration systems and end up in bodies of water, posing a potential threat to aquatic life, or very tiny pieces of manufactured polyethylene plastic that are added as exfoliants to health and beauty products. In this usage, they are replacing natural ingredients that were introduced into cleansers and toothpastes about fifty years ago. Until 2012, few were concerned about microbeads, and there was a profusion of products containing plastic microbeads on the market with very little consumer awareness.

Phenol carbolic acid: Used in skin creams and lotions, phenol carbolic acid can cause circulatory disorders, paralysis, convulsions, and even death.[56]

Propylene glycol: This moisturizer carries fragrance oils in cosmetics. It can cause dermatitis, kidney malfunctions, or liver malfunctions, as well as skin irritation.

Acrylamide: This substance, present in many body creams, is associated with mammary tumors in lab research.

Sodium laurel or lauryl sulfate (SLS): SLS is present in about 90 percent of personal care and cleaning products. SLS breaks down the skin's moisture barrier and enters the skin, and it could allow other chemicals to infiltrate behind it. When SLS combines with other substances, it can become a nitrosamine, a potent carcinogen.

Dioxane: Also known as PEG, polysorbates, lauryl, and ethoxylated alcohol, these substances are usually present in a range of personal care products. Dioxane's carcinogenicity affects nasal passages and hepatic function as reported in studies by the National Cancer Institute in 1978.[57]

Meat

The concept that meat does not induce cancer sounds like a lot of bull to me. Reputable research groups estimate that nearly 35 percent of cancers in Western high-income societies are related to factors such as nutrition and physical activity.[58] More recently, the World Cancer Research Foundation has classified processed meats—including ham, salami, bacon, and sausages—as a group 1 carcinogen. The organization said that "the best prevention of colorectal cancer is the combination of greater physical activity with a fiber-rich and meat products-poor diet."[59] That sounds like Ayurveda.

Red meat has been associated with cancer for decades. Researchers used to wonder why other mammals could eat a diet high in red meat without any adverse health consequences. Eventually they found out that beef, pork, and lamb contain a sugar called Neu5Gc that is naturally produced by other carnivores but not by humans. In other carnivores, the immune system does not kick in when they eat meat, because Neu5Gc is already in their bodies. But when humans eat red meat, the body triggers an immune response to the alien sugar, creating antibodies that cause inflammation and eventually cancer.[60]

Let's consider the potentially dangerous role of antibiotics and hormones given to animal stock in order to increase productivity. About 80 percent of antibiotics sold in the United States are used in meat production. Livestock, poultry, and even farmed fish are given antibiotics to increase their growth and to counteract the unsanitary effects of crowded settings that could promote infection. This subtherapeutic use of antibiotics in raising animals contributes significantly to the rise of antibiotic-resistant bacteria, causing a substantial and growing threat to public health globally. Beef treated with hormones, which account for 75 percent of all cattle, has more estrogenic activity than beef not treated with hormones, creating grave concerns about links with increased risk of cancer.[61]

Dr. S. L. Hazen at the Cleveland Clinic enrolled 113 healthy men and women in a clinical trial to investigate the effects of dietary protein on trimethylamine N-oxide (TMAO), a dietary byproduct formed by gut bacteria during digestion. The chemical is derived in part from nutrients that are abundant in red meat. The study results showed that compared to people eating diets rich in white meat or plant-based protein, those who ate a diet rich in red meat had triple the levels of a chemical linked to heart disease.[62] Prior research has shown that TMAO increases cholesterol deposits in artery walls.[63]

It is equally important to be careful when eating vegetarian food products such as "fake meats" and other products that claim to be healthy, environmentally kind substitutes for beef. These products usually include highly processed, genetically modified soy protein concentrate (containing the herbicide glyphosate, which is toxic for your microbiome), coconut and sunflower oils, and other components that are not real food. Some of those products use genetically engineered yeast to fabricate an artificial blood-heme molecule, creating a blood-like appearance in meat-substitute hamburgers.[64,65]

Over-the-Counter (OTC) Medications

This is a very extensive subject, but in general, if you are suffering depression it is very important to think twice before taking OTC medications. Most individuals assume that OTC medications are safe and free of serious side effects. When taken as directed, most OTC medications are safe for most people. Nevertheless, this is not true for everyone, especially when combined with other OTC drugs or prescription medications. You must try to avoid interactions between antidepressants and other drugs that could prompt an even worse depressive state through their combined effects. Always consult with your specialist before taking an OTC drug.

Let me address one very common OTC drug. Acetaminophen is commonly known as Tylenol, but it is present in many other products, such as Excedrin and Midol, and it is included in many preparations that treat symptoms of colds and flu. Recent studies have shown that acetaminophen, aside from its other reported harmful side effects for organs such as the liver, can also affect mental function. Studies found acetaminophen use to be associated with reduced emotional reactions to both positive and negative stimuli, and acetaminophen can blunt the intensity with which people experience negative events that derive from social, physical, or cognitive sources.[66,67,68]

There are risks of taking other OTC drugs, too, such as nonsteroidal anti-inflammatory drugs, which are consumed as painkillers and are associated with cardiovascular disorders.

This is an important subject, so if you feel concern about these drugs, either discuss them with your specialist or do some research on your own. In Ayurvedic and natural medicinal terms, remember that you have five clinically validated alternatives for natural pain relief: turmeric, ginger, cinnamon, thyme, and arnica.

Dangerous Chemicals Present in Your Drinks or Their Packaging

Water

On average, human beings can live for up to three weeks without food, but they will not survive more than a few days without water. We typically think most of our body is water, when in fact the liquid in question is a solution of water and various electrolytes such as salt. Water dissociates into ions in solution and acquires the capacity to conduct electricity, which is vital for all our bodily functions. We can think of our bodies as hydroelectric systems functioning through the transfer of electrons. To be healthy, we need to maintain the body's electrical systems. Inadequate levels of natural electrolytes or the presence of unnatural substances in our drinking water put our water absorption at risk by altering the body's balance.

One exciting area of research is the form that water molecules take in the body around healthy cells. Recent studies suggest that the cell's outer structural membrane is a semicrystalline matrix. This implies that our trillion-plus body cells could have a resonant frequency specific to each tissue and organ, like a crystal tumbler that rings its own special note when struck. Most people in the world drink municipal tap water, so what could be more imperative than ensuring that water systems provide high-quality, uncontaminated water? Despite the essential role of water for supporting life, a cumulative risk analysis of contaminant occurrence in United States drinking water for the period of 2010–2017 indicates that more than 100,000 lifetime cancer cases could be due to carcinogenic chemicals in tap water. The majority of this risk is due to the presence of arsenic, disinfection byproducts, and radioactive contaminants.[69]

Once upon a time, not too long ago, we humans lived in nature, and we could trust the air we breathed, the land where we grew food, and the water we drew from rivers. Those days are gone, beginning gradually several generations ago when we started living in cities. We moved to a system of mass public sanitation infrastructures, with the consequent accessibility of water that was free of feces and other biological contaminants. Now we find ourselves living in a world where the water, including our tap water, is contaminated by all kinds of toxic chemicals as a result of industrialization, overpopulation, and other factors. These factors affect our body-mind balance, causing acute or chronic effects depending on our body constitution, and the nature of the artificial contaminant, e.g., artificial industrial toxins, fertilizers, disinfectants, radionucleotides, pharmaceuticals, and pesticides, tainting streams, rivers, and oceans worldwide.

"Fruit" Drinks

Scientists at the University of Connecticut revealed in a 2019 report that many popular fruit juices do not contain fruit but are instead composed of water, synthetic sweeteners, and sugar. The FDA does not oblige producers to describe the specific amount of artificial sweetener used in their products, so there is always room for misleading marketing tactics in fruit juice packaging.[70,71] The specific long-term health effects of artificial sweeteners on adults include metabolic syndrome, weight gain, and nonalcoholic fatty liver disease, and the effects on children will likely be the same over the long term.[72]

Coffee

This popular beverage contains the potentially harmful chemical acrylamide, which can form in some foods through high-temperature cooking processes such as frying, roasting, and baking. Acrylamide in food forms from sugars and an amino acid that is naturally present in food; it does not come from food packaging or the environment. Acrylamide is used to make plastics and treat wastewater, among other things. The International Agency for Research on Cancer classifies acrylamide as a "probable human carcinogen." The U.S. National Toxicology Program has classified acrylamide as "reasonably anticipated to be a human carcinogen." The U.S. Environmental Protection Agency classifies acrylamide as "likely to be carcinogenic to humans."[73]

Herbal Drinks

Tea and herbal beverages are well-known, ancient, worldwide traditions acknowledged for their positive health impact. However, recent studies have shown the effects on humans of drinking billions of particles of plastic from tea bags. Plastic and paper tea bags are both sometimes unsafe, since some tea bags and even coffee filters are treated with epichlorohydrin (an industrial solvent and known carcinogen) to reduce the risk of the product tearing during infusion.[74,75]

I am not asking you to change your habit of drinking tea if you like it, but change the way you make it. Just substitute loose tea instead. It requires a bit more work to strain the leaves out, and you will keep enjoying the healthy benefits.

Fluoride

In the United States the fluoridation of drinking water has been approved by the American Medical Association and the WHO, and 75 percent of the population receives fluoridated water from community water systems.[76]

Some U.S. regions have high levels of naturally occurring fluoride in soil, water, and foods, but the fluorides that are added to about 90 percent of municipal water supplies are the silicofluorides, fluorosilicic acid, and sodium fluosilicate, which are byproducts of the aluminum industry.

More than three hundred reports have shown fluoride's toxic effects on the brain. A 2006 National Research Council review suggested that fluoride exposure may be associated with brain damage, endocrine system disruption, and bone cancer.[77] A 2019 study showed an association between maternal fluoride exposure during pregnancy and IQ scores in offspring in Canada, indicating the possible need to reduce fluoride intake during pregnancy.[78]

Despite these findings, people both within and outside the medical community believe water fluoridation is entirely beneficial. However, the ingestion of too much fluoride causes fluorosis, a condition characterized by defects in tooth enamel and brown marks and mottling of the teeth. The U.S. Centers for Disease Control and Prevention reported that 41 percent of U.S. adolescents have fluorosis. Scientific studies have shown that fluoride is a neurotoxin and a hormonal disruptor. High amounts of fluorine may contribute to ADHD symptoms in children, thyroid problems, and other complications such as skeletal fluorosis, causing stiffening and pain of the joints and bones or abdominal pain, nausea, and vomiting.[79] The EPA has been asked to ban fluoridation in

U.S. drinking water, and lawsuits to that effect in states such as California are in progress.

Microplastics in Liquids

Plastic in all shapes and sizes is the most prevalent type of debris found in our oceans and lakes. Recent research on water contamination found microplastics in 90 percent of the table salt brands sampled worldwide. Of 39 salt brands tested, 36 had microplastics in them, according to a new analysis by researchers in South Korea and Greenpeace East Asia. The findings suggest that human ingestion of microplastics via marine products is strongly related to emissions in a given region, and researchers estimate that the average adult consumes approximately two thousand pieces of microplastic per year through salt.[80,81] Microplastics not only contaminate our marine water but also our groundwater systems.[82]

FDA Provides Insufficient Oversight

We have an alarming number of chemicals that are allowed to be added to food and food-contact materials in the United States, either directly or indirectly. An estimated one thousand of these chemicals are used under a "Generally Recognized as Safe" designation, without FDA approval. Despite this framework, there are substantial gaps in the data about probable health effects of food additives. An evaluation of nearly four thousand additives intentionally added to food revealed that for 80 percent of them, there was insufficient information to determine how much could be safely eaten, and only 6.7 percent had reproductive toxicology data.[83]

RECOMMENDATIONS TO DECREASE CHEMICAL EXPOSURE VIA FOOD

It is virtually impossible to avoid potential sources of toxic chemicals, but that does not mean that you cannot take steps to prevent exposure to some of those agents that are contaminating your body both physically and mentally via your water, air, food, and all the indoor chemicals around you. Following are some general eating recommendations to reduce your exposure:

- Resist the marketing pressure to buy unwholesome foods, and prioritize healthy choices of wholesome foods.

- Consume fresh, organic foods, preferably locally grown.

- Always wash all fresh products well, especially if they are not organically grown.

- Consume wild fish instead of conventional or farm-raised fish, which are frequently contaminated with mercury and PCBs.

- Consume certified organic grass-fed meats and dairy, to reduce your exposure to hormones, pesticides, and fertilizers.

- Consume dairy products from cows that have not been exposed to genetically engineered substances, such as recombinant bovine growth hormone.

- A recent study has found that soaking fruits in a solution of one teaspoon of baking soda and three cups of water for two minutes or more will clean the fruits and remove pesticide residues more effectively than other washing methods. After soaking, rinse the fruits in tap water before eating them.[84]

Other recommendations when preparing your food are to avoid certain types of cookware and utensils:

- For cooking use pots, pans, and dishes made of cast iron, stainless steel, or glass instead of those with nonstick or ceramic coatings. Pots and pans with nonstick or ceramic coatings can also leach risky heavy metals like cadmium or lead, especially if they are old.

- Avoid plastic cutting boards, spatulas, and serving utensils; use wooden ones instead.

- Store your food and beverages in glass, rather than plastic, and avoid using plastic wrap.

Concerning your drinking water:

- Learn how much fluoride is in your tap water.

- Filter tap water if it is fluoridated. Reverse osmosis filters remove fluoride from tap water.

- Check labels and make sure the plastic products you purchase are BPA free. "Nontoxic plastic bottles" = BPA/phthalate free.

- Choose ceramic or glass over plastic as often as possible.

DEPRESSION PROMPTED BY SOCIAL MEDIA AND TECHNOLOGY

Through the omnipresence of the internet, we are under the influence of a gigantic invisible "digital brain" changing us into small fragments of the whole. Today's virtual reality transcends space and time, and social media gives us the ability to communicate with people all over the world.

In our world population of 7.75 billion people, there are 5.2 billion mobile subscribers and 9.3 billion mobile connections.[85] How much do all the new social media technologies isolate us from our own sense of presence? Right now, perhaps you are using a mobile phone or a computer allowing you to contact others with the touch of a finger, but perhaps you and all of us are less in contact with ourselves. Can you communicate in the same manner within yourself, or are the distances within becoming even greater? Is it possible for you to really connect with yourself in the same way?

In the United States the pharmaceutical industry bombards audiences with medication advertising, even though in many cases placebos work just as well as Big Pharma drugs. In fact, research shows that in the United States—but apparently not in other countries—the placebo effect is getting stronger.[86] Experts theorize that this might be due to the fact that the United States is one of only two countries worldwide that allow pharmaceutical advertising on TV (the other one being New Zealand). In 2016, the U.S. pharmaceutical industry spent $9.6 billion on advertising. In 2018 the industry spent $3.7 billion on TV ads mostly aimed at people aged 65 and older.[87,88] These advertisement campaigns, which emphasize how taking a tablet can cure an ailment, might be making people more disposed to accept that any tablet—even a drug-free placebo—could help them feel better. Never mind that every drug commercial features a voice speaking rapidly at the end to list the problems and side effects from taking these wonder medications.

It is useful to look at how today's technology affects us, especially with regard to the younger generation, many of whom appear to have an addiction to digital devices. Recent research shows that the more time children and adolescents spend on social media, the more likely they are to feel socially isolated. This is a real challenge for all of us, independent of age. Social media is getting in the way of having meaningful relationships with our loved ones and may lead to feelings of depression and anxiety, health issues that more and more people are facing today at every age.[89]

Electric/Electronic Devices

Cell Phones

These communication devices have become an integral part of modern daily life. According to Statista, there are 3.5 billion mobile phone users in the world today, which accounts for 44 percent of the world's population.[90] Cell phones emit radiofrequency (RF) energy, a form of nonionizing electromagnetic radiation that can be absorbed by human tissue close to the phone. The quantity of RF energy a mobile phone user is exposed to depends on many factors: the specific technology in the phone, the distance between the phone and the user, the degree and type of mobile phone use, and the user's distance from cell phone towers.

The use of mobile phones has been associated with cancer and other conditions. Any increased risk of brain tumors associated with cell phone use is not well established and is still under study. Researchers are concerned about possible increased risks of neurological diseases, physiological addiction, impaired cognition, sleep problems, and behavioral problems, in addition to cancer. We need to carefully evaluate the effect of changed behavior in children and adolescents as a result of their interactions with modern digital technologies.[91]

Frequent exposures to microwave frequencies like those emitted by cell phones could cause mitochondrial abnormality and could harm nuclear DNA as a result of free radicals produced by damaging types of reactive nitrogen (peroxynitrite).[92,93]

Excessive exposure to cell phones and Wi-Fi networks has been linked to chronic diseases such as cardiac arrhythmias, anxiety, depression, autism, Alzheimer's disease, and infertility. "Sleep texting" is now part of a category of behaviors called parasomnia, which include walking and talking while asleep. A recent study published in the *Journal of American College Health* has found that sleep texting is a growing trend among young people. Sleep texting is believed to occur when a person enters the REM sleep stage (characterized by rapid eye movement and dreaming), allowing them to send a message without even waking up to do it.[94]

It is clear that our addictions to smartphones and social media are driving corporate benefit while causing pathological conditions that may link to depression. Personal technology is intended to trigger the same reactions as a drug. Although you may feel pleasure when you take out your cell phone or eat sweet snacks, this sensation is not the same as true happiness. Food manufacturers and electronics corporations both capitalize on the biology of our neurotransmitters such as dopamine and serotonin to entice us to purchase their products.

There is an increasing trend of cell phone addiction and poor psychological and physiological health among today's adolescents. Researchers have noted that when cell phone use functions as an addiction, the behavior is stressful. Studies have postulated that depression and anxiety are positive predictors of smartphone addiction. In light of these adverse effects on adolescents, we must advise them to reduce their cell phone use to the minimum, to avoid addiction. This advice is relevant to all of us who spend significant time on our cell phones or engage at length on social media platforms.

The FDA has endorsed the following steps for reducing exposure to RF energy through cell phone use:

- Reserve cell phones for shorter conversations or for times when a landline phone is not available.

- Use a hands-free device, which places greater distance between the phone and the user's head.[95]

The safe distance to keep away from your telephone, as enumerated in your mobile phone user manual, is based on your phone's specific absorption rate, a measure of how much RF energy your body will absorb from the device when held at a specific distance from your body, typically ranging from five to fifteen millimeters. I advise you to keep the device at a good distance when you are not using it. When carrying your phone, avoid keeping it in your pocket.

As cell phones gain more influence in daily life, they also become potentially more hazardous. Injuries resulting from cell phone use have long been reported in the context of driving-related accidents, but other mechanisms of cell-phone-related injury have been underreported. Many of these injuries occur among people aged thirteen to twenty-nine and are associated with common activities, such as texting while walking.[96]

Microwave Ovens

My advice is that you go microwave-free, or only use a microwave oven in occasional circumstances. Let me share with you three main reasons for my recommendation:

- The mental aspect: using a microwave oven creates a frame of mind that food must be convenient, and you need to prepare and eat it as quickly as possible. I invite you to experiment with getting more involved in the preparation of food, and see if your mood changes. Perhaps it will be not easy at the beginning, but by doing it, you will stimulate the processes of food ingestion, absorption, and assimilation, and as a result you will create a different frame of mind.

- The practical aspect: having a microwave is an invitation to eat processed food containing artificial chemicals such as preservatives, colorants, and highly processed substances that are specifically designed for microwaves.

- The scientific aspect: despite how controversial this subject could be, some studies showed that microwaving protein solutions caused changes in the proteins (unfolding) at a faster speed than when the same foods were cooked with the usual heating process.[97]

Additional studies describe variations in molecules such as phyto-chemicals, vitamins, and minerals. I am sure you have noticed undesirable changes in food when you heated leftovers of pizza, pasta, or even vegetables in your microwave oven; food reheated this way becomes dry, rubbery, and gummy, and it lacks the savory smells and flavors we observe when preparing foods in a slower way. Media sources tell us that today's scientists do not have a clear answer about the effects of micro-waves, but that doesn't mean microwaves are necessarily safe.[98]

The major problem with microwave ovens is not the appliances themselves but the foods that often accompany them. Due to wrong life-styles, most people are using microwaves to cook or heat ultraprocessed food-like packaged products that are not beneficial for their health. It is not the oven's fault that there is a huge difference between steaming fresh vegetables and microwaving an industrially produced frozen TV dinner that is potentially leaching BPAs into your food.[99]

Ayurvedic Recommendations to Reduce Social Media Dependency

Hopefully you are starting to understand that you are usually unaware of your body-mind's essential needs—how the mind moves you in life, and what the perpetual chatter in your mind is really trying to tell you.

How could Ayurveda help you participate more actively in address-ing the many external pressures you face and reducing your condition of depression? For example, consider your mobile phone. Are you the kind of person who gets upset because you forgot your mobile phone at home? And isn't this sometimes a blessing? We do not have to be per-manently attached to our phones. Digital life can occasionally wait for us while we are enjoying a period of time offline.

Let's consider another example, this time related to your emails or text messages. Perhaps it is difficult to disregard the continuous accumulation of emails and other messages. It is not surprising that our fast-moving communication technology has created new mental disorders in parallel with accentuations of the old ones, even to the point of making us feel guilty for not being able to keep up with those pressures. Internet addiction is real, and I am sure if we recorded the actual amount of time we engaged with it, we would be surprised. Your emails and mobile phone calls are traveling through space and air, both of which are very typical of a *vata* constitution—and here again we see how ancient Ayurveda has a useful perspective on modern life. In addition to recording the time we spend online with emails, texts, and web browsing, imagine measuring how much of that time was actually productive and useful.

These external pressures are the ones that exacerbate your *vata* (air/space) qualities by disturbing the natural organic flow of your *prana*, accelerating your mind and nervous system functions, and generating *vata dosha* imbalances. I believe if you master the art of using your phone only rarely, you will dramatically improve your mental, emotional, and physical health. You don't need to react impulsively to all that is going on in the outer world. You can respond from a place of inner peace and awareness—that is, if you need to respond at all to what is often just noise. By working to develop a higher awareness of how certain parts of the mind can be manipulated by external conditions, in this particular case media and technology corporations, you can step forward in your actions, words, and conversations in a manner that is more empowered.

Because contaminants of all kinds are so rampant in our modern world—and right now they are impossible to avoid completely—I strongly recommend that you embrace Ayurvedic lifestyle choices that help to detoxify your body and mind on a regular basis. Under normal circumstances your organs naturally know how to detoxify themselves, but when they become overloaded, contaminants accumulate in a congested way.

....

The more contaminants you are exposed to,
the more a detox may be necessary!

....

If you are looking for an Ayurvedic detox that will cleanse accumulated contaminants from your system, I invite you to return to the previous chapters and put into daily practice the principles outlined to kick-start your return to balance. If you don't feel strong enough to do it by yourself, find a qualified Ayurvedic practitioner who can advise you and support your motivation.

Ayurveda understands the mechanisms underlying *vata*-aggravated conditions, including those in our airy digital era. We can start addressing these conditions by listening to our repetitive mental processes so we can break the loop, allowing the pleasure of mindfulness to guide us from within. Our intrinsic *vata* constitution that embraces connections to air and space can allow us to embrace a new sense of reality. We can become aware of a type of communication that moves you away from a state of separation and depression, due perhaps to the privation of inner and outer love and respect for yourself and others.

Analyzing the Biological Mechanism of Depression

BALANCING BRAIN CHEMISTRY WITH AMINO ACIDS

My aim is that by the end of this chapter (and based on the Ayurvedic tools provided in the previous chapters), you will have a wider perspective on the biological processes that shape the condition of depression, and you will be more motivated to observe and address these issues by yourself. External support can be helpful, but it can also be your crutch. It's time to walk on our own two feet. *Remember, the issues are within your tissues.*

I will be describing here the biological participants in the process of depression based on recent scientific discoveries. We will discuss proteins and amino acids, how the body processes them, how they get converted into neurotransmitters, and how—due to another series of cellular events—they can develop into physical and mental imbalances. These physical imbalances affect the *vata-pitta-kapha* systemic field and finally manifest as mental imbalances of the *sattva-rajas-tamas* systemic field. We will also compare the scientific understanding of these biological processes with ancient Ayurvedic knowledge.

Proteins and Amino Acids

Proteins are constructed from a set of twenty amino acids, eight of which are essential. A complete or whole protein is defined as one that includes an adequate proportion of all eight of the essential amino acids required for your dietary needs. The ones your body cannot produce must be obtained from your daily food.[1]

Proteins are large molecules composed of long chains of amino acids stuck together. They play a crucial role in all our biological processes, and their amino acids are involved in countless important bodily processes. The role of amino acids goes beyond being simply the building blocks of our cells and tissues; they are also fundamental to the synthesis of other proteins, enzymes (biological accelerators of reactions), hormones (messengers to other organs), neurotransmitters (chemical messengers sending information between neurons), membrane receptors (receiving external signals), and much more that takes place within the body to provide us good mental function and stabilization.[2]

We will focus on the role of three amino acids associated with depression. They are the precursors of the neurotransmitters serotonin, norepinephrine, and dopamine, playing a vital role in supporting a balanced mental approach to life.

Here is a wider view of the number of neurons in our bodies and their distribution:

- Brain: sixty-five to ninety billion neurons
  - Cerebral cortex: ten to twenty billion neurons
  - Cerebellum: fifty-five to seventy billion neurons
- Gastrointestinal nervous system: some five hundred million neuron "gut-brain" connections
- Heart: about forty thousand sensory neurons, "heart-brain" links that can sense, feel, learn, think, remember, and harmonize

Scientists are still trying to unravel the networks by which the gut-brain and the heart-brain send messages to the head-brain, how the body feels and harmonizes its needs, and more.[3]

Tryptophan, Phenylalanine, and Tyrosine

Previous chapters described the *prakruti* trilogy *vata-pitta-kapha* and the *manas* trilogy *sattva-rajas-tamas*. Let's consider now the trilogy based on the three amino acids tryptophan, phenylalanine, and tyrosine: where they come from, their functions, and how they play an important role in mental health balance (as precursors of three neurotransmitters). Based on that information we will be able to examine the attributed role of serotonin, norepinephrine, and dopamine (our fourth trilogy) and their influence on mental health and potential contribution to depression.

Tryptophan

This is an essential amino acid with the following main functions:

- Calms anxiety, promotes sleep, reduces headaches
- Precursor to serotonin in the brain
- Competes with five other amino acids to pass through the blood-brain barrier and enter the brain, affecting mental activity
- Stimulates growth hormone
- Synthesizes melatonin (neurohormone)
- Maintains the body's protein balance
- Needs vitamin B6 for conversion to serotonin
- With lysine, carnitine, and taurine, lowers cholesterol and risk of arterial spasms

The FDA recommended daily allowance of tryptophan is 0.29 gm for the average adult. Tryptophan is present in most dietary proteins. It is particularly abundant in chocolate, oats, dried dates, dairy products, eggs, beans, sesame, chickpeas, almonds, walnuts, sunflower seeds, pumpkin seeds, buckwheat, spirulina, peanuts, butternut squash seeds, sea vegetables, wheat, leafy greens, and organic/genetically unmodified soybeans.

Deficiency of tryptophan is observed in connection with depression, insomnia, and chronic fatigue syndrome. An excess is observed in connection with higher blood levels of free fatty acids, intake of salicylates (aspirin), and sleep deprivation.

Phenylalanine

This is an essential amino acid precursor for the following functions:

- Pain reliever
- Converts to tyrosine in the liver, becoming the precursor to catecholamines and dopamine
- Powerful antidepressant; enhances mood, clarity of thought, concentration, and memory; used in the treatment of Parkinson's disease
- Precursor to the hormone thyroxine
- Suppresses appetite
- Major part of collagen formation

Phenylalanine is considered safe in the quantities found in normal foods. However, individuals with the genetic disorder phenylketonuria cannot metabolize this amino acid and must minimize consumption due to the risk of serious health problems. Foods high in protein, including soy products, eggs, seafood, meat, beans, and nuts contain phenylalanine. Eating a variety of protein-rich foods throughout the day will provide you with all the amino acids your body needs, including phenylalanine.[4]

Deficiency of phenylalanine is observed in connection with depression, obesity, cancer, AIDS, and Parkinson's disease.

Caution: phenylalanine should be avoided in cases of high blood pressure, pregnancy, pigmented melanoma, phenylketonuria, lack of phenylalanine hydroxylase, and panic disorder/anxiety attacks.[5]

Tyrosine

This is a nonessential amino acid. It can also be synthesized in the body from the essential amino acid phenylalanine. It plays a structural and functional role at the cell membrane level. Tyrosine's main functions are:

- Metabolism booster, antidepressant
- Precursor of dopamine, norepinephrine, epinephrine, and melanin
- Precursor of thyroxine and growth hormone
- Precursor of alkaloids, phenols, and pigments
- Role in coenzyme Q10 synthesis
- Increases energy
- Improves mental clarity and concentration
- Effective antidepressant for norepinephrine-deficient depressions
- Requires a form of vitamin B6 to be converted into noradrenaline

Deficiency is observed in connection with depression, chronic fatigue syndrome, Gulf War syndrome, hypothyroidism, Parkinson's disease, and drug addiction and dependency. Excess is observed in connection with hyperthyroidism, chronic liver disease, and cirrhosis.[6]

All body-mind biological processes involve molecular reactions and are controlled by specific enzymes requiring the presence of enzymatic cofactors or coenzymes to function properly. Cofactors are nonprotein chemical compounds or "helper" molecules that assist enzymes in their biological action, such as the metal ions magnesium ($Mg2+$), copper ($Cu+$), and manganese ($Mn2+$). Examples of coenzymes include the B vitamins. These molecules are all present in a wholesome diet. A well-balanced diet based on your *prakruti* constitution and wholesome foods will provide all the cofactors and coenzymes you need without intake of vitamin and mineral supplements.

Neurotransmitters

Neurotransmitters are chemical messenger molecules produced within brain cells. They carry, boost, and balance signals between nerve cells

311

and other cells in the body. These messengers can affect an extensive variety of physical and psychological functions, including mood, heart rate, sleep, appetite, and fear. Billions of neurotransmitter molecules work constantly to keep your brain functioning, handling everything from your breathing to your heartbeat to your learning processes and concentration levels.

Although the signals that are carried within each cell are electrical, chemicals such as neurotransmitters play a critical role at the junctions between cells, enabling the transfer of information across the gaps, which are called synapses. The main purpose of a neurotransmitter is to cross the extracellular space and reach the other side of the synapse by binding onto specific proteins, called receptors, that are typically located on the surface of the receiving brain cell.

Think of a neurotransmitter as a neighbor crossing the street while carrying a set of house keys. Receptors are like the doors of the houses on the other side of the street. The neurotransmitter has a key for every house, but only the right key will give access to the right door. When the right neurotransmitter binds to the right receptor, the signal is transmitted across the synapse to the receiving cell, setting up a cascade of chemical reactions within that cell that ultimately results in the continuation of the electrical signal through the cell and farther into the brain. There are trillions of synapses in your brain, each one acting as a critical interface where your body can regulate the chemical and electrical properties of your neural balance (homeostasis) while your brain is hard at work.[7]

Your brain uses various mechanisms to maintain a healthy balance of neurotransmitters and ensure that its response does not get out of hand, especially in situations when it is under neurophysiological stress or pressure. Biomedical science has described more than one hundred known neurotransmitters, some of them originating from amino acids. Getting the most attention by far are dopamine, serotonin, norepinephrine, glutamate, glycine, acetylcholine, and gamma-amino butyric acid. Here our main focus is on serotonin, norepinephrine, and dopamine because these three chemical messengers' roles are more associated with several mental health conditions, including depression and low mood. They also regulate other bodily functions and processes such as sleep, memory, and metabolism.

For more than five decades, the prevailing theory was that depression is caused by a chemical imbalance in the brain—a lack of serotonin. One argument given to justify the serotonin hypothesis is that drugs that elevate serotonin have been shown to help some people with depression. However, the scope of research has expanded significantly to look at the complex array of other factors that may contribute to depression, without denying the important role of serotonin. For example, we would not claim that headaches are the result of aspirin deficiency. Other groups within and outside the psychiatric medical field have even suggested that the whole concept that depression is the result of low serotonin levels is a myth, cleverly perpetuated by pharmaceutical company marketing that has turned depression into a biochemical entity to be exploited financially. We will not dwell on such matters, but we do want to draw attention to the challenges to the view that depression is mainly a chemical imbalance treatable by drugs.[8]

Ongoing studies continue to provide compelling reasons to believe that interactions between serotonin, norepinephrine, and dopamine play a role in the processes of mental health and depression. Recent studies provide more evidence that other neurotransmitters of amino acid origin, such as norepinephrine and DOPA, are associated with the inhibition or decrease of nervous activity.

Let me be clear about one point: neurotransmitters do not act independently. They are always interacting with and affecting each other in a perpetual effort to maintain a careful chemical balance within the body. There are strong links between the serotonin, norepinephrine, and dopamine systems, both structurally and functionally, and research is underway to explore and clarify their functions and how that amazing perpetual biochemical dance works. I will focus my description on recent studies of dopamine, serotonin, and norepinephrine, and I will integrate this information with the Ayurvedic concepts of *prakruti* and *triguna*.

Dopamine, Serotonin, and Norepinephrine

Dopamine:
Inertia, or the "Pleasure/Compulsion/Heavy Molecule"

Dopamine, also called the "pleasure molecule," is produced from its precursor chemical L-DOPA, synthesized in the brain and kidneys. Our body also uses dopamine to create the neurotransmitters norepinephrine and epinephrine.

Dopamine is produced by neurons and cells in the medulla of the adrenal glands. The primary metabolic pathway is:

L-phenylalanine → L-tyrosine → L-DOPA → dopamine

The direct precursor of dopamine, L-DOPA, can be produced indirectly from the essential amino acid phenylalanine or directly from the nonessential amino acid tyrosine. These two amino acids are found in every protein and are readily available in food, with tyrosine being more common.[9]

Although dopamine is also found in many types of food, it cannot cross the very strict blood-brain barrier, the gateway that surrounds and protects our brain. Consequently, it needs to be synthesized inside the brain to play its neuronal role.

In the brain, the role of dopamine is to send signals to other nerve cells; this is why it is called an "excitatory" neurotransmitter. Interestingly, the brain has several distinct dopamine pathways, one of which plays a major role in reward-motivated behavior.

However, the nerve cells do not want to be *over*stimulated; they just want to be excited enough. Consider the case of an overstimulated neuron, increasingly and continuously overexcited. This overstimulation depletes the neuron's functional energy so that it basically tires itself out, which eventually may result in cellular death. To protect themselves from this scenario, neurons have developed a self-defense mechanism called downregulation of the receptors. This means the next time the nerve cell encounters that molecule of dopamine, it will not respond as strongly because it has downregulated its receptors, providing fewer of them for the dopamine to bind to. In lay terms: you get a hit, you get a rush. If that continues, next time you will need a bigger hit to get the same rush, due to downregulation of the receptors. The next time after that you will need an even bigger hit, and this process of craving a bigger and bigger hit continues until a huge hit provides no rush at all. This is how drug users develop increased tolerance to the drugs they use. Once an organism enters that repetitive process, the nerve cells eventually start to die. This process is related to addiction (biochemical changes in the brain after continued substance abuse).

Dopamine is considered to be the "reward or recompense" neurotransmitter that tells your brain you want more. However, every substance or behavior that releases dopamine in the extreme leads to addiction. Dopamine is the molecule that motivates you to pursue your goals and gives you a surge of reinforcing pleasure when attaining them. Self-doubt, procrastination, and lack of enthusiasm are associated with low levels of dopamine. Most types of reward increase the level of dopamine in the brain, and many addictive drugs increase dopamine neuronal activity. Animal studies have shown that animals with small concentrations of dopamine choose to pursue an easier option that provides less reward/food, and animals with higher levels of dopamine apply the effort needed to get a larger amount of food.

In our bodies, dopamine plays the following roles:

- Inside the central nervous system (CNS) it is involved in motor control and in controlling the release of various hormones. These pathways and neuronal cellular groups form a modulatory dopamine system.

- Outside the CNS, dopamine functions largely as a local biochemical messenger. For example:

  - In the blood vessels it inhibits norepinephrine release and acts as a vasodilator.

  - In the kidneys it increases sodium elimination and urine output.

- In the pancreas it reduces insulin production.

- In the gut it reduces gastrointestinal motility and protects the intestinal mucosa.

- In the immune system it reduces the activity of lymphocytes.

Except for the blood vessels, dopamine is produced near to these peripheral systems and exerts its effects on the nearby cells.

Several diseases of the nervous system, such as Parkinson's disease, schizophrenia, ADHD, and restless leg syndrome, are associated with abnormal functions of the dopamine system.[10]

Serotonin:
Truth, or the "Contentment/Clarity/Happiness Molecule"

Now let's consider the neurotransmitter serotonin, derived from the essential amino acid tryptophan, which is largely produced by our gastrointestinal tract, blood platelets, and the CNS. Serotonin is widely thought to be a contributor to feelings of well-being and happiness by sending signals between cells and body organs. While its most well-known functions have to do with brain function and mood, most of the serotonin in your body is found in the digestive system. We can call it the "contentment or serenity" neurotransmitter or the "happiness molecule" that tells our brains we don't need any more, thus reducing food consumption. Serotonin keeps feelings stable and should prevent any major fluctuations in happiness, which is why serotonin deficiency has often been associated with depression.

We previously discussed that around 90 percent of the body's total serotonin is located in the gut, where our microbiome manufactures about 95 percent of the body's supply. Serotonin is secreted when food enters the small intestine, where it helps to stimulate contractions that push food through your intestines. For example, your gut releases extra serotonin when you eat something containing an allergen or harmful microorganisms. The additional serotonin makes the contractions in your gut move faster in order to evacuate the harmful food, usually through vomiting or diarrhea. Low serotonin in your gut is associated with constipation.

The remaining 5 to 10 percent of the body's serotonin is synthesized by neurons of the CNS, where it performs various functions such as the regulation of mood, appetite, and sleep. Serotonin also performs some mental functions, including memory and learning functions. It is thought that modulation of serotonin at the level of neuron cell interaction is the way several classes of pharmacological antidepressants work.

It is important to note that if you take serotonin orally, it will not have a particular action because the molecule cannot cross the blood-brain barrier. However, the amino acid tryptophan and its product 5-HTP (5-hydroxytryptophan), from which serotonin is produced, do cross the blood-brain barrier. These compounds are accessible as dietary supplements and could work to effectively increase serotonin.[11]

For all the above reasons, serotonin is an inhibitory neurotransmitter instead of excitatory; it performs the opposite action of dopamine. Serotonin causes the neighboring neuron to stay silent. You cannot overdose on too much happiness, because serotonin does not injure neurons. But there's one molecule that downregulates serotonin activity, and that is dopamine. So the more pleasure you seek, the unhappier you eventually become. If we include stress in the equation, it will disinhibit dopamine even further, and cortisol (our stress hormone) downregulates the serotonin receptor, making it even harder to generate happiness; as a result, depression may manifest. Now you can understand why some see addiction and depression as two sides of the same coin.

Supplements that are said to increase serotonin include herbs such as arctic root *(Rhodiola rosea)*, brahmi *(Bacopa monnieri)*, curcuma, DHA *(docosahexaenoic acid)*, ginger *(Zingiber officinale)*, ginkgo *(Ginkgo biloba)*, St. John's wort *(Hypericum perforatum)*, oregano oil, and 1-theanine, which is derived from tea leaves. Other products said to boost serotonin include omega-3 essential oils, amino acids, phosphatidylserine, vitamin B6, vitamin B12, and vitamin D.[12]

Norepinephrine:
Action, or the "Acting/Energetic/Desire Molecule"

Norepinephrine (or noradrenaline) is a neurotransmitter found in the brain that is very similar in structure to the hormone neurotransmitter epinephrine (or adrenaline). It is normally essential in activating you for action. Norepinephrine is the main neurotransmitter of your body's sympathetic nervous system—the "triggering" part of your body's autonomic nervous system, which helps to regulate your body systems in response to changing situational demands such as danger or stress.

Norepinephrine also has a broad effect in our bodies (i.e., in the peripheral parts of the nervous system). For that function it is released directly into the blood via the adrenal medulla, and it has an effect on your peripheral nerves when it plays a role in the activation of your body's sympathetic ("prepared to respond") nervous system.

Norepinephrine is the molecule in your brain that influences your level of neurological arousal. It has a generally modulatory effect across a broad range of brain functions, including wakefulness, memory, and alertness, enabling the brain to respond effectively to any challenges or threats it encounters. Norepinephrine is closely related to its hormonal equivalent, epinephrine, which acts not only as a neurotransmitter in the brain but also as a hormone in the body, acting via adrenoreceptors. This action helps to ensure that the body/brain system is ready to deal with physical or emotional stressors and stimulates a specific set of extensive body changes that are generally known as the "fight or flight" responses.

Once it is no longer required within the synaptic extracellular space, transporter mechanisms take norepinephrine back into the cells surrounding the synaptic space. Once within the cell it is recycled or broken down by enzymes.[13]

FACTORS INFLUENCING NEUROTRANSMITTER BALANCE AND POSSIBLY CAUSING DEPRESSION

Your brain needs to obtain the proper neurochemical building blocks, either directly from essential amino acids from your diet, or from carbohydrates and fats, which in the case of tyrosine can be converted into amino acids. Keeping a healthy balance of neurotransmitters requires a wholesome, balanced diet. This involves making sure your brain has sufficient energy supplies, amino acids, and the various vitamins and minerals that are cofactors in the enzymatic pathways. Though there are many foods that contain neurotransmitters and their amino acid precursors, remember that their ability to participate in your brain's response depends on how easily they can cross the blood-brain barrier—the gateway from the body's bloodstream into the brain.

Neurotransmitters like dopamine and serotonin cannot cross the blood-brain barrier because they do not possess the necessary transport mechanisms to get them across. In contrast, their precursor amino acids can sometimes cross the blood-brain barrier. However, since the various amino acids often compete to determine which one gets to cross over and keep the balance, it is the relative levels of the amino acids that are important, not just the absolute levels ingested.

Neurotransmitter Receptors' Role in Body-Mind-Consciousness

In our bodies, each of the many neurotransmitters has its own set of unique receptors to allow the process of neurotransmission. They interact with both extracellular signals and molecules within the cell, affecting cell functions without necessarily entering the cell. In our particular case, these receptors are mostly present in the cellular membrane, to allow them to receive the message transmitted between neurons.[14,15]

Following are some brief descriptions of the receptors involved in the body-mind-consciousness process.

Serotonin Receptors

There are seven families of serotonin receptors modulating functions such as the release of neurotransmitters, including epinephrine, norepinephrine, dopamine, gamma-amino butyric acid, glutamate, and acetylcholine, as well as many hormones. After serotonin interacts with one of its specific receptors, it can even modify nuclear proteins associated with DNA.[16] Serotonin receptors guide and supervise a variety of biological and neurological processes, such as anxiety, aggression, appetite, cognition, learning, memory, mood, nausea, sleep, and thermoregulation.

Serotonin receptors are the target of a variety of pharmaceutical and illicit drugs, including antidepressants, antipsychotics, anorectics, antiemetics, gastroprokinetic agents, antimigraine agents, hallucinogens, and entactogens.[17]

Norepinephrine Receptors (Adrenoreceptors)

These receptors are found on nerve fibers and communicate with many parts of the forebrain. They are targets of the catecholamines, mainly epinephrine and norepinephrine. The adrenergic receptors have two main groups, alpha and beta, with several subtypes.[18]

Dopamine Receptors

Dopamine receptors are implicated in many neurological processes of our CNS, such as motivation, pleasure, cognition, memory, learning, and fine motor control, as well as modulation of neuroendocrine signaling. Abnormal dopamine receptor signaling and dopaminergic nerve functions are implicated in numerous neuropsychiatric disorders. Therefore, dopamine receptors are common neurologic drug targets. Antipsychotics are often dopamine receptor antagonists, and psychostimulants are usually indirect agonists of dopamine receptors. There are at least five subtypes of dopamine receptors. Therefore, a balance between descending controls, both excitatory and inhibitory, can be altered in various discomfort states.[19]

In this chapter we've discussed basic information to give you an idea of how your body-mind functions at a molecular level. By considering the complexity of the roles of the amino acids, their conversion into neurotransmitters, and how neurotransmitters interact with receptors, you can understand how many imbalances originate and then go on to cause disorders such as depression and anxiety.

> *The notion of looking on at life has always been hateful to me. What am I if I am not a participant? In order to be, I must participate.*
>
> —ANTOINE DE SAINT-EXUPÉRY

KOSHAS

Now we will discuss the Ayurvedic concept of *kosha,* a Sanskrit term meaning "bondage," "boundary," "prison," or "limitation." For some scholars the term *kosha* also means error resulting from ignorance.

Centuries ago, when Ayurvedic scholars such as Sushruta studied the anatomy of the physical body, they also studied a more dynamic anatomy based on the understanding of how tissues are created, their functionality, and their interconnection, under the name of five *koshas: annamaya, pranamaya, manomaya, vijnanamaya,* and *anandamaya.* The term *kosha* has been translated as "sheaths"; with all due respect to the scholars, I prefer to describe *koshas* as fields of different energetic qualities. Today we can ponder the *koshas* as a concept, but for the scholars of those days this concept resulted from deep research, described in detail many centuries ago.[20]

A short description of the five *koshas* follows:

- *Annamaya kosha:* the physical body field composed of the five elements and giving form to the being; maintained by food *(anna)*

- *Pranamaya kosha:* the physical body field nourished of *prana* (breathing life force); maintained by yoga activities, e.g., *pranayama* and *asanas*

- *Manomaya kosha:* the mind (senses) or mental field gathering thoughts, feelings, and emotions; maintained through meditation

- *Vijnanamaya kosha:* the subtle knowledge and wisdom field; maintained by developing perception, contemplation, and intuition

- *Anandamaya kosha:* the blissful innermost field of all pervasive knowledge; represented by unending joy, love, peace, and complete happiness

When integrating Ayurveda with Western science, we can conduct an analysis solely using the rational mind, or we can evaluate ideas in light of lived experience in our human bodies. I invite you to use the second perspective when thinking about the *koshas.*

We require carbohydrates, proteins, and fats for daily life. Through the coordinated work of our various bodily organs, these substances provide us their energy, which we use to maintain our metabolic processes. In this particular case, the process of digestion transforms energy from the form of food to another kind of energy integrated into our physical bodies. This is how we derive nourishment at the level of *annamaya kosha.*

The next less dense and more subtle energy provided to our bodies is *pranamaya kosha.* Ayurveda says we are nourished by *prana* through breathing, which involves the integration of oxygen into our tissues and the secretion of combusted materials under the form of another gas (CO_2). In addition, we discussed earlier the effects of molecules of nitric oxide (NO), which are responsible for so many subtle functions and are a breathing force in the real sense of the term.

Food provides energy, allowing us to move and live, responding to different situations in both physical and mental ways. Our actions and emotions come as the result of biochemical reactions that take place in our bodies. Thoughts create emotions, and different emotions create different actions, so that there is a force represented by these biochemical changes in our body. To my understanding, via the participation of *annamaya kosha* and *pranamaya kosha,* this kind of biochemical energy arising from the physiological processes described above is the creational energy that makes it possible for different actions to take place.

This vital energetic force or cellular intelligence, which is able to interconnect all our body systems, is what Ayurveda calls *prana*. It is *prana* that allows the next level of energetic field, *manomaya kosha*, to fully participate. This manifestation of mind-body duality produces physical and mental *ama*, which Ayurveda says is the cause of many kinds of disease (*Ca. Su.* 20/3).

If we move one level down toward *manomaya kosha*, we witness the mental field of perpetual change of thoughts and emotions. We know by now how the interaction of *annamaya kosha* and *pranamaya kosha* allows amino acids and neurotransmitters to participate with *prana* in bringing our mental faculties into manifestation. Gradually we become aware of a more subtle field or level of energy or existence, and we witness our own inability to control some of those reactions, even when they manifest right in front of us.

The three *koshas* above can be found under states of balance and imbalance as a result of our participation or the lack of it. The next two *koshas*—*vijnanamaya kosha*, or field of knowledge and wisdom, and *anandamaya kosha*, represented by endless joy, love, peace, and whole happiness—are much too subtle for the ordinary day-to-day intervention that Ayurveda specializes in. Still, we may consider that life has invited us to work in that direction by becoming aware of our own actions and reactions.

It is important to note that these five *koshas* are always interacting with one another in a bidirectional way at all times. As a result of getting older there is a sense of direction through *annamaya kosha*, and there is the possibility of a retreat of awareness toward *anandamaya kosha*.

What I value enormously about the science of Ayurveda is the way it keeps teaching me to develop my attention and from there to appreciate the fragile relativity of my existence and beliefs. Some Ayurvedic scholars say that by negating or removing each of the *koshas* we can discover our true nature, since they represent levels of ignorance or confusion covering our deeper nature *(atma)*. They say the purpose of our existence is to experience that cosmic self by understanding the *koshas* and then separating them. Perhaps we do not all like to address these issues in our daily life as a result of our lack of acceptance of our own fragility, ignorance, egocentrism, and sense of mortality. Only in difficult times, when we can either see ourselves dying or other people dying around us, do we believe we might one day die. Otherwise, due to our need to believe in our own continuity, we keep avoiding the possibility of our death.

As a scientist my education was based on quantifying what I was able to see. I related only to analytical processes and became overidentified with my role. Gradually, through the practice of Ayurvedic principles, I started observing my inability to quantify and understand everything. By focusing my attention on that part of myself, a connection with a deeper part of myself slowly emerged. I started taking proper care of myself and of the life around me. I felt a connection with the earth when seeing myself as just a minuscule part of nature compared to the universe. At moments like that, the duality disappears, even if only for a small fraction of time. Even now as I write these words, I am trying to compare myself to that reality instead of realizing that I am part of it. But I keep trying.

You, too, could start trying to move with joy toward the unknown: yourself!

Ayurvedic Psychology and Psychotherapy

AYURVEDIC PSYCHOLOGY'S UNIQUE BASIS FOR TREATMENT OF DEPRESSION

So far we have focused on Ayurvedic protocols that often mirror or correlate to modern Western medicine. Where this correspondence is not evident, we have explored the rationale and efficacy behind Ayurveda's use of specific protocols or treatments (e.g., *pranayamas, panchakarma*). The protocols elucidated so far have focused on physical and mental food as the source of healing and lifestyle adjustments that aim to accelerate the restoration of balance Ayurvedic treatments have focused on.

In this chapter, I want to introduce you to the realm of Ayurveda's unique tool kit for treating depression and other conditions of the mind, expressed through Ayurvedic psychology and psychotherapy, for which there is no corresponding canon of work in Western medicine.

· · · · · · · ·

Ayurvedic psychology and psychotherapy's foundational basis is rooted in the core treatises of the Indian philosophy of Vedanta.

· · · · · · · ·

These texts have been available to us for thousands of years as epic tales of challenge, adversity, heroism, and euphoric triumph, but we in the West have remained largely ignorant of their powerful healing properties.

So far we have focused on how the general field of Ayurvedic medicine is a holistic psychological and physical treatment system, treating both mental *(manas)* and physical *(sharira)* imbalances. Now we will explore unique components of Ayurvedic psychology, which provide a fascinating and effective range of treatments and protocols that separate it from mainstream Western approaches to the treatment of depression and other mental conditions.

For this section of the book, it is relevant to introduce the ancient Ayurvedic concept of identification, also known as *maya,* as a support to the holistic approach of self-observation or psychological treatments. *Maya* is derived from the Sanskrit *maa,* meaning "measure," and *yaa,* meaning "experience." It concerns what we can measure and experience as reality. However, reality varies from person to person; it is a product of cause and effect, time and space, and is always changing.

You do not need to read Sanskrit or know the contents of *Charaka Samhita* to practice and benefit from the many health, diet, and lifestyle protocols we have covered in previous chapters. In the hands of a skilled Ayurvedic physician, you will be guided in the right direction based on your *prakruti, vikruti,* and *manas prakruti.* All of Ayurveda's concepts and procedures are set out in detailed texts that have guided physicians for centuries, irrespective of the Ayurvedic knowledge of the patient.

In Ayurvedic psychology, however, we must delve deeper into the origins of Ayurveda to understand the psychological treatment components of this system. It is not possible to avoid the core philosophical texts because these texts *are* the material used to treat mental conditions.

. . . .

The words are the medicine.

. . . .

Epic tales are the device used. These stunning narratives are embedded in the core philosophical texts, which are taught and used today much as they were centuries ago in India. These narratives seek to connect us to the principle that the original nature of mind is undisturbed, clear, and full of equanimity and that this state is achievable through practices to remove ignorance and misconceptions that fill it through desire, aversion, ego, and misplaced fears. They are road maps detailing the challenges and missteps we all face along the way, and they shine light on pathways away from the imbalances we are experiencing.

To appreciate this fully, it is necessary to remember Ayurveda's view of the mind and consciousness. The medical scholars say most diseases, including mental imbalances, result from improper use of our senses, which affects our choices and subsequent behaviors (*Ca. Su.* 1/54). This principle is expounded throughout the epics in various forms: the origins of disputes (with others and within oneself), the impact of outcomes determined either by chance or other factors, and so on.

We will briefly examine the key texts and provide some insight into each. This is a vast and profoundly rich subject area, and my aim here is to draw your attention and pique your interest to explore this more yourself.

First I want to address the matter of fate, fatalism, or determinism, with respect to Ayurveda's approach to any type of imbalance or ill health of the mind and body. I often hear that ancient philosophies are "highly deterministic" of the human condition. We often hear someone say, "Oh, that's karma," when something that seems inevitable happens, or "Oh, that's my dharma," when there is something we would like to do for others. So, the question arises in Ayurveda: are there predispositions of *manas* constitutions such that we have fixed, rigid mental states we are destined to occupy?

Ayurveda says no: we start with a clean mental sheet. However, the mental state of humans is generally flexible. We can be passionate *(rajas)* or ignorant *(tamas)*, and in some cases we would like to do good *(sattva)*. Nevertheless, Ayurveda says that, despite our changing state of mind, there is one main quality that prevails in each person—if they do not make efforts to rebalance. This can be evaluated according to the frequency of that quality. For example, if someone manifests mostly with qualities of passion, despite bouts of both ignorance and goodness, then that person can be considered to primarily be of *rajasic* nature.

Here, in seeking to determine a person's main mental quality, incorporating Vedic psychology could be a productive element of interaction between a physician and a patient when assessing patterns of physical and mental activities that may give rise to factors affecting our mental health, and that help define the predominant *manas* constitution. By putting into practice some of the Ayurvedic methodologies described here, you can learn how to observe these patterns. Gradually you actively participate in the process of observing the recurrent patterns of the mind, the range of your emotions, and perhaps the extent of your misperceptions, all of which is difficult to acknowledge in our ordinary lives without support mechanisms and techniques specific to self-observation. In becoming this observer of patterns, one sees what needs to change in order to bring oneself to a more balanced mental and physical state.

To achieve that state, we need to understand how the entire body-mind-consciousness system operates, not just how different parts of the body operate irrespective of one another and disconnected from the mind. This is fully in keeping with Ayurveda's holistic approach to the patient.

I am addressing this specific subject matter not as a psychologist or a psychiatrist but as a medical scientist, an Ayurvedic doctor, and someone who, as a result of some deeply traumatic accidents, was instructed to embark upon a lifelong regime of antidepressants and painkillers—which I rejected for an alternative path that puts me in front of you here today.

Before focusing on how Ayurveda perceives our psychological framework, let me briefly return to our framework of the Western perspective on mental imbalances as a point of reference.

CLASSIFYING DEPRESSION

Depression is defined as a group of mental disorders associated with a decrease in the quality of a person's mood, causing impairments in daily life. Specifically, the American Psychiatric Association defines major depressive disorder as a common and serious medical illness that negatively affects how you feel, the way you think, and how you act.[1] To refresh, the main types of depression can be broadly classified as:

- Major depressive disorder or clinical depression: persistently depressed mood, fatigue, lack of motivation and focus, feeling guilty, suicidal thoughts, changes in body weight and sleep
- Persistent depressive disorder: mild but lasts for two years or longer
- Bipolar disorder: mood episodes range from intense high energy with an "up" mood to "low" depressive moods
- Premenstrual dysphoric disorder: signs appear a week or two before the period starts and usually go away two to three days after the period starts
- Postpartum depression: occurs in the weeks or months after giving birth
- Seasonal affective disorder: often occurs during winter months and when there is less sunlight
- Situational depression or stress response syndrome: occurs due to trouble managing stressful life events, e.g., death, divorce
- Atypical depression: a depressed mood that can brighten or become cheerful in response to positive events

These diagnoses can be treated by two types of medical professionals:

- Psychiatrists are trained medical doctors, licensed to write prescriptions. Many of their patients will be on medication such as antidepressants as part of a management program aiming to reduce or contain the manifestations of their condition.
- Psychologists specialize in the study of mind and behavior or in the treatment of mental, emotional, and behavioral disorders. Treatment focuses on psychotherapeutic approaches.

Despite some of the previously described limitations of the Western approach to the treatment of depression, it is relevant to acknowledge the contribution of 150 years of Western psychology protocols, supported by the scientific discoveries of how body and mind function as a result of advances in biomedical technology.

AYURVEDIC METHODS FOR TREATMENT OF DEPRESSION

- Psychotherapy *(sattvavajaya):* literally translates to "uplifting of the mind from the depressive condition."[2] Ayurveda says the lack of connection or proper contact with our senses is one of the principal causes of physical and mental diseases (*Ca. Su.* 16/13–19).

- Rational therapy *(yukti vyapasrya):* analyzes the origin of the imbalance based on your *tridosha* and plans how to reestablish balance through the support of suitable therapies, medicines, diet, and lifestyle changes.[3]

- Faith therapy *(daiva vyapasrya):* psychological treatment where the patient embraces treatments of a spiritual dimension, such as prayer, chanting songs or mantras, or *poojas* (a combination of meditation, austerity, and chanting). These methods are often described as spiritual treatments, and their efficacy lies in the profound impact on the body-mind-consciousness system. For example, the resonance created by correctly chanting certain mantras affects specific organs while pacifying the mind.[4]

- Yogic techniques: a practical tool to control and pacify the mind, described earlier.[5]

Charaka Samhita describes treatments involving internal and external application of medication:

- Purification of body-mind toxins, pacifying and removing the cause; *panchakarma (sodhana)*

- Pacification of the disease by procedures involving internal medication *(samana)*

- Minor surgical procedures to battle mental disease (*Ca. Su.*11/46)

Ayurvedic scholars understood that psychological disorders and physical illness can occur at the same time in the same individual, and they developed protocols for the observation of the patient's psychological history and physical-mental constitution. The present mental state is determined by a combination of observation, palpation, and inquiring about the patient's lifestyle, diet, habits, and environment to get a complete understanding of the patient's *prakruti*, *vikruti*, and *manas prakruti* natures.

Ayurvedic Psychopathology

Behind each disorder there is a specific biological origin, prompting physical and mental imbalances that aggravate your *prakruti*. This is due to factors such as lifestyle, diet, heredity, stress, and environmental changes and adaptations. All of these could generate unmetabolized, undigested particles of both physical and mental nature, i.e., *ama*. In terms of your physical body, this aggravation challenges different tissues and organs depending on your *prakruti* in the following ways:

- *Vata* predominance affects mostly the colon.

- *Pitta* predominance affects the intestines.

- *Kapha* predominance affects the stomach.

Ayurvedic treatises say *ama* accumulation provokes gradual imbalances from the cellular level up through the organ level, targeting the *doshas* of the individual that are particularly weak and lodging in places where *ama* can create more imbalance. This type of place is called *khavaigunya*, or "weak or defective space." The innumerable nerve cells and fibers, and the countless pathways between networks transmitting nerve impulses to the different parts of the body, are directly connected to the original factors responsible for the process of *khavaigunya*. How many times under stressful conditions do we experience a recurrence of lower back pain, right on cue, or irritable bowel syndrome, or migraines? The Ayurvedic concept stating that any existing defective or weak space in your physical body—resulting from previous physical trauma, chronic disease, or hereditary influence, for example—becomes a place where aggravated *doshas* can easily lodge, incubate, and generate dysfunctional conditions also applies to your mind.

In your body-mind system, everything is interconnected. As a consequence, if you are living in a state of repressed emotions, this can be toxic, and these repressed emotions could end up lodging in a weak space in your mind, creating mental imbalances. The physical is the mental.

Nurturing a Supportive State of Mind

Because the mind and body are one, *ama* is also affected by our quality of consciousness and can be treated by increasing *sattva* qualities in our lives while being careful not to overindulge in *rajas* and *tamas*. *Sattva* is the principle of trust and clarity of perception. *Rajas* is the principle of action and movement. *Tamas* is the principle of inertia, heaviness, and decay. Each of these three *gunas* has a place in our lives, although *ama* shares qualities with *rajas* and *tamas*, not *sattva*. Consequently, when trying to clear accumulated *ama*, it is important to grow *sattva* and to be mindful to balance *rajas* and *tamas*. Here are some suggestions for how to achieve this in your life:

- *Rajas* is balanced with the practice of compassion and patience.

- *Tamas* is counteracted by practicing selflessness and generosity.

- *Sattva* is stimulated by peace obtained via spiritual practice, cultivating unconditional love and contentment.

One does not need Ayurveda to understand the impact that cultivating a deeper respect and appreciation for yourself will have on your condition of depression. Patterns of reinforcing disapproval and even hate toward yourself can only be damaging to the healing process. It is time to accept deep within yourself: you have to give those patterns up. It is my deep personal conviction that once we have that internal acceptance that enough is enough, then we can recuperate our body's intelligence in a relatively well-managed way, starting with rebalancing at the cellular level.

Certain mental conditions could be of organic or functional character. Some types of depression could be functional if we consider the function of the *doshas*. *Vata dosha* (space/air) is primarily responsible for the flow of breath that nourishes the brain, the nervous system, and the rest of the tissues in the body by carrying with it the oxygenation required to facilitate cellular function. The function of *prana vata* is to fill space and maintain life. In that way, *vata*—via *prana*—can generate harm at the level of nerve tissues, leading to organic or functional disorders that diminish these functions, as is observed in the case of depression disorders.[6] Classical Ayurvedic texts describe various disorders under the name of psychosis.[7]

What Is Really Going On?

Under conditions of depression, one major mechanism is present: inertia. Do you recognize that feeling when you feel depressed—you wish you could run but you can only shuffle along? Mentally, you are speeding up, full of energy, but physically, you feel lethargic. These are the qualities of the *tamasic* state, and they are what we observe under conditions of depression. *Tamas* is characterized by inertia. We previously discussed how *tamasic* food and depression go hand in hand by disturbing our balance at many physical and mental levels. In certain conditions, such as overeating or reheating leftover or stale food, what was once *sattvic* food can turn *tamasic*. According to Ayurveda, foods that represent these features lose their Ayurvedic energy *(prana)* and therefore end up acting in a toxic way, making the body and mind lethargic and accelerating the decline into a less refined state of consciousness, finally ending in a state of depression.

These *tamasic* foods are not just about the quality *(guna)* and type of food. Remember, food is affected by how and where we prepare and eat it and the quantity in which we consume it. Any food that is overeaten turns *tamasic* in the long term. The best way to avoid food becoming *tamasic* is to consider three factors—moderation, moderation, and moderation—in the way we nourish both our body and our mind.

Psychophysiology vs. Psychopathology

Ayurvedic scholars specified that food with a light quality *(sattvic)* does not possess psychopathological elements and is considered to be psychophysiological. In contrast, both *rajasic* and *tamasic* foods are considered to have psychopathological elements when eaten in excess or in wrong ways. The Ayurvedic concept sees imbalance or the disease process as starting from the subtle, psychic level and from there influencing the physiology. Both negative and positive emotions have a direct effect on the body. Stress and anger will reduce a person's immunity. If such a status persists, it will set in motion the imbalance process on the somatic level. Mainstream medicine has come to terms with these facts and now recognizes them in the concept of psychoneuroimmunology.

Table 14.1. Organs and emotions

ORGAN	POSITIVE EMOTION	NEGATIVE EMOTION
Heart	Love and compassion	Grief
Lungs	Inspiration	Sorrow
Liver	Discrimination and judgment	Anger
Gallbladder	Collection and accumulation	Hate
Spleen	Protection	Attachment and greed
Kidney	Energy and vitality	Fear and insecurity
Colon	Absorption—essential/ nonessential	Nervousness

Ayurvedic Psychotherapy and Psychiatry

Ayurvedic psychotherapy has a philosophical foundation. As Charaka wrote, mental restraint or "mind control" can be achieved through spiritual knowledge, philosophical allegory, fortitude, remembrance, and concentration (*Ca. Su.* 8/17). Ayurveda adopts a complete psychosomatic-spiritual approach that attempts to maintain balanced mental health and to rebalance a healthy body state if there is any impairment.

. . . .

Ayurveda's allegorical approach to psychotherapy uses the epic tales from the foundational texts of the Vedic traditions and Hinduism as a source of treatment. The Ayurvedic psychotherapist is, in one sense, a storyteller, connecting the fortunes of the heroes and villains of these epic tales to the patient's own experiences.

. . . .

Indian Epics as Psychotherapeutic Treatment

The Ayurvedic description of the *triguna* of the mind—*sattva, rajas,* and *tamas*—can be restated as balance, arrogance, and indolence, respectively. Let us describe the concept of Ayurvedic psychotherapy by presenting parts of the epics Bhagavad Gita, Mahabharata, and Ramayana, for two main purposes:

- To remind you that mental health difficulties, including depression, have been present since the beginning of civilization. What is novel in Ayurvedic psychotherapy is the use of epic narratives to treat these difficulties.

- To empower you by helping you develop awareness of your potential to address your depression by ways other than antidepressive medication. The stories in many cases reflect a parallel description of your experience. They are also a timeline of outbreak and resolution, portrayed through a variety of protagonists who correspond to us.

Bhagavad Gita

The Bhagavad Gita or "Song of God" is one of the most influential treatises in Eastern philosophy. The Bhagavad Gita depicts the unity of truth-realization between humankind and nature, allowing the perfect balance of mind-body-consciousness. In India, psychotherapy has existed for a very long time interlinked with social norms, structures, and obligations in spiritual practices and rites, which were incorporated in Ayurveda, yoga, Buddhism, and other spiritual paths. The Bhagavad Gita, part of the Hindu epic Mahabharata, is a message of transcendent wisdom and selfless action aimed at inspiring people and providing a psychotherapy guide to Hindus.[8]

Ayurveda recommends addressing self-control of the mind. This is considered to be one of the most difficult tasks to undertake, requiring a combination of desire, willpower, and dedication, as described in the Bhagavad Gita by Lord Krishna. The Gita says balance of body-mind-consciousness can be attained through practice and detachment, by directing the thought processes *(cintya)*, substitution of ideas *(vicarya)*, channeling beliefs *(uhya)*, improving the objectives *(dhyeya)*, and proper guidance and advice for making right decisions *(samkalpa)*. These practices are considered valuable in terms of achieving self-examination and deriving motivation to observe situations, feelings, and emotions from another angle or perspective.

Mahabharata

The Mahabharata is considered one of the greatest epics of world literature, with several fascinating philosophical dialogues. The Gita represents chapters 25–42 of the Mahabharata, which has one hundred thousand verses. When looking at treatment of depression, the Mahabharata is a great textbook of psychopathology, and the Bhagavad Gita describes various aspects of psychotherapeutic assessments and interventions.

In this epic, the protagonists are prince Arjuna and the blue god Lord Krishna, the most revered deity of Hinduism. The main story revolves around two branches of a family who are in a war for the throne.

The real role of the Gita, to my understanding as a student of these classical texts, is to free you from a sense of guilt in your own framework and to resolve depression, guilt, shame, and blame by supplying vitality and self-esteem. It invites the person to calmly dig deeper into his or her own self and to develop an understanding of their own functioning by engaging in deep observation of the inner self.[9,10]

....

*The central theme of psychological inner observation is
seeing the expression of conflict related to the lack of acceptance
of aspects of the self. In several of these theories, distress arises
as a result of an internal disagreement with an external
obligation. By striking a compromise between the two,
acceptance and adaptation are promoted.*

....

The Gita involves Arjuna's successful resolution of conflicts between parts of the *triguna* forces described earlier, or in simpler words, one's inner battle.

Ramayana

Each god in the Hindu pantheon represents an aspect of our enlightened mind. This is how the dynamics of devotion and higher intelligence, of spirit and ego, of faith and ignorance come into form. In the epic known as Ramayana, the venerated Hanuman, one of the most popular Hindu gods, is represented as an enormous monkey (a mind that constantly jumps from thought to thought) of great physical strength, inner self-control, persistence, and dynamism, but with an inability to fully realize his potential to fight, fly, and perform great actions.

In the story, Hanuman was enlisted to locate Lord Rama's wife Queen Sita, who had been kidnapped by King Ravana and taken to Sri Lanka. Heading an army as a general, Hanuman, who had lost all memory of his full powers, needed a member of his company, named Jambavan, to remind him about them. Despite all the many ordeals described in the Ramayana, Hanuman fulfills his potential, conquers all obstructions, and achieves the task.[11,12]

The epic story shows us how to find courage and healing when dealing with difficult times, i.e., grief and loss, in the following three ways:

- We all have the tendency to label ourselves as the body-mind-ego we think we are, as a result of not knowing our real nature. A person with low self-esteem can relate to Hanuman and feel supported and cheered since he represents the one who opens up to the power of higher life forces, i.e., *prana*, that strengthens the mind by increasing our perseverance.

- Most patients who have lost confidence and who feel unable to meet life's challenges also believe they have the power to change their lives, but they feel they have temporarily lost the knowledge of their own strength or abilities, perhaps through illness or denying reality. Like Hanuman, they have to clear this indecision and move toward the realization of their true potential.

- To the specialists, this story stresses the impact of helpful intervention, as practiced by Jambavan. Just as Hanuman lost his way, the job of a therapist (like Jambavan) consists of empowering the patient to address challenges obstructing restoration of confidence.

Obviously Ayurvedic psychotherapy predates Freud, Jung, and many others. Mythologist Joseph Campbell said stories are important for the human race because they represent an archetypal adventure—the story of a child becoming a youth, or the awakening to a new world that begins at adolescence—that would help to provide a model for navigating these developmental stages.[13]

I suggest you discover more aspects of your inner self and the condition of depression through Indian philosophy by reading these two ancient classics of literature and enjoying their profound contents. Take them just as a couple of enjoyable reads, and perhaps you will be surprised to discover the similarities between the teachings of the Gita and psychology. You may come to realize how these ancient texts captured the essence of our physical and mental imbalances.

Ayurvedic Psychiatry

Ayurvedic practitioners integrated psychiatry into their discipline thousands of years ago. The various volumes of *Charaka Samhita* show that Ayurvedic doctors organized their science of mental health and disease after rejecting the ancient belief that mental imbalances were induced by demonic influences, instead associating them with our five senses. They proved that mental imbalances often originate from definite causes, and there exist definite measures to combat them. The importance of psychiatry in the Ayurvedic system is supported by texts showing the origins, expansion, and therapeutics of a system of treating mental imbalances. Ayurveda describes life as the multifaceted combination of body, senses, mind, and soul (*Ca. Su.* 1/42), showing that whatever affects life *(ayu)* will affect all the other components, and treatments for rebalancing will be addressed accordingly.

Ayurveda says negative feelings are emotional toxins that can accumulate in the mind. If they are not properly eliminated from the body they can manifest as chronic mental imbalances such as anxiety, depression, and insomnia. If this condition is further ignored, it turns into more serious permanent mental disorders.

Mind is one of the bedrocks of the imbalances having its own constitution.

—*Ca. Su.* 1/55, 1/57

SUMMARY

Today, there are many types of therapies used in the depression treatments we are accustomed to, such as cognitive behavioral therapy addressing changes in thoughts and behavior, interpersonal therapy tackling changes in interpersonal responses and behavior, and psychodynamic therapy changing awareness. In all of them, the practitioners are trying to create changes in order to help the patient overcome their depression. The main feature of the Ayurvedic approach is the different approach to redressing imbalances. Ayurveda invites the patient to overcome the condition of depression by acceptance of what it is, rather than what we want it to be, and by very actively participating in self-awareness.

The Ayurvedic knowledge of the mind, body, and mental well-being, and its classifications of mental imbalances, can be integrated with modern psychology and psychiatry approaches. The profound conceptualization of the *tridosha* and *triguna* is a useful tool to combine with modern concepts and approaches for the management and ultimate cure of depression. By integrating them, the millions of individuals suffering from depression will have access to a more well-rounded form of support, which may release them from drug dependencies by facilitating their active participation in their treatment.[14,15,16]

The examination of mental *(manas)* qualities is emphasized through evaluation of psychic personality *(manas prakruti)* via the questionnaire included in this book. I recommend you take this evaluation from time to time. It will allow you to correlate your previously completed body constitution test (body *prakruti*) with the always-changing mind constitution *(manas prakruti)*. The *manas prakruti* evaluation is a valuable tool for a better understanding of how your mind-body works in particular life phases. Rather than falling victim to our stressful or depressive thoughts, the evaluation gives you a framework for observing the state of your mind and becoming less vulnerable to the moods, distractions, or identifications of the moment. Instead, you can awaken to nature bringing you back to your core again and again, moving away from *maya*. In that way, you can visualize how your mind-body-consciousness system works, bringing awareness to your daily actions and reactions, either as the person dealing with depression or as the therapist.

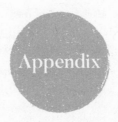

Food Recommendations
for Your *Dosha*

Pitta-Type Main Constitution: Foods That Are Recommended

INTEGRATE NEW FOODS ONE AT A TIME OVER A PERIOD OF TWO TO THREE WEEKS.	
Fruits (mostly when sweet)	Apples, apricots, berries, cherries, coconut, dates, figs, grapes (red), limes, mangoes, melons, oranges, papayas, pears, pineapples, plums, pomegranates, prunes, raisins, raspberries, strawberries, tangerines, watermelon
Vegetables	Artichokes, avocados, beets (cooked), bitter melon, broccoli (steamed), brussels sprouts, cabbage, carrots, cauliflower (steamed), celery, cilantro, coriander, cucumber, fennel, green beans, Indian asparagus (shatavari), Jerusalem artichokes, kale, ladies' fingers (okra), leafy greens, leeks (cooked), lettuce, mushrooms, olives (black), onions (cooked), parsley, parsnips, peas, peppers (sweet), potatoes (sweet), prickly pear (leaves), pumpkin, radishes (cooked), sprouts, watercress, zucchini (courgette)

INTEGRATE NEW FOODS ONE AT A TIME OVER A PERIOD OF TWO TO THREE WEEKS.	
Grains	Barley, cereal (dried), couscous, durum flour, oat bran, oats (cooked), pasta, rice, rice cakes/crackers, sago, sprouted wheat bread, tapioca, wheat
Legumes	Black beans, black-eyed peas, chickpeas, green gram (mung beans), kidney beans, lentils (red and brown), peas (dried), pinto beans, red mung beans (adzuki beans), soybeans, split peas, tofu (and other soy products)
Dairy products	Butter (unsalted), cheese (soft, not mature, unsalted), cottage cheese, cow's milk, ghee, goat cheese (soft, unsalted), goat's milk, ice cream, yogurt (fresh, plain)
Animal products	Chicken, eggs (white only), fish (freshwater), rabbit, shrimp, turkey (white meat), venison
Condiments	Black pepper, chutney (mango), coriander leaves, lime pickle, mango pickle (sweet)
Nuts and seeds (in moderation)	Almonds, coconut, flax seed, popcorn (unsalted), pumpkin seeds, sunflower seeds
Oils (in moderation)	Coconut, corn, flaxseed, ghee, olive, safflower, sunflower
Beverages	Almond milk, aloe vera juice, apple cider, apricot juice, black tea, cherry juice, cool dairy drinks, grain coffee, grape juice, mango juice, orange juice, peach nectar, pear juice, pomegranate juice, prune juice, rice milk, soymilk, vegetable broth
Herbs	Alfalfa, basil (fresh), blackberries, borage, burdock, cardamom, chamomile, chicory, comfrey, coriander (cilantro), curry leaves, dandelion, echinacea, false daisy (bhringaraj), fennel, goldenseal, hibiscus, hops, Indian madder (manjistha), Indian pennywort (gotu kola), jasmine, lavender, lemon balm, licorice, mint, neem, nettle, parsley, passionflower, peppermint, puncture vine (gokshura), red clover, sarsaparilla, spearmint, tarragon, violet, wintergreen, yarrow

INTEGRATE NEW FOODS ONE AT A TIME OVER A PERIOD OF TWO TO THREE WEEKS.	
Spices and flavorings	Black pepper, caraway, cinnamon, coriander, cumin, dill, fennel, ginger (fresh), Indian gooseberry (amalaki), lemongrass, saffron, sandalwood, turmeric, vanilla
Sweeteners	Barley malt, maple syrup, rice syrup, sugar cane
Food supplements (if required)	Aloe vera juice, barley green, brewer's yeast, essential fatty acids, minerals (calcium, magnesium, zinc), spirulina
Consult your physician if you have food allergies or intolerances to the above food items.	

Pitta-Type Main Constitution: Foods to Avoid

REDUCE INTAKE OR AVOID GRADUALLY, ESPECIALLY DRIED FOODS. AVOID QUICK CHANGES, PARTICULARLY IF THE FOOD HAS BEEN PART OF YOUR REGULAR DIET FOR A LONG TIME.	
Fruits (when sour or green)	Apples, apricots, bananas, berries, cherries, cranberries, grapefruit, grapes, kiwis, lemons, mangoes, oranges, peaches, persimmons, pineapples, plums, rhubarb, strawberries, tamarind
Vegetables	Beet greens, beets (raw), burdock root, corn (fresh), daikon radish, eggplant, garlic, German turnip (kohlrabi), green chilies, horseradish, leeks (raw), mustard greens, olive (green), onion (raw), peppers (hot), prickly pear (fruit), radishes (raw), spinach, tomatoes, turnip greens, turnips
Grains	Bread (with yeast), buckwheat, corn, millet, muesli, oats (dry), rice (brown), rye
Legumes	Black lentils (urad dal), pigeon peas (tur dal), soy sauce
Dairy products	Butter (salted), buttermilk, cheese (ripe), sour cream, yogurt (with fruit)
Animal products	Beef, duck, egg yolk, fish, lamb, pork

REDUCE INTAKE OR AVOID GRADUALLY, ESPECIALLY DRIED FOODS. AVOID QUICK CHANGES, PARTICULARLY IF THE FOOD HAS BEEN PART OF YOUR REGULAR DIET FOR A LONG TIME.	
Condiments	Chili pepper, chocolate, horseradish, kelp, ketchup, lemon, mango pickle (spicy), mayonnaise, mustard, salt (in excess), seaweed, tahini, vinegar
Nuts and seeds	Brazil nuts, cashews, hazelnuts, peanuts, pecans, pine nuts, pistachios, sesame seeds, walnuts
Oils	Almond, corn, safflower, sesame
Beverages	Alcohol (strong and wine), apple cider, berry juice (sour), caffeinated drinks, carbonated drinks, carrot juice, cherry juice (sour), chocolate milk, coffee, cranberry juice, grapefruit juice, iced tea, icy-cold drinks, lemonade, papaya juice, pineapple juice, tomato juice
Herbs	Basil (fresh or dried), bay leaf, bishop's seed (ajwain), eucalyptus, ginseng, hawthorn, hyssop, marjoram, oregano, pennyroyal, rosehip, rosemary, sage, sassafras, thyme
Spices and flavorings	Allspice, anise, asafoetida (hing), cayenne, cinnamon, clove, fenugreek, garlic, ginger (dried), juniper berries, long pepper (pippali), mace, mustard seeds, nutmeg, paprika, poppy seeds, star anise
Sweeteners	Industrial fructose, white sugar, molasses
Consult your physician if you have food allergies or intolerances to the above food items.	

Vata-Type Main Constitution: Foods That Are Recommended

INTEGRATE NEW FOODS ONE AT A TIME OVER A PERIOD OF TWO TO THREE WEEKS.	
Fruits (most sweet fruit)	Apples (red), apricots, bananas (ripe), berries, cherries, coconut, dates (fresh), figs (fresh), grapefruit, grapes, kiwis, lemons, limes, mangoes, melons, oranges, papayas, peaches, pineapples, plums, prunes (soaked), raisins (soaked), rhubarb, strawberries

INTEGRATE NEW FOODS ONE AT A TIME OVER A PERIOD OF TWO TO THREE WEEKS.	
Vegetables	Asparagus, avocados, beets, cabbage (cooked), carrots, cauliflower, cucumber, fennel, green beans, ladies' fingers (okra), leafy greens, leeks, parsnips, peas (cooked), pumpkin, radishes, spinach, sprouts, squash, sweet potatoes, turnip greens, zucchini (courgette)
Grains	Oats (cooked), pasta, rice (brown, wild, white), whole-wheat cereals
Legumes	Black lentils (urad dal), green gram (mung beans), pigeon peas (tur dal), red lentils, red mung beans (adzuki beans), tofu (and other soy products)
Dairy products	Butter, buttermilk, cheese (soft), cottage cheese, cow's milk, diluted yogurt (lassi), ghee, goat cheese, goat's milk
Animal products	Chicken, duck, eggs, fish (salmon, sardines, tuna), seafood, shrimp, turkey
Condiments	Black pepper, chutney (mango), lemons, lime pickle, limes, mango pickle, mustard, salt, soy sauce, tahini, tamari, vinegar
Nuts and seeds (in moderation)	Almonds, Brazil nuts, cashews, coconut, hazelnuts, macadamia nuts, pine nuts, pistachios, pumpkin seeds, sesame seeds, sunflower seeds, walnuts
Oils	Most oils, but particularly ghee, olive, and sesame in moderation
Beverages	Juices: apricot, carrot, grape, grapefruit, mango, orange, papaya, peach nectar, pineapple; alcohol (beer, white wine), almond milk, aloe vera juice, apple cider, soymilk (warm), vegetable juices and broths

INTEGRATE NEW FOODS ONE AT A TIME OVER A PERIOD OF TWO TO THREE WEEKS.	
Herbs (including teas)	Bala, basil, bay leaf, bishop's seed (ajwain), black myrobalan (haritaki), catmint (catnip), chamomile, chicory, clove, comfrey, elderflower, eucalyptus, fennel, ginger, ginseng, hawthorn, Indian asparagus (shatavari), Indian ginseng (ashwagandha), Indian pennywort (gotu kola), lavender, licorice, marjoram, mint, Mukul myrrh tree (guggul), oat straw, oregano, parsley, pennyroyal, peppermint, rosehip, rosemary, saffron, sage, sarsaparilla, spearmint, tarragon, thyme, valerian, wintergreen
Spices and flavorings	Allspice, almond extract, anise, asafoetida (hing), black pepper, cardamom, cinnamon, cloves, coriander, cumin, dill, fennel, fenugreek, garlic, ginger, juniper berries, lemongrass, long pepper (pippali), mustard seeds, nutmeg, orange blossom oil (neroli), orange peel, paprika, poppy seeds, saffron, salt, turmeric, vanilla
Sweeteners	Barley malt, honey, molasses, rice syrup, unrefined sugar (jaggary)
Food supplements (if required)	Aloe vera, bee pollen, essential fatty acids, minerals (calcium, copper, iron, magnesium, zinc), royal jelly, spirulina
Consult your physician if you have food allergies or intolerances to the above food items.	

Vata-Type Main Constitution: Foods to Avoid

REDUCE INTAKE OR AVOID GRADUALLY, ESPECIALLY DRIED FOODS. AVOID QUICK CHANGES, PARTICULARLY IF THE FOOD HAS BEEN PART OF YOUR REGULAR DIET FOR A LONG TIME.	
Fruits	Apples (raw), cranberries, dates (dried), figs (dried), pears, persimmons, pomegranates, prunes (dried), raisins (dried); most dried fruits

REDUCE INTAKE OR AVOID GRADUALLY, ESPECIALLY DRIED FOODS. AVOID QUICK CHANGES, PARTICULARLY IF THE FOOD HAS BEEN PART OF YOUR REGULAR DIET FOR A LONG TIME.

Vegetables	Artichokes, bitter melon, broccoli, brussels sprouts, burdock root, cabbage (raw), cauliflower (raw), celery, corn (fresh), dandelion greens, eggplant, German turnip (kohlrabi), horseradish, kale, mushrooms, olives (green), onions (raw), peppers (sweet and hot), potatoes (white), radishes (raw), tomatoes (raw), turnips, wheatgrass sprouts
Grains	Barley, bread (with yeast), buckwheat, cereal (cold, dry, or puffed), corn, couscous, millet, muesli, oat bran, oats (dried), rice cakes/crackers, rye, sago, tapioca, wheat bran; most dry, light grains
Legumes	Black beans, black-eyed peas, chickpeas, kidney beans, lentils (brown or yellow), lima beans, peas (dried), pinto beans, soybeans, white beans
Dairy products	Powdered milk, yogurt (plain, cold, frozen, or with fruit)
Animal products	Lamb, pork, rabbit, venison
Condiments	Horseradish
Nuts and seeds	Suitable in moderation
Oils	Flaxseed
Beverages (avoid cold)	Alcohol (strong), apple juice, black tea, caffeinated or carbonated drinks, chocolate milk, coffee, cold dairy drinks, cranberry juice, iced tea, icy-cold drinks, pear juice, pomegranate juice, soymilk (cold), tomato juice
Herbs	Basil, blackberries, borage, burdock, cornsilk, dandelion, ginseng, hibiscus, hops, nettle, red clover, yarrow

REDUCE INTAKE OR AVOID GRADUALLY, ESPECIALLY DRIED FOODS. AVOID QUICK CHANGES, PARTICULARLY IF THE FOOD HAS BEEN PART OF YOUR REGULAR DIET FOR A LONG TIME.	
Spices	Caraway (Persian cumin)
Sweeteners	Industrial fructose, white sugar

Consult your physician if you have food allergies or intolerances to the above food items.

Kapha-Type Main Constitution: Foods That Are Recommended

INTEGRATE NEW FOODS ONE AT A TIME OVER A PERIOD OF TWO TO THREE WEEKS.	
Fruits	Apples, apricots, berries, cherries, cranberries, figs, grapes, lemons, limes, peaches, pears, persimmons, pomegranates, prunes, raisins, strawberries
Vegetables (in season)	Artichokes, asparagus, beet greens, beets, bitter melon, broccoli, brussels sprouts, cabbage, carrots, cauliflower, celery, corn, eggplant, fennel, German turnip (kohlrabi), green beans, green chilies, horseradish, Jerusalem artichokes, kale, ladies' fingers (okra), leafy greens, leeks, lettuce, mixed-bean sprouts, mushrooms, mustard greens, onions, parsley, peas, peppers (sweet and hot), potato (white), radish, spinach, squash, tomatoes, turnip greens, turnips, watercress, wheatgrass sprouts
Grains	Barley, buckwheat, cereal (cold, dry, or puffed), corn, couscous, crackers, durum flour, millet, muesli, oat bran, oats (dried), rice (basmati and wild), rye, sago, sprouted wheat, tapioca, wheat bran
Legumes	Black beans, black-eyed peas, chickpeas, lentils (red and brown), lima beans, mung beans (green gram), peas (dried), pigeon peas (tur dal), pinto beans, red mung beans (adzuki beans), soymilk, split peas, sprouts, tofu (hot)

INTEGRATE NEW FOODS ONE AT A TIME OVER A PERIOD OF TWO TO THREE WEEKS.	
Dairy products	Buttermilk, cottage cheese (from skimmed goat's milk), goat cheese (fresh unsalted), goat's milk (skimmed)
Animal products	Chicken (white meat), eggs, fish (freshwater), rabbit, shrimp, turkey (white meat), venison
Condiments	Black pepper, chili pepper, chutney (mango), coriander leaves, garlic, horseradish, mustard (without vinegar), seaweed
Nuts and seeds	Flaxseed, popcorn (without salt or butter), pumpkin seeds, sunflower seeds
Oils	Almond, corn, ghee, sesame, sunflower
Beverages	Aloe vera juice, apple cider, apple juice, apricot juice, berry juice, black tea (spiced), carrot juice, cherry juice, cranberry juice, grape juice, mango juice, peach nectar, pear juice, pineapple juice, pomegranate juice, prune juice, soymilk (warm and spiced), vegetable juices and broths
Herbs	Alfalfa, angelica, basil, bay leaf, beleric (bibhitaki), bergamot, bishop's seed (ajwain), blackberries, burdock, chamomile, chicory, comfrey, dandelion, ginseng, hibiscus, hyssop, Indian asparagus (shatavari), jasmine, lavender, lemon balm, licorice, long pepper (pippali), Mukul myrrh tree (guggul), mustard, nettle, passionflower, pennyroyal, peppermint, raspberry, red clover, sage, sarsaparilla, sassafras, slippery elm, spearmint, thyme, valerian, wintergreen, yarrow

INTEGRATE NEW FOODS ONE AT A TIME OVER A PERIOD OF TWO TO THREE WEEKS.	
Spices and flavorings	Allspice, anise, asafoëtida (hing), black pepper, caraway, cardamom, cayenne, cinnamon, cloves, coriander, cumin, curry leaves, dill, fennel, fenugreek, garlic, ginger, juniper berries, lemongrass, mace, marjoram, mint, mustard seeds, nutmeg, orange peel, oregano, paprika, parsley, peppermint, poppy seeds, rosemary, saffron, salt, spearmint, star anise, tarragon, thyme, turmeric, vanilla
Sweeteners	Honey (raw, not processed)
Food supplements (if required)	Aloe vera, bee pollen, essential fatty acids, minerals (calcium, copper, iron, magnesium, zinc), royal jelly

Consult your physician if you have food allergies or intolerances to the above food items.

Kapha-Type Main Constitution: Foods to Avoid

REDUCE INTAKE OR AVOID GRADUALLY, ESPECIALLY DRIED FOODS. AVOID QUICK CHANGES, PARTICULARLY IF THE FOOD HAS BEEN PART OF YOUR REGULAR DIET FOR A LONG TIME.	
Fruits	Avocados, bananas, coconut, dates, figs (fresh), grapefruit, kiwis, limes, mangoes, melons, oranges, papayas, pineapples, plums, rhubarb, tamarind, watermelon
Vegetables	Cucumber, olives (black and green), parsnips, potatoes (sweet), pumpkin, squash, tomatoes (raw), zucchini (courgette)
Grains	Bread (with yeast), oats (cooked), pancakes, pasta, rice (brown and white), rice cakes, wheat
Legumes	Black lentils (urad dal), kidney beans, soy products, soybeans, tofu (cold)

REDUCE INTAKE OR AVOID GRADUALLY, ESPECIALLY DRIED FOODS. AVOID QUICK CHANGES, PARTICULARLY IF THE FOOD HAS BEEN PART OF YOUR REGULAR DIET FOR A LONG TIME.	
Dairy products	Butter, cheese (soft and hard), cow's milk, ice cream, sour cream, yogurt (plain, frozen, or with fruit)
Animal products	Beef, chicken (dark meat), duck, fish (saltwater), lamb, pork, salmon, sardines, seafood, tuna, turkey (dark meat)
Condiments	Chocolate, chutney (sweet), kelp, ketchup, lime pickle, mango pickle, mayonnaise, salt, soy sauce, tahini, vinegar
Nuts and seeds	Almonds, Brazil nuts, cashews, coconut, filberts, hazelnuts, peanuts, pecans, pine nuts, pistachios, sesame, walnuts
Oils	Coconut, flaxseed, olive, safflower, sesame, walnut
Beverages	Alcohol (strong, beer, sweet wines), almond milk, caffeinated beverages, carbonated drinks, cherry juice, chocolate milk, cold dairy drinks, grapefruit juice, iced tea, lemonade, orange juice, papaya juice, rice milk, soymilk, tomato juice
Herbs	Rosehip
Spices	Industrially produced spices (combined with salt)
Sweeteners	Barley malt, fructose, jaggary, maple syrup, molasses, rice syrup, white sugar

Consult your physician if you have food allergies or intolerances to the above food items.

Adapted from Food Guidelines for Basic Constitutional Types.
Copyright © 1994, 2008 The Ayurvedic Institute and Vasant Lad, MASc. All Rights Reserved.

GLOSSARY OF SANSKRIT TERMS

abhyanga: Body massage.

agni: Fire; digestion; transformation of food into energy.

ahara: Food.

ahararasa: Nutrients.

ahimsa: Nonviolence.

ama: Undigested food; undigested nutrients.

amasaya: Stomach.

amla: Sour.

apana: Control of the sphincters; induces elimination.

arsa: Blood.

asana: Physical posture in hatha yoga practice.

ashtanga: Possessing eight limbs or components.

asti: Bones.

atma: The Self, Soul, Consciousness, true essence.

Ayurveda: Sanskrit for the science of life or the science of living. *Ayur* means "life," and *veda* means "knowledge" or "science."

basti: Enema.

bheda: Development of complications; sixth stage of disease.

brumana: Restorative.

chakra: "Wheel" or "disk." There are seven chakras, which are considered to be the seven conductors of bodily energy. Their balance or imbalance affects your overall health.

dhamani: Artery.

dhatus: The seven basic types of bodily tissues.

dinacharya: Daily duties.

dipana: Digestive; appetizer.

doshas: The three psychophysiological functional principles of the body.

drava: Liquid.

dravya: Substance; drug.

dravyaguna: Pharmacology.

guna: Attribute or quality.

guru: Heavy.

indriya: Sense organs.

janma: Birth, nascence.

kapha: One of the three *doshas*.

kasaya: Astringent.

katu: Sharp; pungent.

kaya: Physiology; metabolism.

kayachikitsa: Internal medicine.

khamala: Excretions.

kitta: Waste products.

kleda: Liquefaction; hydration; associated with *kapha dosha*.

kledaka: Moistens food in the stomach.

kosha: Bondage; boundary; prison; limitation.

kriyakala: Stage of pathogenesis.

laghu: Light.

lavana: Salty.

lekhana: Emaciating.

madhura: Sweet.

majja: Bone marrow.

mala: Impurity; waste product.

manas: Mind, can be individual or universal.

manovasada: Depression.

mansa: Muscular tissue.

medas: Adipose tissue.

medoroga: Obesity.

mutra: Urine.

nasya: Medication through the nose.

nidana: Pathology; causative factors.

ojas: A vital, subtle essence that promotes and sustains physical vitality, mental clarity, and overall health.

pachaka: A *pitta* subtype that aids digestion.

pachana: Digestion; that which promotes digestion.

panchakarma: The five methods of eliminating excess *doshas* or *ama*.

panchamahabhutas: The five basic elements.

pitta: One of the three *doshas*.

prabhava: Special dynamic efficacy or property of a substance.

prakopa: Excitation of the *doshas*; second stage of disease.

prakriti: The prime material energy of which all matter is composed.

prakruti: Biological constitution of an individual.

prana: Vital force for life existence; primarily taken in through the breath.

prasara: Delocalization and spreading of the *doshas*; third stage of disease.

prthivi: Earth.

purisha: Feces.

purvarupa: Prodromes.

rajas: One of the three qualities of consciousness; principle of kinetic energy.

rakta: Blood.

raktamoksa: Bloodletting or blood cleansing.

rasa: Nutrient fluid; plasma.

rasayana: Rejuvenation therapy; science of longevity.

ritucharya: Seasonal duties.

rochana: Appetizing.

roga: Disease.

rupa: Symptoms.

samadosha: *Ama* combined with *dosha*.

samana: Separates nutrients and waste; removes waste.

samavaya: Inherence.

samhitas: Classic Ayurvedic texts.

samprapti: Pathogenesis.

samsamana: Palliative.

samshodhana: Curative purification.

sanchaya: Accumulation of the *doshas*; first stage of disease.

sattva: One of the three qualities of consciousness; principle of equilibrium; essence.

sharira: Body; anatomy.

siras: Veins.

sloka: Poetic form used in Sanskrit.

snehana: Oleation therapy.

snigdha: Unctuous.

srotami: Channels.

srotas: Channel.

sthana: Position; rank; place.

sthana samsraya: Localization of vitiated *dosha*; fourth stage of disease.

sthoulya: Thick; solid; strong; big; bulky.

sthula: Gross.

sukra: Semen.

sutra: Rule or aphorism in Sanskrit literature.

sveda: Sweat.

svedana: Sudation therapy.

tamas: One of the three qualities of consciousness; principle of inertia.

tejas: Essence of fire (*agni*) and *pitta dosha* leading all body fires.

tikta: Bitter.

udana: Carries the air out; induces speech; effort.

ushna: Hot.

vaidya: Ayurvedic doctor.

vamana: Vomiting.

vata: One of the three *doshas*.

veda: Knowledge; science; when capitalized, refers to the Vedas, ancient scriptures in India.

vikruti: State of imbalance of your primary constitution.

vipaka: Taste of the ingested material after digestion.

virechana: Purgation.

virya: Energy; power or potency of a substance, i.e., food, medicinal herb.

vruddhi: Increase of a *dosha* or substance; aggravation.

vyakti: Manifestation of a disease; fifth stage of disease.

yakrut : Liver.

NOTES

INTRODUCTION: THE ORIGINS OF AYURVEDA

1 World Health Organization, *WHO Global Report on Traditional and Complementary Medicine 2019*, 2019, https://apps.who.int/iris/handle/10665/312342.

CHAPTER 2: INTRODUCTION TO AYURVEDA FOR THE FIRST-TIME READER

1 D. Rosenthal, "Two Concepts of Consciousness," *Philosophical Studies* 49 (1986): 329–59.

2 D. Frawley and N. S. Rajaram, *Hidden Horizons: Unearthing 10,000 Years of Indian Culture* (Amdvad, India: Swaminarayan Aksharpith, 2007).

3 B. Avari, *India: The Ancient Past* (London: Routledge, 2007).

4 R. K. Sharma and Bhagwan Dash, eds., *Charaka Samhita of Agnivesa*, 3rd ed. (Varanasi, India: Chowkhamba Sanskrit Series Office, 1998), 3: 341–42.

5 Suśruta, *An English Translation of the Sushruta Samhita: Based on Original Sanskrit Text*, trans. K. L. Bhishagratna, 2nd ed. (Varanasi, India: Chowkhamba Sanskrit Series Office, 1963).

6 M. S. Valiathan, *The Legacy of Sushruta* (Hyderabad, India: Orient Longman, 2007).

7 B. Chatterjee and J. Pancholi, "Prakriti-Based Medicine: A Step towards Personalized Medicine," *Ayu* 32, no. 2 (2011): 141–46, https://doi.org/10.4103/0974-8520.92539.

8 M. Stiles, *Yoga Sutras of Patanjali* (San Francisco: Weiser Books, 2001).

9 World Health Organization, *Constitution of the World Health Organization* (New York: World Health Organization, 1948), www.who.int/governance/eb/who_constitution_en.pdf.

10 G. J. Larson. *Classical Sāṃkhya: An Interpretation of Its History and Meaning* (Delhi, India: Motilal Banarsidass Publishers, 1969).

11 P. Kramer and P. Bressan, "Our (Mother's) Mitochondria and Our Mind," *Perspectives on Psychological Science* 13, no. 1 (January 2018): 88–100.

12 A. Pyle et al., "Extreme-Depth Re-sequencing of Mitochondrial DNA Finds No Evidence of Paternal Transmission in Humans," *PLoS Genetics* 11, no. 5 (May 14, 2015): https://doi.org/10.1371/journal.pgen.1005040.

13 S. Sharan and V. Pathak, "Concepts of *Panchamahabhut* at Elemental Level," *World Journal of Pharmaceutical and Medical Research* 3, no. 7 (2017): 80–89.

14 R. Walgate, "Particle Physics: Where Now with Superstrings?" *Nature* 322 (1986): 592–93.

15 Editorial staff, "How Your Lungs Get the Job Done," *Each Breath* (blog), American Lung Association, July 20, 2017, www.lung.org/blog/how-your-lungs -work.

16 C. King, "The Central Enigma of Consciousness," *Nature Proceedings* (2008), https://doi.org/10.1038/npre.2008.2465.1.

17 Caroline Park et al., "Stress, Epigenetics and Depression: A Systematic Review," *Neuroscience and Biobehavioral Reviews* 102 (2019): 139–52.

18 M. I. Lind and F. Spagopoulou, "Evolutionary Consequences of Epigenetic Inheritance," *Heredity* 121 (2018): 205–9, www.nature.com/articles/s41437 -018-0113-y.

19 R. R. Kanherkar et al., "Epigenetic Mechanisms of Integrative Medicine," *Evidence-Based Complementary and Alternative Medicine* 2017 (2017): https://doi.org/10.1155/2017/4365429.

CHAPTER 3: FUNDAMENTALS OF AYURVEDA

1 W. H. Sheldon, S. S. Stevens, and W. B. Tucker, *The Varieties of Human Physique* (New York: Harper and Brothers, 1940).

2 H. Gardner, *Multiple Intelligences: New Horizons* (New York: Basic Books, 2010).

3 H. Liiv et al., "Anthropometry, Somatotypes, and Aerobic Power in Ballet, Contemporary Dance, and Dancesport," *Medical Problems of Performing Artists* 28, no. 4 (December 2013): 207–11.

4 H. Sharma, "Ayurveda: Science of Life, Genetics, and Epigenetics," *Journal of Research in Ayurveda* 37, no. 2 (April–June 2016): 87–91.

5 B. Dash and R. K. Sharma, eds., *Charaka Samhita* (Varanasi, India: Chaukhambha Orientalia, 1995).

6 R. Svoboda, *Prakruti: Your Ayurvedic Constitution* (Twin Lakes, WI: Lotus Press, 1988).

7 B. Prasher et al., "Whole Genome Expression and Biochemical Correlates of Extreme Constitutional Types Defined in Ayurveda," *Journal of Translational Medicine* 6 (2008): 48.

8 B. Patwardhan and G. Bodeker, "Ayurvedic Genomics: Establishing a Genetic Basis for Mind-Body Typologies," *Journal of Alternative and Complementary Medicine* 14, no. 5 (2008): 571–76.

9 N. P. Mahalle et al., "Association of Constitutional Type in Ayurveda with Cardiovascular Risk Factors, Inflammatory Markers and Insulin Resistance," *Journal of Ayurveda and Integrative Medicine* 3, no. 3 (2012): 150–57.

10 R. M. Palmer, A. G. Ferrige, and S. Moncada, "Nitric Oxide Release Accounts for the Biological Activity of Endothelium-Derived Relaxing Factor," *Nature* 327, no. 6122 (June 11–17, 1987): 524–26.

11 C. Farah et al., "Nitric Oxide Signalling in Cardiovascular Health and Disease," *Nature Reviews Cardiology* 15 (2018): 292–316.

12 V. N. Sumantran and P. P. Nair, "Can the Vagus Nerve Serve as Biomarker for *Vata Dosha* Activity?" *Journal of Ayurveda and Integrative Medicine* 10, no. 2 (2019): 146–51, https://doi.org/10.1016/j.jaim.2019.04.003.

13 K. E. Barrett et al., *Ganong's Review of Medical Physiology*, 26th ed. (New York: McGraw-Hill Education, 2019).

14 Srikantha K. R. Murthy, *Ashtanga Hridayam* (Varanasi, India: Chowkhamba Krishnadas Academy, 2010), 1: 156.

CHAPTER 4: MENTAL CONSTITUTION *(MANAS PRAKRUTI)*

1 S. K. Pandya, "Understanding Brain, Mind and Soul: Contributions from Neurology and Neurosurgery," *Mens Sana Monographs* 9, no. 1 (2011): 129–49.

2 V. Lad, *Ayurveda: The Science of Self-Healing: A Practical Guide* (Twin Lakes, WI: Lotus Press, 2009).

3 D. Frawley, *Ayurveda and the Mind: The Healing of Consciousness* (Twin Lakes, WI: Lotus Press, 1996).

4 E. W. Silvertooth, "Special Relativity," *Nature* 322, no. 6080 (1986): 590.

5 S. S. Bagali, "Review: Concept of *Manas Prakruti* as Described in *Charaka Samhita*," *Journal of Ayurveda and Integrated Medical Sciences* 1, no. 3 (2016): 81–86.

CHAPTER 5: AYURVEDA AND THE MIND: HOW AYURVEDA TREATS DEPRESSION

1 Sri Ajai Kumar Chawcharia, *One Hundred Eight Vedic Upanishads* (Varanasi, India: Chaukhamba Surbharti Prakashan, 2010).

2 G. B. Feld and J. Born, "Neurochemical Mechanisms for Memory Processing during Sleep: Basic Findings in Humans and Neuropsychiatric Implications," *Neuropsychopharmacology* 45 (2020): 31–44, https://doi.org/10.1038/s41386-019-0490-9.

3 R. R. McCrae et al., "Person-Factors in the California Adult Q-Set: Closing the Door on Personality Trait Types?" *European Journal of Personality* 20, no. 1 (2006): 29–44.

4 S. K. Pandya, "Understanding Brain, Mind and Soul: Contributions from Neurology and Neurosurgery," *Mens Sana Monographs* 9, no. 1 (2011): 129–49.

CHAPTER 6: IMPROVEMENT THROUGH LIFESTYLE CHANGES: GENERAL RECOMMENDATIONS

1 "Adult Prevalence of Mental Illness—Adults with Any Mental Illness (AMI) 2020," Mental Health America, www.mhanational.org/issues/mental-health -america-prevalence-data#two.

2 "Youth with at Least One Major Depressive Episode (MDE) in the Past Year 2020," Mental Health America, www.mhanational.org/issues /mental-health-america-prevalence-data#five.

3 R. Sharma, "A Review on Role of Ayurveda in the Management of Stress," *International Journal of Ayurveda and Pharma Research* 6, no. 1 (2018): 59–61.

4 R. Sharma et al., "Herbal and Holistic Solutions for Neurodegenerative and Depressive Disorders: Leads from Ayurveda," *Current Pharmaceutical Design* 24, no. 22 (2018): 2597–2608.

5 M. Wittmann et al., "Circadian Rhythms and Depression," *Fortschritte der neurologie-psychiatrie* 86, no. 5 (May 2018): 308–18.

6 P. Angerer et al., "Night Work and the Risk of Depression," *Deutsches Ärzteblatt International* 114, no. 24 (2017): 404–11.

7 H. M. Francis et al., "A Brief Diet Intervention Can Reduce Symptoms of Depression in Young Adults—A Randomised Controlled Trial," *PLOS ONE* 14, no. 10 (2019): e0222768, https://doi.org/10.1371/journal.pone.0222768.

8 M. P. Mattson, V. D. Longo, and M. Harvie, "Impact of Intermittent Fasting on Health and Disease Processes," *Ageing Research Reviews* 39 (October 2017): 46–58.

9 F. Madeo et al., "Caloric Restriction Mimetics against Age-Associated Disease: Targets, Mechanisms, and Therapeutic Potential," *Cell Metabolism* 29, no. 3 (March 5, 2019): 592–610.

10 S. Kvam et al., "Exercise as a Treatment for Depression: A Meta-analysis," *Journal of Affective Disorders* 202 (September 15, 2016): 67–86.

11 M. Wegner et al., "Systematic Review of Meta-analyses: Exercise Effects on Depression in Children and Adolescents," *Frontiers in Psychiatry* 11 (2020), https://doi.org/10.3389/fpsyt.2020.00081.

12 S. Kvam et al., "Exercise as a Treatment for Depression: A Meta-analysis," *Journal of Affective Disorders* 202 (September 15, 2016): 67–86.

13 Neha P. Gothe et al., "Yoga Effects on Brain Health: A Systematic Review of the Current Literature," *Brain Plasticity* 5, no. 1 (2019): 105–22.

14 R. Govindaraj et al., "Yoga and Physical Exercise—A Review and Comparison," *International Review of Psychiatry* 28, no. 3 (2016): 242–53.

15 R. Tejvani et al., "Effect of Yoga on Anxiety, Depression and Self-Esteem in Orphanage Residents: A Pilot Study," *Ayu* 37, no. 1 (2016): 22–25.

16 S. G. Wankhede, V. D. Udhan, and P. Shinde, "Assessment of Long-Term Yoga Training as a Complementary Therapeutic Measure for Anxiety, Depression, and Psychological Distress in Healthy Individuals," *National Journal of Physiology, Pharmacy and Pharmacology* 10, no. 2 (2020): 99–103.

17 B. H. Smith, G. Esat, and A. Kanojia, "School-Based Yoga for Managing Stress and Anxiety," in *Promoting Mind-Body Health in Schools: Interventions for Mental Health Professionals*, ed. C. Maykel and M. A. Bray, Applying Psychology in the Schools series (Washington, DC: American Psychological Association, 2020), 201–16.

18 R. Chandra, "Benefits of Yoga from HEAD to TOE (Based on Scientific Research)," FITSRI, November 6, 2019, https://fitsri.com/yoga/benefits-of-yoga.

19 P. Sengupta, "Health Impacts of Yoga and Pranayama: A State-of-the-Art Review," *International Journal of Preventive Medicine* 3, no. 7 (2012): 444–58.

20 H. Sharma, "Meditation: Process and Effects," *Ayu* 36, no. 3 (2015): 233–37, https://doi.org/10.4103/0974-8520.182756.

21 Quinn A. Conklin et al., "Insight Meditation and Telomere Biology: The Effects of Intensive Retreat and the Moderating Role of Personality," *Brain, Behavior, and Immunity* 70 (May 2018): 233–45.

22 M. Merrow, K. Spoelstra, and T. Roenneberg, "The Circadian Cycle: Daily Rhythms from Behavior to Genes," *EMBO Reports* 6, no. 10 (2005): 930–35.

23 Y. Li et al., "The Role of Microbiome in Insomnia, Circadian Disturbance and Depression," *Frontiers in Psychiatry* 9 (2018), https://doi.org/10.3389/fpsyt.2018.00669.

24 L. E. Cardona-Sanclemente, "Stress: The Role of Catecholamines in Atherosclerosis and Cardiovascular Diseases" (presentation, Global Holistic Health Summit, Bangalore, India, January 2003).

25 L. A. Peccoralo et al., "The Health Benefits of Resilience," in *Nutrition, Fitness, and Mindfulness: An Evidence-Based Guide for Clinicians*, ed. J. Uribarri and J. Vassalotti, Nutrition and Health series (Cham, Switzerland: Humana Press, 2020), 189–201.

26 Ariel Shensa et al., "Emotional Support from Social Media and Face-to-Face Relationships: Associations with Depression Risk among Young Adults," *Journal of Affective Disorders* 260 (January 2020): 38–44.

27 Ziggi Ivan Santini et al., "Social Disconnectedness, Perceived Isolation, and Symptoms of Depression and Anxiety among Older Americans (NSHAP): A Longitudinal Mediation Analysis," *Lancet Public Health* 5 (2020): e62–70.

28 M. H. Teicher, "Childhood Maltreatment Hampers Interpersonal Distance and Social Touch in Adulthood," *American Journal of Psychiatry* 177, no. 1 (2020): 4–6.

29 M. C. Marrone and R. Coccurello, "Dietary Fatty Acids and Microbiota-Brain Communication in Neuropsychiatric Diseases," *Biomolecules* 10, no. 1 (2020): 12.

30 Isak Sundberg, "Exploring Links between Melatonin, Inflammation and Depression" (doctoral dissertation, Uppsala University, 2019).

31 T. Chen et al., "Butyrate Suppresses Demyelination and Enhances Remyelination," *Journal of Neuroinflammation* 16, no. 165 (2019), https://doi.org/10.1186/s12974-019-1552-y.

32 A. Mooventhan, L. Nivethitha, "Scientific Evidence-Based Effects of Hydrotherapy on Various Systems of the Body," *North American Journal of Medical Sciences* 6, no. 5 (2014): 199–209.

33 Nikolai A. Shevchuk, "Adapted Cold Shower as a Potential Treatment for Depression," *Medical Hypotheses* 70, no. 5 (2008): 995–1001.

34 E. Grodzinsky and M. Sund Levander, "Thermoregulation of the Human Body," in *Understanding Fever and Body Temperature*, ed. E. Grodzinsky and M. Sund Levander (Cham, Switzerland: Palgrave Macmillan, 2020), 49–65.

35 C. M. Bleakley and G. W. Davison, "What Is the Biochemical and Physiological Rationale for Using Cold-Water Immersion in Sports Recovery? A Systematic Review," *British Journal of Sports Medicine* 44 (2010): 179–87.

36 N. A. Shevchuk and S. Radoja, "Possible Stimulation of Anti-tumor Immunity Using Repeated Cold Stress: A Hypothesis," *Infectious Agents and Cancer* 2 (2007), https://doi.org/10.1186/1750-9378-2-20.

37 G. A. Buijze et al., "The Effect of Cold Showering on Health and Work: A Randomized Controlled Trial," *PLOS ONE* 11, no. 9 (2016): e0161749.

CHAPTER 7: ARE YOU JUST DEPRESSED BACTERIA?

1 M. Simrén et al., "Intestinal Microbiota in Functional Bowel Disorders: A Rome Foundation Report," *Gut* 62 (2013): 159–76.

2 S. M. Henning et al., "Health Benefit of Vegetable/Fruit Juice-Based Diet: Role of Microbiome," *Scientific Reports* 7 (2017), https://doi.org/10.1038/s41598-017-02200-6.

3 P. I. Costea et al., "Enterotypes in the Landscape of Gut Microbial Community Composition," *Nature Microbiology* 3, no. 1 (2018): 8–16, https://doi.org/10.1038/s41564-017-0072-8.

4 P. Turnbaugh et al., "The Human Microbiome Project," *Nature* 449 (2007): 804–10.

5 "Interview: On Location in Tanzania with Martin Blaser," Gut Check: Exploring Your Microbiome, Coursera, www.coursera.org/learn/microbiome.

6 Jose C. Clemente et al., "The Microbiome of Uncontacted Amerindians," *Science Advances* 1, no. 3 (April 2015): e1500183.

7   M. H. Mohajeri et al., "The Role of the Microbiome for Human Health: From Basic Science to Clinical Applications," *European Journal of Nutrition* 57 (supplement 1, May 2018): 1–14.

8   J. Walter, I. Martínez, and D. J. Rose, "Holobiont Nutrition: Considering the Role of the Gastrointestinal Microbiota in the Health Benefits of Whole Grains," *Gut Microbes* 4, no. 4 (2013): 340–46.

9   I. Martínez et al., "Gut Microbiome Composition Is Linked to Whole Grain-Induced Immunological Improvements," *The ISME Journal* 7, no. 2 (2013): 269–80.

10 I. C. L. van den Munckhof et al., "Role of Gut Microbiota in Chronic Low-Grade Inflammation as Potential Driver for Atherosclerotic Cardiovascular Disease: A Systematic Review of Human Studies," *Obesity Reviews* 19, no. 12 (2018): 1719–34.

11 Y. K. Kim and C. Shin, "The Microbiota-Gut-Brain Axis in Neuropsychiatric Disorders: Pathophysiological Mechanisms and Novel Treatments," *Current Neuropharmacology* 16, no. 5 (2018): 559–73.

12 M. K. Zinöcker and I. A. Lindseth, "The Western Diet–Microbiome-Host Interaction and Its Role in Metabolic Disease," *Nutrients* 10, no. 3 (2018): 365.

13 Mingyue Cheng and Kang Ning, "Stereotypes about Enterotype: The Old and New Ideas," *Genomics, Proteomics and Bioinformatics* 17, no. 1 (February 2019): 4–12.

14 T. G. Dinan and J. F. Cryan, "Gut Microbiota: A Missing Link in Psychiatry," *World Psychiatry* 19, no. 1 (2020): 111–12.

15 G. V. R. Born et al., "Factors Influencing the Transendothelial Accumulation of Atherogenic Plasma Proteins in Artery Walls," *Clinical Hemorheology and Microcirculation* 37, no. 1–2 (2007): 9–18.

16 Linoy Mia Frankiensztajn, Evan Elliott, and Omry Koren, "The Microbiota and the Hypothalamus-Pituitary-Adrenocortical (HPA) Axis, Implications for Anxiety and Stress Disorders," *Current Opinion in Neurobiology* 62 (2020): 76–82.

17 B. Kuo et al., "Genomic and Clinical Effects Associated with a Relaxation Response Mind-Body Intervention in Patients with Irritable Bowel Syndrome and Inflammatory Bowel Disease," *PLOS ONE* 12, no. 2 (2017): e0172872.

18 Richard T. Liu, "The Microbiome as a Novel Paradigm in Studying Stress and Mental Health," *American Psychologist* 72, no. 7 (2017): 655–67.

19 Claudia Welch, *Balance Your Hormones, Balance Your Life* (Philadelphia: Da Capo Press, 2011).

20 V. Lazar et al., "Aspects of Gut Microbiota and Immune System Interactions in Infectious Diseases, Immunopathology, and Cancer," *Frontiers in Immunology* 9 (2018): 1830, https://doi.org/10.3389/fimmu.2018.01830.

21 Hartmut Wekerle, "The Gut-Brain Connection: Triggering of Brain Auto-immune Disease by Commensal Gut Bacteria," *Rheumatology* 55 (2016): ii68–ii75.

22 M. E. M. Obrenovich, "Leaky Gut, Leaky Brain?" *Microorganisms* 6, no. 4 (2018): 107, https://doi.org/10.3390/microorganisms6040107.

23 Y. Wang and L. H. Kasper, "The Role of Microbiome in Central Nervous System Disorders," *Brain, Behavior, and Immunity* 38 (2014): 1–12.

24 A. Evrensel and M. D. Ceylan, "The Gut-Brain Axis: The Missing Link in Depression," *Clinical Psychopharmacology and Neuroscience* 13, no. 3 (2015): 239–44.

25 Chong-Su Kim et al., "Probiotic Food Consumption Is Associated with Lower Severity and Prevalence of Depression: A Nationwide Cross-Sectional Study," *Nutrition* 63–64 (2019): 169–74.

26 C. A. Calarge et al., "Gut Permeability and Depressive Symptom Severity in Unmedicated Adolescents," *Journal of Affective Disorders* 246, no. 1 (2019): 586–94.

CHAPTER 8: CARING FOR YOUR DEPRESSION: AYURVEDIC BODY TREATMENTS

1 Kaviraj Kunja Lal Bhishagratna, "The Medicinal Use of Sneha (Oleaginous Substances)," in *Sushruta Samhita*, vol. 4, *Cikitsasthana*, www.wisdomlib.org /hinduism/book/sushruta-samhita-volume-4-cikitsasthana/d/doc142947 .html.

2 B. A. Lohith, *A Text Book of Panchakarma* (Varanasi, India: Chaukambha Orientalia, 2016).

3 Arun Kumar Pandey and Rajesh Kumar Mishra, "*Nasya* and Ayurveda: A Classical Review Based on Ancient Ayurvedic Treatise," *International Journal of Unani and Integrative Medicine* 3, no. 4 (2019): 103–9.

4 Kapil A. Pandya and Jani Jalpa, "Achievements through *Panchakarma* in Clinical Management and Future Prospects," *Journal of Ayurveda and Integrated Medical Sciences* 3, no. 2 (2018): 62–65.

5 Rohit Sharma et al., "Herbal and Holistic Solutions for Neurodegenerative and Depressive Disorders: Leads from Ayurveda," *Current Pharmaceutical Design* 24, no. 22 (2018): 2597–2608.

6 A. Atara et al., "An Ayurvedic Management of Nasal Polyposis," *Indian Journal of Otolaryngology and Head and Neck Surgery* 71 (2019): 1876–84.

7 K. S. Praveen Kumar et al., "Different Types of *Nasya* Karma in Current Practice—A Review," *European Journal of Biomedical and Pharmaceutical Sciences* 6, no. 13 (2019): 225–28.

8 Gurdip Singh, "*Nasya* Therapy—A Pharmacological Route for Drug Delivery to Brain," *Journal of Ayurveda Physicians and Surgeons* 5, no. 3 (2018): 76.

9 D. Frawley, S. Ranade, and A. Lele, *Ayurveda and Marma Therapy: Energy Points in Yogic Healing* (Twin Lakes, WI: Lotus Press, 2003).

10 Durve Anisha and Vasant Lad, *Marma Points of Ayurveda* (Albuquerque, NM: Ayurvedic Press, 2016).

11 Xiao Nan Lv et al., "Aromatherapy and the Central Nerve System (CNS): Therapeutic Mechanism and Its Associated Genes," *Current Drug Targets* 14, no. 8 (2013): 872–79.

12 S. Taavoni et al., "The Effect of Aromatherapy Massage on the Psychological Symptoms of Postmenopausal Iranian Women," *Complementary Therapies in Medicine* 21, no. 3 (2013): 158–63.

13 A. Moussaieff et al., "Incensole Acetate, an Incense Component, Elicits Psychoactivity by Activating TRPV3 Channels in the Brain," *The FASEB Journal* 22, no. 8 (2008): 3024–34.

14 A. Moussaieff et al., "Incensole Acetate, a Novel Anti-inflammatory Compound Isolated from Boswellia Resin, Inhibits Nuclear Factor-Kappa B Activation," *Molecular Pharmacology* 72, no. 6 (2007): 1657–64.

15 D. Frawley, *Wisdom of the Ancient Seers: Mantras of the Rig Veda* (Salt Lake City: Morson Publishing, 1992).

16 G. Oster, "Auditory Beats in the Brain," *Scientific American* 229, no. 4 (1973): 94–102.

17 Pierre Stocker, "Psycho-Acoustic Medicine: Science behind Sound Healing for Serotonin, Neurotransmitters and Health," www.pierrestocker.com.

18 Bill Harris, "The Science behind Holosync® and Other Neurotechnologies," www.strategies-for-managing-change.com/support-files/scienceofholosync.pdf.

19 K. S. Kumar et al., "Classification of Electrophotonic Images of Yogic Practice of Mudra through Neural Networks," *International Journal of Yoga* 11, no. 2 (2018): 152–56.

20 Gertrud Hirschi, *Mudras: Yoga in Your Hands* (Newburyport, MA: Weiser Books, 2016).

21 V. V. Kuchewar, M. A. Borkar, and M. A. Nisargandha, "Evaluation of Antioxidant Potential of *Rasayana* Drugs in Healthy Human Volunteers," *Ayu* 35, no. 1 (2014): 46–49.

22 Claudia Welch, "Oil Pulling: Miracle or Myth?" https://drclaudiawelch.com/oil-pulling-miracle-or-myth/.

23 Smitha Sammith Shetty et al., "Effect of Oil Pulling on Oral Health—A Microbiological Study," *Research Journal of Pharmacy and Technology* 12, no. 1 (2019): 1–4.

24 A. Tokinobu et al., "Effects of Tongue Cleaning on Ayurvedic Digestive Power and Oral Health-Related Quality of Life: A Randomized Cross-Over Study," *Complementary Therapies in Medicine* 36 (2018): 9–13.

25 Narek Israelyan, "Effects of Neuronal Serotonin and Slow-Release 5-HTP on Gastrointestinal Motility in a Mouse Model of Depression," *Gastroenterology* 157, no. 2 (2019): 507–21.

26 S. T. Hosseinzadeh et al., "Psychological Disorders in Patients with Chronic Constipation," *Gastroenterology and Hepatology from Bed to Bench* 4, no. 3 (2011): 159–63.

27 Agrawal Lokesh et al., "Therapeutic Potential of Serotonin 4 Receptor for Chronic Depression and Its Associated Comorbidity in the Gut," *Neuropharmacology* 166 (April 2020): 107969, https://doi.org/10.1016/j.neuropharm .2020.107969.

CHAPTER 9: AYURVEDIC MASTERY OF FOOD, DIET, AND NUTRITION

1 J. B. Ward and S. J. Keely, "Oxygen in the Regulation of Intestinal Epithelial Transport," *Journal of Physiology* 592, no. 12 (2014): 2473–89.

2 V. Lad, *Textbook of Ayurveda: Fundamental Principles* (Albuquerque, NM: Ayurveda Press, 2002).

3 Baghwan Dash et al., *Charaka Samhita* (Varanasi , India: Chowkhamba Sanskrit Series Office, 2009), 1: 43.

4 "Healthy Diet," World Health Organization, October 23, 2018, www.who.int /news-room/fact-sheets/detail/healthy-diet.

5 Andrea T. da Poian and Miguel Castanho, *Integrative Human Biochemistry* (New York: Springer, 2015).

6 A. K. Agrawal, C. R. Yadav, and M. S. Meena, "Physiological Aspects of *Agni*," *Ayu* 31, no. 3 (2010): 395–98.

7 K. Shastri and G. Chaturvedi, eds., *Charaka Samhita* (Varanasi, India: Chaukhamba Bharti Academy, 2004), 461.

8 Shastri Ambicadutt, *Sushruta Samhita* (Varanasi, India: Chaukhamba Sanskrit Sansthan, 2005), 88.

9 B. K. Brandley and R. L. Schnaar, "Cell-Surface Carbohydrates in Cell Recognition and Response," *Journal of Leukocyte Biology* 40, no. 1 (1986): 97–111.

10 L. E. Cardona-Sanclemente, "Role of Potentially Atherogenic Plasma Proteins, Catecholamines, Angiotensin, and Other Factors in the Development of Cardiovascular Diseases" (presentation given at Hrydayam: National Seminar on Preventive Cardiology, Trivendrum, India, 2003).

11 L. E. Cardona-Sanclemente and G. V. R. Born, "Increase by Adrenaline or Angiotensin II on the Uptake of Low-Density Lipoprotein and Fibrinogen by

Aortic Walls in Unrestrained Conscious Rats," *British Journal of Pharmacology* 117 (1996): 1089–94.

12 C. J. Crespo et al., "Television Watching, Energy Intake and Obesity in US Children: Results from the Third National Health and Nutrition Examination Survey," *Archives of Pediatrics and Adolescent Medicine* 155 (2001): 360–65.

13 L. Lien et al., "Consumption of Soft Drinks and Hyperactivity, Mental Distress, and Conduct Problems among Adolescents in Oslo, Norway," *American Journal of Public Health* 96, no. 10 (2006): 1815–20.

14 L. E. Cardona-Sanclemente and G. V. R. Born, "Adrenaline Increases the Uptake of Low-Density Lipoprotein in Carotid Arteries," *Atherosclerosis* 96 (1992): 215–18.

15 V. V. Subrahmanya Sastri, *Tridosha Theory*, Kottakkal Ayurveda Series 18 (Kerala, India: Kottakal, 2002).

16 M. Wittmann et al., "Circadian Rhythms and Depression," *Fortschritte der neurologie-psychiatrie* 86, no. 5 (2018): 308–18.

17 P. Angerer et al., "Night Work and the Risk of Depression," *Deutsches Ärzteblatt International* 114, no. 24 (2017): 404–11.

18 C. Peterson et al., "Therapeutic Uses of Triphala in Ayurvedic Medicine," *Journal of Alternative and Complementary Medicine* 23, no. 8 (2017): 607–14.

19 M. S. Baliga et al., "Scientific Validation of the Ethnomedicinal Properties of the Ayurvedic Drug Triphala: A Review," *Chinese Journal of Integrative Medicine* 18, no. 12 (2012): 946–54.

20 S. Prasad and S. K. Srivastava, "Oxidative Stress and Cancer: Chemopreventive and Therapeutic Role of Triphala," *Antioxidants* 9 (2020): 72.

21 V. Lad, *Textbook of Ayurveda: Fundamental Principles* (Albuquerque, NM: Ayurveda Press, 2002), 245–50.

22 L. E. Cardona-Sanclemente, "Effect of *Allium sativum* (Garlic) Supplementation on Plasma Lipoproteins and Cholesterol Metabolism in a Hyperlipidemic Rat Model" (presentation given at Svastha International Ayurveda Conference, London, 2007).

23 M. S. Valiathan, *The Legacy of Caraka* (Chennai, India: Orient Longman, 2003), 30–33.

24 L. E. Cardona-Sanclemente, "Effects of Diet on Lipid Profile and Protein Levels in Different Kinds of Long-Term Vegetarian Diets and a Control Group" (master's thesis, Valle University, 1979).

25 L. E. Cardona-Sanclemente, "Decrease of Plasma Cholesterol Levels Induced by Vegetarian Diets in a Normal Adult Population" (presentation given at Svastha International Ayurveda Conference, London, 2007).

26 J. I. Harland, J. Buttriss, and S. Gibson, "Achieving Eatwell Plate Recommendations: Is This a Route to Improving Both Sustainability and Healthy Eating?" *Nutrition Bulletin* 37, no. 4 (2012): 324–43.

27 Denise de Ridder et al., "Healthy Diet: Health Impact, Prevalence, Correlates, and Interventions," *Journal of Psychology and Health* 32, no. 8 (2016): 907–41.

28 M. Molendijk et al., "Diet Quality and Depression Risk: A Systematic Review and Dose-Response Meta-analysis of Prospective Studies," *Journal of Affective Disorders* 226 (2018): 346–54.

29 Courtney Davis et al., "Definition of the Mediterranean Diet: A Literature Review," *Nutrients* 7, no. 11 (2015): 9139–53.

30 R. S. Opie, "A Modified Mediterranean Dietary Intervention for Adults with Major Depression: Dietary Protocol and Feasibility Data from the SMILES Trial," *Nutritional Neuroscience* 21, no. 7 (2017): 487–501.

31 C. Lassale et al., "Healthy Dietary Indices and Risk of Depressive Outcomes: A Systematic Review and Meta-analysis of Observational Studies," *Molecular Psychiatry* 24 (2019): 965–86.

32 Lee Ga Bin, Kim Hyeon Chang, and Jung Sun Jae, "Association between Depression and Disease-Specific Treatment," *Journal of Affective Disorders* 260, no. 1 (2020): 124–30.

33 K. D. Pett et al., "Ancel Keys and the Seven Countries Study: An Evidence-Based Response to Revisionist Histories," August 1, 2017, www.truehealthinitiative.org/wp-content/uploads/2017/07/SCS-White-Paper.THI_.8-1-17.pdf.

34 D. Grotto and E. Zied, "The Standard American Diet and Its Relationship to the Health Status of Americans," *Nutrition in Clinical Practice* 25, no. 6 (2010): 603–12.

35 M. J. Gibney, "Dietary Guidelines: A Critical Appraisal," *Journal of Human Nutrition and Dietetics* 3, no. 4 (1990): 245–54.

CHAPTER 10: AYURVEDIC HERBAL PROGRAMS FOR YOUR TYPE OF DEPRESSION

1 N. H. Aboelsoud, "Herbal Medicine in Ancient Egypt," *Journal of Medicinal Plants Research* 4, no. 2 (2010): 82–86.

2 M. M. Pandey, S. Rastogi, and A. K. Rawat, "Indian Traditional Ayurvedic System of Medicine and Nutritional Supplementation," *Evidence-Based Complementary and Alternative Medicine* 2013 (2013): 376327, https://doi.org/10.1155/2013/376327.

3 M. Ekor, "The Growing Use of Herbal Medicines: Issues Relating to Adverse Reactions and Challenges in Monitoring Safety," *Frontiers in Pharmacology* 4 (2014): 177.

4 Jon C. Tilburt and Ted J. Kaptchuk, "Herbal Medicine Research and Global Health: An Ethical Analysis," *Bulletin of the World Health Organization* 86, no. 8 (2008): 594–99.

5 M. R. Rahman et al., "A Review Study on the Traditional Plants Has Potential Antidepressant Property," *MedCrave Online Journal of Cell Science and Report* 4, no. 5 (2017): 138–45.

6 Talha Jawaid, Roli Gupta, and Zohaib Ahmed Siddiqui, "A Review on Herbal Plants Showing Antidepressant Activity," *International Journal of Pharmaceutical Sciences and Research* 2 (2011): 3051–60.

7 Nawab John Dar and Muzamil Ahmad, "Neurodegenerative Diseases and *Withania somnifera* (L.)," *Journal of Ethnopharmacology* 256 (June 28, 2020): 112769.

8 K. Chandrasekhar, J. Kapoor, and S. Anishetty, "A Prospective, Randomized Double-Blind, Placebo-Controlled Study of Safety and Efficacy of a High-Concentration Full-Spectrum Extract of Ashwagandha Root in Reducing Stress and Anxiety in Adults," *Indian Journal of Psychological Medicine* 34, no. 3 (2012): 255–62.

9 K. N. Chengappa et al., "Randomized Placebo-Controlled Adjunctive Study of an Extract of *Withania somnifera* for Cognitive Dysfunction in Bipolar Disorder," *Journal of Clinical Psychiatry* 74, no. 11 (2013): 1076–83.

10 Zohre Fathinezhad et al., "Depression and Treatment with Effective Herbs," *Current Pharmaceutical Design* 25, no. 6 (2019): 738–45.

11 Deepali Mathur et al., "The Molecular Links of Re-emerging Therapy: A Review of Evidence of Brahmi *(Bacopa monnieri),*" *Frontiers in Pharmacology* 7, no. 44 (2016): 1–15.

12 T. Simpson, M. Pase, and C. Stough, "*Bacopa monnieri* as an Antioxidant Therapy to Reduce Oxidative Stress in the Aging Brain," *Evidence-Based Complementary and Alternative Medicine* (2015): 615384, https://doi.org/10.1155/2015/615384.

13 Sachi Petrohilos, "Curcumin and Depression: Review," *Journal of the Australian Traditional-Medicine Society* 23, no. 2 (2017): 88.

14 Q. X. Ng et al., "Clinical Use of Curcumin in Depression: A Meta-analysis," *Journal of the American Medical Directors Association* 18, no. 6 (2017): 503–8.

15 S. Rathore et al., "Curcumin: A Review for Health Benefits," *International Journal of Research and Review* 7, no. 1 (2020): 273–90.

16 Jayesh Sanmukhani et al., "Efficacy and Safety of Curcumin in Major Depressive Disorder: A Randomized Controlled Trial," *Phytotherapy Research* 28, no. 4 (2014): 579–85.

17 Eleonora Hay et al., "Therapeutic Effects of Turmeric in Several Diseases: An Overview," *Chemico-Biological Interactions* 310 (2019): 108729.

18 L. Fusar-Poli et al., "Curcumin for Depression: A Meta-analysis," *Critical Reviews in Food Science and Nutrition* (2019), https://doi.org/10.1080/10408 398.2019.1653260.

19 S. Saha and S. Ghosh, "*Tinospora cordifolia:* One Plant, Many Roles," *Ancient Science of Life* 31, no. 4 (2012): 151–59, https://doi.org/10.4103 /0257-7941.107344.

20 K. Antul et al., "Review on Pharmacological Profile of Medicinal Vine: *Tinospora cordifolia,*" *Current Journal of Applied Science and Technology* 35, no. 5 (2019): 1–11.

21 Saeideh Jalali et al., "A System Pharmacology Study for Deciphering Antidepression Activity of *Nardostachys jatamansi,*" *Current Drug Metabolism* 19, no. 5 (2018): 469–76.

22 Liwen Wang et al., "Antidepressant Effects and Mechanisms of the Total Iridoids of *Valeriana jatamansi* on the Brain-Gut Axis," *Planta Medica* 86, no. 3 (2020): 172–79.

23 Debjit Bhowmik et al., "Traditional Indian Herbs Punarnava and Its Medicinal Importance," *Journal of Pharmacognosy and Phytochemistry* 1, no. 1 (2012): 52–57.

24 Lili Dai et al., "Safety and Efficacy of Saffron (*Crocus sativus* L.) for Treating Mild to Moderate Depression: A Systematic Review and Meta-analysis," *Journal of Nervous and Mental Disease* 208, no. 4 (2020): 269–76, https://doi .org/10.1097/NMD.0000000000001118.

25 H. A. Hausenblas et al., "Saffron(*Crocus sativus* L.) and Major Depressive Disorder: A Meta-analysis of Randomized Clinical Trials," *Journal of Integrative Medicine* 11, no. 6 (2013): 377–83.

26 A. A. Noorbala et al., "Hydro-alcoholic Extract of *Crocus sativus* L. versus Fluoxetine in the Treatment of Mild to Moderate Depression: A Double-Blind, Randomized Pilot Trial," *Journal of Ethnopharmacology* 97, no. 2 (2005): 281–84.

27 Kalaivani Selvaraj et al., "*Asparagus racemosus*—A Review," *Systematic Reviews in Pharmacy* 10, no. 1 (2019): 87–89.

28 Shashi Alok et al., "Plant Profile, Phytochemistry and Pharmacology of *Asparagus racemosus* (Shatavari): A Review," *Asian Pacific Journal of Tropical Disease* 3, no. 3 (2013): 242–51.

29 Negar Jamshidi and Marc M. Cohen, "The Clinical Efficacy and Safety of Tulsi in Humans: A Systematic Review of the Literature," *Evidence-Based Complementary and Alternative Medicine Journal* 2017 (2017): 9217567, https://doi .org/10.1155/2017/9217567.

30 J. Martins and S. Brijesh, "Phytochemistry and Pharmacology of Antidepressant Medicinal Plants: A Review," *Biomedicine and Pharmacotherapy* 104 (August 2018): 343–65.

31 Bingli Cheng et al., "Complementary and Alternative Medicine for the Treatment of Insomnia: An Overview of Scientific Evidence from 2008 to 2018," *Current Vascular Pharmacology* 17 (2019), https://doi.org/10.2174/157016111 7666190506111239.

32 Sibylle Meier et al., "Effects of a Fixed Herbal Drug Combination (Ze 185) to an Experimental Acute Stress Setting in Healthy Men—An Explorative Randomized Placebo-Controlled Double-Blind Study," *Phytomedicine* 39 (2018): 85–92.

33 Peter Houghton, ed., *Valerian: The Genus* Valeriana (London: Routledge, 2017).

34 E. Toolika, N. P. Bhat, and S. K. Shetty, "A Comparative Clinical Study on the Effect of Tagara (*Valeriana wallichii* DC.) and Jatamansi (*Nardostachys jatamansi* DC.) in the Management of Anidra (Primary Insomnia)," *Ayu* 36, no. 1 (2015): 46–49.

35 Amritpal Singh Saroya and Jaswinder Singh, "Neuropharmacology of *Valeriana* Genus," in *Pharmacotherapeutic Potential of Natural Products in Neurological Disorders* (Singapore: Springer, 2018), 179–86.

36 Durgavati Yadav, Shivani Srivastava, and Yamini Bhusan Tripathi, "*Acorus calamus:* A Review," *International Journal of Scientific Research in Biological Sciences* 6, no. 4 (2019): 62–67.

37 Pulok Kumar Mukherjee et al., "*Acorus calamus:* Scientific Validation of Ayurvedic Tradition from Natural Resources," *Journal of Pharmaceutical Biology* 45, no. 8 (2007): 651–66.

38 N. Titova et al., "'Levodopa Phobia': A Review of a Not Uncommon and Consequential Phenomenon," *npj Parkinson's Disease* 4, no. 31 (2018): https://doi.org /10.1038/s41531-018-0067-z.

39 M. Shreevathsa, B. Ravishankar, and R. Dwivedi, "Anti-depressant Activity of *Mamsyadi kwatha:* An Ayurvedic Compound Formulation," *Ayu* 34, no. 1 (2013): 113–17.

40 R. Valecha and D. Dhingra, "Behavioral and Biochemical Evidences for Antidepressant-Like Activity of *Celastrus paniculatus* Seed Oil in Mice," *Basic and Clinical Neuroscience* 7, no. 1 (2016): 49–56.

41 Amit Mukherjee et al., "Potency of *Nasya* Karma," *Journal of Drug Delivery and Therapeutics* 9, no. 6-s (2019): 261–66.

42 S. Rayees and F. Malik, "*Withania somnifera:* From Traditional Use to Evidence Based Medicinal Prominence," in *Science of Ashwagandha: Preventive and Therapeutic Potentials*, ed. S. Kaul and R. Wadhwa (Cham, Switzerland: Springer, 2017), 81–103.

43 K. Simon Yeung et al., "Herbal Medicine for Depression and Anxiety: A Systematic Review with Assessment of Potential Psycho-oncologic Relevance," *Phytotherapy Review* 32, no. 5 (2018): 865–91.

44 Natalia da Silva Leitao Peres et al., "Medicinal Effects of Peruvian Maca *(Lepidium meyenii):* A Review," *Food and Function* 11 (2020): 83–92.

45 L. Stojanovska et al., "Maca Reduces Blood Pressure and Depression in a Pilot Study in Postmenopausal Women," *Climacteric* 18, no. 1 (2015): 69–78.

46 Qin Xiang Ng, Nandini Venkatanarayanan, and Collin Yih Xian Ho, "Clinical Use of *Hypericum perforatum* (St. John's Wort) in Depression: A Meta-analysis," *Journal of Affective Disorders* 210, no. 1 (2017): 211–21.

47 Seungyeop Lee and Dong-Kwon Rhee, "Effects of Ginseng on Stress-Related Depression, Anxiety, and the Hypothalamic–Pituitary–Adrenal Axis," *Journal of Ginseng Research* 41, no. 4 (October 2017): 589–94.

48 X. Huang et al., "Neuroprotective Effects of Ginseng Phytochemicals: Recent Perspectives," *Molecules* 24 (2019): 2939.

49 V. M. Ghamchini et al., "The Effect of Chamomile Tea on Anxiety and Depression in Cancer Patients Treated with Chemotherapy," *Journal of Young Pharmacists* 11, no. 3 (2019): 309–12.

50 Mohsen Adib-Hajbaghery and Seyedeh Nesa Mousavi, "The Effects of Chamomile Extract on Sleep Quality among Elderly People: A Clinical Trial," *Complementary Therapies in Medicine* 35 (December 2017): 109–14.

51 J. D. Amsterdam et al., "A Randomized, Double-Blind, Placebo-Controlled Trial of Oral *Matricaria recutita* (Chamomile) Extract Therapy for Generalized Anxiety Disorder," *Journal of Clinical Psychopharmacology* 29, no. 4 (2009): 378–82.

52 Effati Daryani et al., "Effect of Lavender Cream with or without Footbath on Anxiety, Stress and Depression of Women in Postpartum: A Clinical Randomized Controlled Trial," *Iranian Journal of Obstetrics, Gynecology and Infertility* 20, no. 10 (2017): 52–61.

53 Kecia-Ann Blissett, Victora Chima, and Melinda S. Lantz, "From Stress to Serenity: The Use of Aromatherapy to Engage Patients in Care," *American Journal of Geriatric Psychiatry* 26, no. 3 (2018): S119.

54 A. Abdelhalim et al., "Antidepressant, Anxiolytic and Antinociceptive Activities of Constituents from *Rosmarinus officinalis*," *Journal of Pharmacy and Pharmaceutical Sciences* 18, no. 4 (2015): 448–59.

55 Raphaelle Sousa Borges et al., "Review: *Rosmarinus officinalis* Essential Oil: A Review of Its Phytochemistry, Anti-inflammatory Activity, and Mechanisms of Action Involved," *Journal of Ethnopharmacology* 229, no. 30 (January 2019): 29–45.

56 K. Simon Yeung et al., "Review: Herbal Medicine for Depression and Anxiety: A Systematic Review with Assessment of Potential Psycho-oncologic Relevance," *Phytotherapy Research* 32, no. 5 (May 2018): 865–91.

57 A. K. Nadkarni, *Indian Materia Medica* (Mumbai, India: Popular Prakashan, 2005), 1: 236.

58 Christine Nazarenus, *Medical Cannabis Handbook for Healthcare Professionals* (New York: Springer, 2020).

59 L. John Horwood et al., "Cannabis and Depression: An Integrative Data Analysis of Four Australasian Cohorts," *Drug and Alcohol Dependence* 126, no. 3 (December 2012): 369–78.

60 K. Hodgson et al., "Cannabis Use, Depression and Self-Harm: Phenotypic and Genetic Relationships," *Addiction* 115, no. 3 (2020): 482–92.

61 Anna-Karin Danielsson et al., "Cannabis Use, Depression and Anxiety: A 3-Year Prospective Population-Based Study," *Journal of Affective Disorders* 193, no. 15 (March 2016): 103–8.

62 Yih-Ing Hser et al., "Reductions in Cannabis Use Are Associated with Improvements in Anxiety, Depression, and Sleep Quality, but Not Quality of Life," *Journal of Substance Abuse Treatment* 81 (October 2017): 53–58.

CHAPTER 11: APPLY THE AYURVEDIC MASTERY OF FOOD, DIET, AND NUTRITION FOR YOUR DEPRESSION

1 DW Documentary, "Better Brain Health," March 5, 2020, www.youtube.com/watch?v=TLpbfOJ4bJU.

2 M. Heather et al., "A Brief Diet Intervention Can Reduce Symptoms of Depression in Young Adults—A Randomized Controlled Trial," *PLOS ONE* 14, no. 10 (2019), https://doi.org/10.1371/journal.pone.0222768.

3 A. Majumdar, *Ayurveda: The Ancient Science of Healing* (Delhi, India: Macmillan, 2004).

4 Tom P. Heath et al., "Human Taste Thresholds Are Modulated by Serotonin and Noradrenaline," *Journal of Neuroscience* 26, no. 49 (December 2006): 12664–71.

CHAPTER 12: DEPRESSION, FOOD CONTAMINATION, AND SOCIAL MEDIA

1 Sara Goodman, "Tests Find More Than 200 Chemicals in Newborn Umbilical Cord Blood," *Scientific American,* December 2, 2009, www.scientificamerican.com/article/newborn-babies-chemicals-exposure-bpa/.

2 Åke Bergman et al., eds., *State of the Science of Endocrine Disrupting Chemicals 2012* (Geneva, Switzerland: United Nations Environment Programme and the World Health Organization, 2013).

3 Melissa Denchak, "Water Pollution: Everything You Need to Know," Natural Resources Defense Council, May 14, 2018, www.nrdc.org/stories/water-pollution-everything-you-need-know.

4 Gustavo Oliveira and Susanna Hecht, "Sacred Groves, Sacrifice Zones and Soy Production: Globalization, Intensification and Neo-nature in South America," *Journal of Peasant Studies* 43, no. 2 (2016): 251–85.

5 Veslemøy Andersen, *Genetically Modified and Irradiated Food: Controversial Issues: Facts versus Perceptions* (London: Elsevier, 2020).

6 Kelly Crowe, "Food Cravings Engineered by Industry," *CBC News*, March 6, 2013, www.cbc.ca/news/health/food-cravings-engineered-by-industry-1.1395225.

7 "45 Alarming Statistics on Americans' Sugar Consumption and the Effects of Sugar on Americans' Health," TheDiabetesCouncil.com, last reviewed July 10, 2018, www.thediabetescouncil.com/45-alarming-statistics-on-americans-sugar-consumption-and-the-effects-of-sugar-on-americans-health/.

8 M. B. Abou-Donia et al., "Splenda Alters Gut Microflora and Increases Intestinal p-Glycoprotein and Cytochrome p-450 in Male Rats," *Journal of Toxicology and Environmental Health* 71, no. 21 (2018): 1415–29.

9 J. Suez et al., "Artificial Sweeteners Induce Glucose Intolerance by Altering the Gut Microbiota," *Nature* 514, no. 7521 (2014): 181–86.

10 P. Shankar, S. Ahuja, and K. Sriram, "Non-nutritive Sweeteners: Review and Update," *Nutrition* 29, no. 11–12 (2013): 1293–99.

11 Volker Bornemann et al., "Intestinal Metabolism and Bioaccumulation of Sucralose in Adipose Tissue in the Rat," *Journal of Toxicology and Environmental Health, Part A* 81, no. 18 (2018): 913–23.

12 D. Dhurandhar, V. Bharihoke, and S. Kalra, "A Histological Assessment of Effects of Sucralose on Liver of Albino Rats," *Morphologie* 102, no. 338 (September 2018): 197–204.

13 S. S. Schiffman and K. I. Rother, "Sucralose, a Synthetic Organochlorine Sweetener: Overview of Biological Issues," *Journal of Toxicology and Environmental Health, Part B: Critical Reviews* 16, no. 7 (2013): 399–451.

14 A. K. Choudhary and Y. Y. Lee, "Neurophysiological Symptoms and Aspartame: What Is the Connection?" *Nutritional Neuroscience* 21, no. 5 (2018): 306–16.

15 G. N. Lindseth et al., "Neurobehavioral Effects of Aspartame Consumption," *Research in Nursing and Health* 37, no. 3 (2014): 185–93.

16 James S. Ruff et al., "Compared to Sucrose, Previous Consumption of Fructose and Glucose Monosaccharides Reduces Survival and Fitness of Female Mice," *Journal of Nutrition* 145, no. 3 (March 2015): 434–41.

17 A. Knüppel et al., "Sugar Intake from Sweet Food and Beverages, Common Mental Disorder and Depression: Prospective Findings from the Whitehall II Study," *Scientific Reports* 7, no. 1 (2017): 6287.

18 Beatriz Merino et al., "Review: Intestinal Fructose and Glucose Metabolism in Health and Disease," *Nutrients* 12, no. 1 (2020): 94.

19 Daniel J. Reis et al., "The Depressogenic Potential of Added Dietary Sugars," *Medical Hypotheses* 134 (January 2020): 109421, https://doi.org/10.1016/j.mehy.2019.109421.

20 C. L. Frankenfeld et al., "High-Intensity Sweetener Consumption and Gut Microbiome Content and Predicted Gene Function in a Cross-Sectional Study of Adults in the United States," *Annals of Epidemiology* 25, no. 10 (2015): 736–42.

21 Zehra Kazmi et al., "Monosodium Glutamate: Review on Clinical Reports," *International Journal of Food Properties* 20, suppl. 2 (2017): 1807–15.

22 Mark A. D'Andrea and G. Kesava, "Adverse Health Complaints of Adults Exposed to Benzene after a Flaring Disaster at the BP Refinery Facility in Texas City, Texas," *Disaster Medicine and Public Health Preparedness* 12, no. 2 (April 2018): 232–40.

23 Madar Talibov, "Benzene Exposure at Workplace and Risk of Colorectal Cancer in Four Nordic Countries," *Cancer Epidemiology* 55 (August 2018): 156–61.

24 J. Yoon, W. S. Kwak, and Y. Ahn, "A Brief Review of Relationship between Occupational Benzene Exposure and Hematopoietic Cancer," *Annals of Occupational and Environmental Medicine* 30, no. 33 (2018).

25 Diane Roberts Stoler, "Trans Fats: Bad for Your Brain," *The Resilient Brain* (blog), *Psychology Today*, June 25, 2015, www.psychologytoday.com/us/blog/the-resilient-brain/201506/trans-fats-bad-your-brain.

26 Di Li et al., "Prospective Association between Trans Fatty Acid Intake and Depressive Symptoms: Results from the Study of Women's Health across the Nation," *Journal of Affective Disorders* 264, no. 1 (March 2020): 256–62.

27 Tina Ljungberg, Emma Bondza, and Connie Lethin, "Review: Evidence of the Importance of Dietary Habits Regarding Depressive Symptoms and Depression," *International Journal of Environmental Research and Public Health* 17, no. 5 (2020): 1616.

28 Thaddeus T. Schug and Linda S. Birnbaum, "Endocrine-Disrupting Chemicals," in *Environmental Toxicants: Human Exposures and Their Health Effects*, 4th ed., ed. Morton Lippmann and George D. Leikauf (Hoboken, NJ: John Wiley and Sons, 2020), 535–54.

29 N. Meyer and A. C. Zenclussen, "Immune Cells in the Uterine Remodeling: Are They the Target of Endocrine Disrupting Chemicals?" *Frontiers in Immunology* 11 (2020): 246.

30 "Pesticide Residue Monitoring Program Reports and Data," U.S. Food and Drug Administration, updated September 13, 2019, www.fda.gov/food/pesticides/pesticide-residue-monitoring-program-reports-and-data.

31 "Total Diet Study," U.S. Food and Drug Administration, updated February 23, 2018, www.fda.gov/food/science-research-food/total-diet-study.

32 Michele A. La Merrill, "Consensus on the Key Characteristics of Endocrine-Disrupting Chemicals as a Basis for Hazard Identification," *Nature Reviews Endocrinology* 16 (2020): 45–57.

33 Mariangela Martini, Victor G. Corces, and Emilie F. Rissman, "Epigenetic Mechanisms That Promote Transgenerational Actions of Endocrine Disrupting Chemicals: Applications to Behavioral Neuroendocrinology," *Hormones and Behavior* 119 (March 2020): 104677.

34 Karin B. Michels et al., "In Utero Exposure to Endocrine-Disrupting Chemicals and Telomere Length at Birth," *Environmental Research* 182 (March 2020): 109053.

35 S. K. Bopp, R. Barouki, W. Brack, et al., "Current EU Research Activities on Combined Exposure to Multiple Chemicals," *Environment International* 120 (2018): 544–62, https://doi.org/10.1016/j.envint.2018.07.037.

36 Jiuyong Xu et al., "Comparative Cytotoxic Effects of Five Commonly Used Triazole Alcohol Fungicides on Human Cells of Different Tissue Types," *Journal of Environmental Science and Health, Part B* (2020), https://doi.org/10.1080/03601234.2019.1709377.

37 F. Perera et al., "Bisphenol A Exposure and Symptoms of Anxiety and Depression among Inner City Children at 10-12 Years of Age," *Environmental Research* 151 (2016): 195–202.

38 Lauren Zanolli, "Bisphenol: What to Know about the Chemicals in Water Bottles and Cans," *The Guardian*, May 24, 2019, www.theguardian.com/us-news/2019/may/24/bisphenols-bpa-everyday-toxics-guide.

39 Melanie H. Jacobson et al., "Urinary Bisphenols and Obesity Prevalence among U.S. Children and Adolescents," *Journal of the Endocrine Society* 3, no. 9 (September 2019): 1715–26.

40 H. Serra et al., "Evidence for Bisphenol B Endocrine Properties: Scientific and Regulatory Perspectives," *Environmental Health Perspectives* 127, no. 10 (October 16, 2019), https://doi.org/10.1289/EHP5200.

41 I. Shiue, "Urinary Heavy Metals, Phthalates and Polyaromatic Hydrocarbons Independent of Health Events Are Associated with Adult Depression: USA NHANES, 2011–2012," *Environmental Science and Pollution Research* 22 (2015): 17095–103.

42 L. P. Bustamante-Montes et al., "Prenatal Exposure to Phthalates Is Associated with Decreased Anogenital Distance and Penile Size in Male Newborns," *Journal of Developmental Origins of Health and Disease* 4, no. 4 (2013): 300–306.

43 "History and Use of Per- and Polyfluoroalkyl Substances (PFAS)," Interstate Technology Regulatory Council, February 7, 2020, https://pfas-1.itrcweb.org /fact_sheets_page/PFAS_Fact_Sheet_History_and_Use_April2020.pdf.

44 "DuPont vs. the World: Chemical Giant Covered Up Health Risks of Teflon Contamination across Globe," *Democracy Now!,* January 23, 2018, www .democracynow.org/2018/1/23/dupont_vs_the_world_chemical_giant.

45 R. W. Lash, "Diabetes and Pregnancy—An Endocrine Society Clinical Practice Guideline Publication Note," *Journal of Clinical Endocrinology and Metabolism* 103, no. 11 (2018): 4042.

46 A. Wouter, Stefan Gebbink, and P. J. van Leeuwen, "Environmental Contamination and Human Exposure to PFASs near a Fluorochemical Production Plant: Review of Historic and Current PFOA and GenX Contamination in the Netherlands," *Environment International* 137 (2020): 105583.

47 A. M. Leung, E. N. Pearce, and L. E. Braverman, "Perchlorate, Iodine and the Thyroid," *Best Practice and Research: Clinical Endocrinology and Metabolism* 24, no. 1 (2010): 133–41.

48 S. G. Khambadkone et al., "Nitrated Meat Products Are Associated with Mania in Humans and Altered Behavior and Brain Gene Expression in Rats," *Molecular Psychiatry* 25 (2020): 560–71.

49 L. E. Arnold, N. Lofthouse, and E. Hurt, "Artificial Food Colors and Attention-Deficit/Hyperactivity Symptoms: Conclusions to Dye For," *Neurotherapeutics* 9, no. 3 (2012): 599–609.

50 "Hair Dyes," American Cancer Society, updated December 5, 2019, www .cancer.org/cancer/cancer-causes/hair-dyes.html.

51 Carolyn E. Eberle et al., "Hair Dye and Chemical Straightener Use and Breast Cancer Risk in a Large US Population of Black and White Women," *International Journal of Cancer,* December 3, 2019, https://doi.org/10.1002 /ijc.32738.

52 Sarah Jackson, "95 Percent of Baby Foods Tested Contain Toxic Metals, New Report Says," *NBC News,* October 17, 2019, www.nbcnews.com/health /kids-health/new-report-95-percent-baby-foods-tested-contain-toxic-metals-n1068306.

53 Sandra Rainieri and Alejandro Barranco, "Microplastics, a Food Safety Issue?" *Trends in Food Science and Technology* 84 (February 2019): 55–57.

54 B. Chuberre et al., "Mineral Oils and Waxes in Cosmetics: An Overview Mainly Based on the Current European Regulations and the Safety Profile of These Compounds," *Journal of the European Academy of Dermatology and Venereology* 33, no. 57 (November 2019): 5–14.

55 "Should People Be Concerned about Parabens in Beauty Products?" *Earthtalk* (column), *Scientific American,* October 6, 2014, www.scientificamerican.com /article/should-people-be-concerned-about-parabens-in-beauty-products/.

56 P. P. Giri et al., "Acute Carbolic Acid Poisoning: A Report of Four Cases," *Indian Journal of Critical Care Medicine* 20, no. 11 (2016): 668–70.

57 S. Wilbur, D. Jones, J. F. Risher, et al., *Toxicological Profile for 1,4-Dioxane,* chap. 3, "Health Effects" (Atlanta, GA: Agency for Toxic Substances and Disease Registry, 2012), www.ncbi.nlm.nih.gov/books/NBK153671.

58 M. Wiseman, "The Second World Cancer Research Fund/American Institute for Cancer Research Expert Report: Food, Nutrition, Physical Activity, and the Prevention of Cancer: A Global Perspective," *Proceedings of the Nutrition Society* 67, no. 3 (2008): 253–56.

59 Federico J. A. Pérez-Cueto and Wim Verbeke, "Consumer Implications of the WCRF's Permanent Update on Colorectal Cancer," *Meat Science* 90, no. 4 (April 2012): 977–78.

60 Annie N. Samraj et al., "A Red Meat-Derived Glycan Promotes Inflammation and Cancer Progression," *Proceedings of the National Academy of Sciences* 112, no. 2 (January 13, 2015): 542–47.

61 Consumer Reports, "The Overuse of Antibiotics in Food Animals Threatens Public Health," November 9, 2012, https://advocacy.consumerreports .org/press_release/the-overuse-of-antibiotics-in-food-animals-threatens -public-health-2/.

62 Z. Wang et al., "Impact of Chronic Dietary Red Meat, White Meat, or Non-meat Protein on Trimethylamine N-oxide Metabolism and Renal Excretion in Healthy Men and Women," *European Heart Journal* 40, no. 7 (February 14, 2019): 583–94.

63 "Eating Red Meat Daily Triples Heart Disease-Related Chemical," *NIH Research Matters,* January 8, 2019, www.nih.gov/news-events/nih-research -matters/eating-red-meat-daily-triples-heart-disease-related-chemical.

64 F. B. Hu, B. O. Otis, and G. McCarthy, "Can Plant-Based Meat Alternatives Be Part of a Healthy and Sustainable Diet?" *Journal of the American Medical Association* 322, no. 16 (2019): 1547–48.

65 Laura Reiley, "Impossible Burger: Here's What's Really in It," *Washington Post,* October 23, 2019, www.washingtonpost.com/business/2019/10/23/an -impossible-burger-dissected/.

66 G. R. Durso, A. Luttrell, and B. M. Way, "Over-the-Counter Relief from Pains and Pleasures Alike: Acetaminophen Blunts Evaluation Sensitivity to Both Negative and Positive Stimuli," *Psychological Science* 26, no. 6 (2015): 750–58.

67 C. I. Ghanem et al., "Acetaminophen from Liver to Brain: New Insights into Drug Pharmacological Action and Toxicity," *Pharmacological Research* 109 (2016): 119–31.

68 Suneil Agrawal and Babak Khazaeni, *Acetaminophen Toxicity* (Treasure Island, FL: StatPearls Publishing, 2020).

69 Sydney Evans, Chris Campbell, and Olga V. Naidenko, "Cumulative Risk Analysis of Carcinogenic Contaminants in United States Drinking Water," *Heliyon* 5 (2019): e02314, https://doi.org/10.1016/j.heliyon.2019.e02314.

70 A. Sylvetsky, K. I. Rother, and R. Brown, "Artificial Sweetener Use among Children: Epidemiology, Recommendations, Metabolic Outcomes, and Future Directions," *Pediatric Clinics of North America* 58, no. 6 (2011): 1467–80, xi.

71 J. L. Harris et al., *Children's Drink Food Advertising to Children and Teens Score*, UConn Rudd Center for Food Policy and Obesity, October 2019, http://uconnruddcenter.org/files/Pdfs/FACTS2019.pdf.

72 Sandee LaMotte, "Top 34 Bestselling 'Fruit' Drinks for Kids Deemed Unhealthy," *CNN Health*, updated October 16, 2019, www.cnn.com/2019/10/16/health/children-fruit-drinks-report-wellness/index.html.

73 "Acrylamide and Cancer Risk," American Cancer Society, revised February 11, 2019, www.cancer.org/cancer/cancer-causes/acrylamide.html.

74 Rob Picheta, "A Single Tea Bag Can Leak Billions of Pieces of Microplastic Into Your Brew," *CNN Health*, September 27, 2019, www.cnn.com/2019/09/27/health/microplastics-tea-bags-study-scn-scli-intl/index.html.

75 Laura M. Hernandez et al., "Plastic Teabags Release Billions of Microparticles and Nanoparticles into Tea," *Environmental Science and Technology* 53, no. 21 (2019): 12300–12310.

76 "Water Fluoridation Data and Statistics," Centers for Disease Control and Prevention, last reviewed January 13, 2020, www.cdc.gov/fluoridation/statistics/reference_stats.htm.

77 National Research Council, *Fluoride in Drinking Water: A Scientific Review of EPA's Standards* (Washington, DC: National Academies Press, 2006), 205.

78 R. Green et al., "Association between Maternal Fluoride Exposure during Pregnancy and IQ Scores in Offspring in Canada," *JAMA Pediatrics* 173, no. 10 (2019): 940–48.

79 Humayun Kabir, Ashok Kumar Gupta, and Subhasish Tripathy, "Fluoride and Human Health: Systematic Appraisal of Sources, Exposures, Metabolism, and Toxicity," *Critical Reviews in Environmental Science and Technology* 50, no. 11 (2020): 1116–93.

80 E. E. Burns and A. B. A. Boxall, "Microplastics in the Aquatic Environment: Evidence for or Against Adverse Impacts and Major Knowledge Gaps," *Environmental Toxicology and Chemistry* 37, no. 11 (2018): 2776–96.

81 Laura Parker, "Planet or Plastic? Microplastics Found in 90 Percent of Table Salt," *National Geographic,* October 17, 2018, www.nationalgeographic.com /environment/2018/10/microplastics-found-90-percent-table-salt-sea-salt/.

82 Samuel V. Panno et al., "Microplastic Contamination in Karst Groundwater Systems," *Groundwater* 57, no. 2 (2019): 189–96.

83 Lars Noah, "Legal Aspects of the Food Additive Approval Process," appendix A in *Enhancing the Regulatory Decision-Making Approval Process for Direct Food Ingredient Technologies,* Institute of Medicine (Washington, DC: National Academies Press, 1999).

84 Tianxi Yang et al., "Effectiveness of Commercial and Homemade Washing Agents in Removing Pesticide Residues on and in Apples," *Journal of Agricultural and Food Chemistry* 65, no. 44 (2017): 9744–52.

85 "How Many Smartphones Are in the World?" BankMyCell, www.bankmycell .com/blog/how-many-phones-are-in-the-world.

86 A. H. Tuttle et al., "Increasing Placebo Responses over Time in U.S. Clinical Trials of Neuropathic Pain," *Pain* 156, no. 12 (2015): 2616–26.

87 L. M. Schwartz and S. Woloshin, "Medical Marketing in the United States, 1997–2016," *Journal of the American Medical Association* 321, no. 1 (2019): 80–96.

88 Statista, *TV Advertising in the U.S.* (Hamburg, Germany: Stroer Content Group, 2019).

89 Brian A. Primack et al., "Social Media Use and Perceived Social Isolation among Young Adults in the U.S.," *American Journal of Preventive Medicine* 53, no. 1 (2017): 1–8.

90 S. O'Dea, "Number of Smartphone Users Worldwide from 2016 to 2021," Statista, February 28, 2020, www.statista.com/statistics/330695/number-of -smartphone-users-worldwide/.

91 L. Hardell, "Effects of Mobile Phones on Children's and Adolescents' Health: A Commentary," *Child Development* 89, no. 1 (2018): 137–40.

92 J. S. Beckman and W. H. Koppenol, "Nitric Oxide, Superoxide, and Peroxynitrite: The Good, the Bad, and the Ugly," *American Journal of Physiology* 271, no. 5, part 1 (1996): C1424–37.

93 H. Ischiropoulos et al., "Peroxynitrite-Mediated Tyrosine Nitration Catalyzed by Superoxide Dismutase," *Archives of Biochemistry and Biophysics* 298, no. 2 (1992): 431–37.

94 Elizabeth B. Dowdell and Brianne Q. Clayton, "Interrupted Sleep: College Students Sleeping with Technology," *Journal of American College Health* 67, no. 7 (2019): 640–46.

95 Z. Naeem, "Health Risks Associated with Mobile Phone Use," *International Journal of Health Sciences (Qassim)* 8, no. 4 (2014): V–VI.

96 R. Povolotskiy et al., "Head and Neck Injuries Associated with Cell Phone Use," *JAMA Otolaryngology—Head and Neck Surgery* 146, no. 2 (2020): 122–27.

97 Fatih Oz, Mevlüde Kizil, and Tuğba Çelik, "Effects of Different Cooking Methods on the Formation of Heterocyclic Aromatic Amines in Goose Meat," *Journal of Food Processing and Preservation* 40, no. 5 (2016): 1047–53.

98 Juming Tang, "Unlocking Potentials of Microwaves for Food Safety and Quality," *Journal of Food Science* 80, no. 8 (2015): E1776–93.

99 Kanishka Bhunia et al., "Migration of Chemical Compounds from Packaging Polymers during Microwave, Conventional Heat Treatment, and Storage," *Comprehensive Reviews in Food Science and Food Safety* 12, no. 5 (2013): 523–45.

CHAPTER 13: ANALYZING THE BIOLOGICAL MECHANISM OF DEPRESSION

1 Amanda Gomes Almeida Sá, Yara Maria Franco Moreno, and Bruno Augusto Mattar Carciofi, "Plant Proteins as High-Quality Nutritional Source for Human Diet," *Trends in Food Science and Technology* 97 (March 2020): 170–84.

2 Krishnarao Appasani, *Optogenetics: From Neuronal Function to Mapping and Disease Biology* (Cambridge: Cambridge University Press, 2017).

3 Ismael Palacios-García and Francisco J. Parada, "Measuring the Brain-Gut Axis in Psychological Sciences: A Necessary Challenge," *Frontiers in Integrative Neuroscience* 13 (2020), https://doi.org/10.3389/fnint.2019.00073.

4 George M. Kapalka, *Nutritional and Herbal Therapies for Children and Adolescents: A Handbook for Mental Health Clinicians* (Cambridge, MA: Elsevier, 2010).

5 "Phenylalanine," WebMD, last reviewed May 29, 2019, www.webmd.com /vitamins-and-supplements/phenylalanine-uses-and-risks#.

6 S. N. Young, "L-tyrosine to Alleviate the Effects of Stress?" *Journal of Psychiatry and Neuroscience* 32, no. 3 (2007): 224.

7 James McIntosh, "What Is Serotonin and What Does It Do?" Medical News Today, last reviewed February 2, 2018, www.medicalnewstoday.com /articles/232248.

8 Irving Kirsch, *The Emperor's New Drugs: Exploding the Antidepressant Myth* (New York: Basic Books, 2010).

9 J. Meiser, D. Weindl, and K. Hiller, "Complexity of Dopamine Metabolism," *Cell Communication and Signaling* 11, no. 1 (2013): 34.

10 "What Is Dopamine?" WebMD, last reviewed June 19, 2019, www.webmd .com/mental-health/what-is-dopamine#1.

11 Scott T. Brady et al., *Basic Neurochemistry: Principles of Molecular, Cellular, and Medical Neurobiology*, 8th ed. (Cambridge, MA: Elsevier, 2012).

12 Rahul Costa-Pinto and Dashiell Gantner, "Macronutrients, Minerals, Vitamins and Energy," *Anaesthesia and Intensive Care Medicine* 21, no. 3 (March 2020): 157–61.

13 Anne I. Turner, "Psychological Stress Reactivity and Future Health and Disease Outcomes: A Systematic Review of Prospective Evidence," *Psychoneuroendocrinology* 114 (2020): 104599.

14 McGill University, "Brain Signaling Proteins Hit the Road Running: New Study of Brain Neurotransmitter Receptor Has Implications for Drug Discovery," *Science Daily*, April 30, 2019, www.sciencedaily.com/releases/2019/04/190430121731.htm.

15 C. J. Watson, H. A. Baghdoyan, and R. Lydic, "Neuropharmacology of Sleep and Wakefulness," *Sleep Medicine Clinics* 5, no. 4 (2010): 513–28.

16 Eva Friedel and Andreas Heinz, "Genetic, Epigenetic, and Environmental Factors in Serotonin-Associated Disease Condition," chap. 7 in *Handbook of the Behavioral Neurobiology of Serotonin*, 2nd ed., ed. Christian P. Müller and Kathryn A. Cunningham, 923–40; vol. 21 of *Handbook of Behavioral Neuroscience* (Cambridge, MA: Elsevier, 2020).

17 Alan Frazer and Julie G. Hensler, *Basic Neurochemistry: Molecular, Cellular and Medical Aspects*, 6th ed. (Philadelphia: Lippincott-Raven, 1999).

18 Juliana Akinaga, J. Adolfo García-Sáinz, and André S. Pupo, "Updates in the Function and Regulation of α1-adrenoceptors," *British Journal of Pharmacology* 178, no. 14 (2019): 2343–57.

19 A. Mishra, S. Singh, and S. Shukla, "Physiological and Functional Basis of Dopamine Receptors and Their Role in Neurogenesis: Possible Implication for Parkinson's Disease," *Journal of Experimental Neuroscience* 12 (2018): 1179069518779829.

20 *Taittiriya Upanishad* 2.2.1.

CHAPTER 14: AYURVEDIC PSYCHOLOGY AND PSYCHOTHERAPY

1 "What Is Depression?" American Psychiatric Association, last reviewed January 2017, www.psychiatry.org/patients-families/depression/what-is-depression.

2 Divya Kajaria, "An Introduction to Sattvavajaya: Psychotherapy in Ayurveda," *Unique Journal of Ayurvedic and Herbal Medicine* 1, no. 1 (2013): 10–13.

3 S. S. Bagali, U. C. Baragi, and R. A. Deshmukh, "Concept of Sattvavajayachikitsa (Psychotherapy)," *Journal of Ayurveda and Integrated Medical Sciences* 1, no. 1 (2016): 56–63.

4 G. Oster, "Auditory Beats in the Brain," *Scientific American* 229, no. 4 (1973): 94–102.

5 C. C. Streeter et al., "Treatment of Major Depressive Disorder with Iyengar Yoga and Coherent Breathing: A Randomized Controlled Dosing Study," *Journal of Alternative and Complementary Medicine* 23, no. 3 (2017): 201–7.

6 V. Lad, *Ayurvedic Perspective of Selected Pathologies*, 2nd ed. (Albuquerque, NM: Ayurvedic Press, 2012).

7 M. G. Ramu and B. S. Venkataram, "*Manovikara* (Mental Disorders) in Ayurveda," *Ancient Science of Life* 4, no. 3 (1984): 165–73.

8 Eknath Easwaran, trans., *The Bhagavad Gita*, 2nd ed. (Tomales, CA: Nilgiri Press, 2007).

9 Alf Hildebidle, *Freud's Mahabharata* (New York: Oxford University Press, 2018).

10 Indrajit Bandyopadhyay, *Evolutionary Psychology in Mahabharata* (Lulu.com, 2013).

11 Vanamali Gita Yogashram, *Hanuman: The Devotion and Power of the Monkey God* (New Delhi, India: Aryan Books International, 2010).

12 N. N. Wig, "Hanuman Complex and Its Resolution: An Illustration of Psychotherapy from Indian Mythology," *Indian Journal of Psychiatry* 46 (2004): 25–28.

13 Joseph Campbell and Bill Moyers, *The Power of Myth* (New York: Anchor Books, 1991).

14 J. Langford, "Ayurvedic Psychotherapy: Transposed Signs, Parodied Selves," *Political and Legal Anthropology Review* 21, no. 1 (1998): 84–98.

15 J. Langford, *Fluent Bodies: Ayurvedic Remedies for Postcolonial Imbalances* (Durham, NC: Duke University Press, 2002).

16 C. Lang and E. Jansen, "Appropriating Depression: Biomedicalizing Ayurvedic Psychiatry in Kerala, India," *Medical Anthropology* 32, no. 1 (2013): 25–45.

INDEX

ABOUT THE AUTHOR

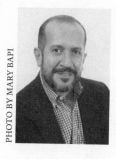

THE MEDICAL AND SCIENTIFIC career of L. Eduardo Cardona-Sanclemente, DSc, PhD, MSc, spans professorships and senior scientific research posts at some of Europe's most distinguished medical schools and universities in England, France, and Italy.

After graduating in medical sciences, he completed his master's degree in clinical biochemistry and his PhD in the mechanism of neurotransmitters. For his *docteur d'état* (doctor of science) thesis in physiopathology of nutrition at Sorbonne University in Paris, he was awarded the highest distinction: *très honorable.* Dr. Cardona-Sanclemente has also been studying and practicing integrative medicine for decades, and he holds a master's degree in Ayurvedic medicine from Middlesex University, London, with rigorous internships at AVP Hospital Coimbatore in Tamil Nadu, India, and in Udupi, India, where he also held visiting professorships.

He is certified by the National Ayurvedic Medical Association (USA) to practice as an Ayurvedic doctor, and he presided for several years as the research committee director of the Ayurvedic Professional Association (UK).

Dr. Cardona-Sanclemente resides in Berkeley, California, where he is a consultant engaged in enhancing awareness of the value of Ayurveda and integrative medicine in the Bay Area, specifically in developing programs for minorities, alongside his clinical work. He has been an international conference speaker for more than thirty years, addressing allopathic, Ayurvedic, and integrative medical topics.

About North Atlantic Books

North Atlantic Books (NAB) is an independent, nonprofit publisher committed to a bold exploration of the relationships between mind, body, spirit, and nature. Founded in 1974, NAB aims to nurture a holistic view of the arts, sciences, humanities, and healing. To make a donation or to learn more about our books, authors, events, and newsletter, please visit www.northatlanticbooks.com.

North Atlantic Books is the publishing arm of the Society for the Study of Native Arts and Sciences, a 501(c)(3) nonprofit educational organization that promotes cross-cultural perspectives linking scientific, social, and artistic fields. To learn how you can support us, please visit our website.